Irritability in Pediatric Psychopathology

Irritability in Pediatric Psychopathology

Edited by Amy Krain Roy
Melissa A. Brotman
and
Ellen Leibenluft

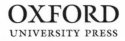

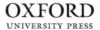

Oxford University Press is a department of the University of Oxford. It furthers
the University's objective of excellence in research, scholarship, and education
by publishing worldwide. Oxford is a registered trade mark of Oxford University
Press in the UK and certain other countries.

Published in the United States of America by Oxford University Press
198 Madison Avenue, New York, NY 10016, United States of America.

Library of Congress Cataloging-in-Publication Data
Names: Roy, Amy Krain, editor. | Brotman, Melissa A., 1975– editor. |
Leibenluft, Ellen, 1953– editor.
Title: Irritability in pediatric psychopathology / edited by Amy Krain Roy,
Melissa A. Brotman, and Ellen Leibenluft.
Description: New York, NY : Oxford University Press, [2019] |
Includes bibliographical references.
Identifiers: LCCN 2018051654 (print) | LCCN 2018053047 (ebook) |
ISBN 9780190846824 (UPDF) | ISBN 9780190846831 (EPUB) |
ISBN 9780190846800 (hardcover : alk. paper)
Subjects: | MESH: Irritable Mood | Affective Symptoms—psychology |
Child Behavior Disorders—diagnosis | Child | Adolescent
Classification: LCC RJ503.3 (ebook) | LCC RJ503.3 (print) | NLM WS 350.6 |
DDC 618.92/89—dc23
LC record available at https://lccn.loc.gov/2018051654

1 3 5 7 9 8 6 4 2
Printed by Sheridan Books, Inc., United States of America

{ CONTENTS }

SECTION IV Clinical Presentation

SECTION V Treatment

{ CONTRIBUTORS }

Robert R. Althoff, MD, PhD
Departments of Psychiatry, Pediatrics, and Psychological Science
Larner College of Medicine at the University of Vermont
Burlington, Vermont

Merelise Ametti, MPH
Departments of Psychiatry, Pediatrics, and Psychological Science
Larner College of Medicine at the University of Vermont
Burlington, Vermont

Pablo Vidal-Ribas Belil, MSc
Mood Brain and Development Unit, Emotion and Development Branch
National Institute of Mental Health
Bethesda, Maryland

Melissa A. Brotman, PhD
Emotion and Development Branch
National Institute of Mental Health
Bethesda, Maryland

M. Catalina Camacho, BA
Center for Neuroscience
University of Pittsburgh School of Medicine
Pittsburgh, Pennsylvania

Rachel E. Christensen, BS
Department of Psychiatry and Human Behavior
Bradley Hospital and Brown University
East Providence, Rhode Island

Kimberly R. Cimino, MA
Child Study Center
Yale University School of Medicine
New Haven, Connecticut

Taylor N. Day, MS
Department of Psychology
Florida State University
Tallahassee, Florida

Mariah DeSerisy, MA
Department of Psychology
Fordham University
Bronx, New York

Christen M. Deveney, PhD
Department of Psychology
Wellesley College
Wellesley, Massachusetts

Daniel P. Dickstein, MD
Department of Psychiatry and Human Behavior
Bradley Hospital and Brown University
East Providence, Rhode Island

Meridith L. Eastman, PhD
Virginia Institute for Psychiatric and Behavioral Genetics
Virginia Commonwealth University
Richmond, Virginia

Theresa R. Gladstone, BA
Child Study Center
Yale University School of Medicine
New Haven, Connecticut

Joshua Golt, BS
Department of Psychiatry
University of Pittsburgh School of
  Medicine
Pittsburgh, Pennsylvania

Emily Hirsch, MA
Department of Psychology
Fordham University
Bronx, New York

Leslie Hulvershorn, MD
Department of Psychiatry
Indiana University School of Medicine
Indianapolis, Indiana

Soonjo Hwang, MD
Department of Psychiatry
University of Nebraska Medical Center
Omaha, Nebraska

Cynthia Kiefer, MA
Department of Psychology
San Diego State University
San Diego, California

Ellen Leibenluft, MD
Emotion and Development Branch
National Institute of Mental Health
Bethesda, Maryland

Carolyn L. Marsh, BA
Child Study Center
Yale University School of Medicine
New Haven, Connecticut

Carla A. Mazefsky, PhD
Department of Psychiatry
University of Pittsburgh School of
  Medicine
Pittsburgh, Pennsylvania

Ashlee A. Moore, BS
Virginia Institute for Psychiatric and
  Behavioral Genetics
Center for Clinical and Translational
  Research
Virginia Commonwealth University
Richmond, Virginia

Susan B. Perlman, PhD
Department of Psychiatry
University of Pittsburgh School of
  Medicine
Pittsburgh, Pennsylvania

Michael Potegal, PhD, LP
Program in Occupational Therapy
University of Minnesota
Minneapolis, Minnesota

Roxann Roberson-Nay, PhD
Virginia Institute for Psychiatric and
  Behavioral Genetics
Virginia Commonwealth University
Richmond, Virginia

Amy Krain Roy, PhD
Department of Psychology
Fordham University
Bronx, New York

Giovanni Abrahão Salum, MD, PhD
Department of Psychiatry
Universidade Federal do Rio
  Grande do Sul
Porto Alegre, Brazil

Valerie Scelsa, MA
Department of Psychology
Miami University
Oxford, Ohio

Joel Stoddard, MD
Department of Psychiatry
University of Colorado School of
   Medicine
Aurora, Colorado

**Argyris Stringaris, MD, PhD,
FRCPsych**
Mood Brain and Development Unit,
   Emotion and Development Branch
National Institute of Mental Health
Bethesda, Maryland

Denis G. Sukhodolsky, PhD
Child Study Center
Yale University School of Medicine
New Haven, Connecticut

Lauren S. Wakschlag, PhD
Department of Medical Social Sciences
Northwestern University
Chicago, Illinois

Jillian Lee Wiggins, PhD
Department of Psychology
San Diego State University
San Diego State University/University
   of California San Diego Joint
   Doctoral Program in Clinical
   Psychology
San Diego, California

Irritability in Pediatric Psychopathology

Introduction

Amy Krain Roy, Melissa A. Brotman, and Ellen Leibenluft

According to the Merriam-Webster dictionary, irritability is defined as "quick excitability to annoyance, impatience or anger" (www.merriam-webster.com) While young children may exhibit transient irritable mood when hungry or tired, when children present with irritability that is chronic, persistent, impairing, and greater than that of their peers, it becomes a symptom of clinical concern. This latter form of pediatric irritability is one of the most common reasons for referral for evaluation and treatment (Collishaw, Maughan, Natarajan, & Pickles, 2010; Peterson, Zhang, Santa Lucia, King, & Lewis, 1996) and is the focus of this edited volume. Indeed, such irritability is a transdiagnostic concept, appearing in the diagnostic criteria for several disorders including generalized anxiety disorder (GAD), oppositional defiant disorder (ODD), and major depressive disorder (MDD) in children. It is also common in other disorders such as attention deficit/hyperactivity disorder (ADHD) and autism. Thus, a complete understanding of pediatric irritability requires comprehensive investigations from both disorder-specific and transdiagnostic perspectives.

Over the past 15 years, significant advances have been made in our understanding of pediatric irritability, in part due to the increased focus on examining transdiagnostic dimensions of normal versus abnormal functioning, as reflected in the National Institute of Mental Health's (NIMH) Research Domain Criteria (RDoC). For example, studies indicate that chronic irritability is not diagnostic of pediatric bipolar disorder, but rather its longitudinal associations are with anxiety and unipolar depressive disorders (Stringaris, Cohen, Pine, & Leibenluft, 2009; Stringaris & Goodman, 2009; Vidal-Ribas, Brotman, Valdivieso, Leibenluft, & Stringaris, 2016). Further, irritability is associated with significant long-term consequences, such as suicidality (Orri et al., 2018; Pickles et al., 2010) and decreased educational and income levels in adulthood (Copeland, Shanahan, Egger, Angold, & Costello, 2014; Stringaris et al., 2009). Innovations in technology such as functional near-infrared spectroscopy (fNIRS) (Perlman, Luna, Hein, & Huppert,

2014) provide us with methods to obtain reliable neural and physiological data in young children, allowing for a broader developmental perspective. Advances in the assessment of irritability, such as the development of the Affective Reactivity Index (ARI; Stringaris et al., 2012), the Multidimensional Assessment Profile of Disruptive Behavior (MAP-DB) survey, and the Disruptive Behavior Diagnostic Observation Schedule (DB-DOS) standardized clinical observation (Wakschlag et al., 2014; Wakschlag, Briggs-Gowan, et al., 2008; Wakschlag, Hill, et al., 2008), allow for greater consistency in the assessment of irritability across studies, with the ultimate aim of introducing more standardized measures into clinical practice. Despite these advances, however, numerous unanswered questions remain. In particular, while RDoC constructs in the Negative Valence system, such as threat and frustrative nonreward have directly informed research and theoretical models of irritability (Brotman, Kircanski, Stringaris, Pine, & Leibenluft, 2017), more work is needed to elucidate specific mechanisms that can inform predictive models of longitudinal outcomes and guide novel treatment development. We designed this edited volume to provide the reader with the current state of the empirical literature on pediatric irritability with the aim of inspiring directions for future work.

Historical Context

While irritability has always been considered a symptom of clinical syndromes such as ODD and MDD in children, there has been a dramatic surge in the empirical study of pediatric irritability over the past two decades (Brotman et al., 2017; Leibenluft, 2017; Wakschlag et al., 2018). This increased interest developed in response to a rise in juvenile bipolar disorder (BD) diagnoses in the United States at the end of the last century and in the early 2000s (Blader & Carlson, 2007; Moreno et al., 2007). At that time, several influential researchers argued that bipolar disorder presents differently in children than in adults. Specifically, they suggested that children with pediatric bipolar disorder exhibit chronic irritability rather than discrete hypomanic or manic episodes (Biederman et al., 2004). Others proposed that children have both very short-duration daily cycles and very long-duration (e.g., multiple-year) episodes (Geller, Tillman, Bolhofner, & Zimerman, 2008). In response to this, often termed the "pediatric bipolar disorder controversy," researchers at the NIMH began a line of research to answer the question of whether children with nonepisodic, impairing irritability have BD or another clinical condition (Leibenluft, 2011). Evidence from epidemiological and longitudinal studies suggested that children presenting with irritability in the absence of discrete mood episodes did not exhibit BD as adults (Leibenluft, 2011). Additional data from familial, neuroimaging, behavioral, and physiological studies further supported the existence of two distinct phenotypes: a "narrow phenotype" characterized by the hallmark symptoms of adult BD (namely, discrete episodes of mania and depression) and a "broad phenotype" (later termed severe mood dysregulation [SMD]), characterized by chronic irritability (Brotman et al., 2017; Leibenluft, 2011, 2017). However, while this broad phenotype held great empirical interest, it was not a diagnosis found in the *Diagnostic and Statistical Manual of Mental Disorders* (DSM), suggesting that there was a group of highly impaired children who were understudied and did not have a clear nosological "home."

Consequently, in 2013, with the publication of the fifth edition of the DSM (DSM-5; American Psychiatric Association [APA], 2013), came a new diagnosis, disruptive mood dysregulation disorder (DMDD), that was established to provide such a home. Initial studies reanalyzing previously obtained data (Althoff et al., 2016; Copeland, Angold, Costello, & Egger, 2013) raised questions about this new diagnosis regarding significant overlap with other diagnoses, particularly ODD; low interrater reliability; low prevalence; and poor longitudinal stability (Althoff et al., 2016; Axelson et al., 2012; Freeman, Youngstrom, Youngstrom, & Findling, 2016; Fristad et al., 2016; Margulies, Weintraub, Basile, Grover, & Carlson, 2012; Mayes et al., 2015; Mayes, Waxmonsky, Calhoun, & Bixler, 2016; Mitchell et al., 2016; Roy, Lopes, & Klein, 2014; Stringaris, 2011). While establishing a diagnosis that accurately captures chronic irritability in children is important in terms of informing when to treat and which treatment to use, more work is needed to determine empirically supported thresholds for key DMDD symptoms of irritable mood and temper outbursts. For example, how frequent should outbursts be to be considered clinically impairing, and how might this differ depending on the age or sex of the child? Furthermore, as we know, irritability is evident in other disorders besides DMDD including ODD, intermittent explosive disorder (IED), ADHD, and autism, and thus transdiagnostic and dimensional investigations are needed if we are to develop a comprehensive model of pediatric irritability. For example, recent work has examined unique and overlapping neural correlates in irritability and anxiety (Kircanski et al., 2018). In summary, while advances have been made in the nosological classification of children with chronic irritability, there is still considerable work to be done to ensure that such impaired youth are assessed accurately and treated successfully.

Book Content

The aim of this book is to provide clinicians, clinical researchers, trainees, and students with a comprehensive overview of the current research on pediatric irritability. We approach the topic from multiple perspectives and disciplines, including child psychiatry, clinical psychology, developmental psychology, and neuroscience. We have arranged the book into five sections, each of which is made up of chapters written by preeminent scholars in the field from across the globe.

The first section, Perspectives on Assessment and Measurement, provides the reader an overview of the definition and prevalence of pediatric irritability, current assessment methods and their empirical support, and novel behavioral and psychophysiological indicators of irritability in youth. While significant advances have been made in the clinical assessment of pediatric irritability, including brief measures such as the ARI and extensive assessments such as the MAP-DB, more work is needed to validate these measures in diverse populations of children across ages, gender, settings (i.e., outpatient vs. inpatient), and informant (clinician, parent, teacher, child self-report). This will allow for improved estimates of irritability in community and clinical samples, as well as more targeted interventions and measurement of outcomes. For example, detailed assessment can be used to identify familial- or context-dependent factors that can be addressed in treatment. Physiological assessments of associated traits such as frustration intolerance are currently only conducted in the laboratory. However, with further development and validation, they have the potential to be used clinically to identify correlates of irritability that can be targeted specifically in treatment (e.g., precision medicine).

The second section, Developmental Considerations, reviews the literature on the development of pediatric irritability from preschool age through adolescence and young adulthood. These reviews highlight the serious longitudinal consequences of pediatric irritability, including development of anxiety and mood disorders and even suicidal behavior. Additionally, we include a chapter on temper tantrums that is unique in that it examines this behavioral manifestation of irritability from sociological, developmental, behavioral, and neuroscience perspectives. While tantrums are universal expressions of frustration and anger in young children, certain characteristics, such as persistence into middle and later childhood, can indicate emotion regulation deficits and psychopathology. This section highlights the need for longitudinal investigations to truly capture the developmental consequences of irritability and temper tantrums in childhood.

The third section, Etiological Mechanisms, summarizes the current state of the research on genetic factors and neural dysfunction contributing to pediatric irritability. Emerging evidence supports the role of genetic factors in pediatric irritability. However, more work is needed to investigate the interaction of genetic and environmental factors, perhaps working through epigenetic mechanisms, to better inform our etiological understanding and treatment selection. There is a growing literature suggesting neurobiological deficits in two primary domains, reward and threat processing. While these have typically been examined as distinct domains, evidence suggests that children with significant irritability exhibit alterations in reward pathways involving both frontostriatal circuits and corticolimbic threat circuits. Further work is needed in larger samples, using more complex modeling approaches, to tease apart the contribution of these neural pathways and associated behavioral deficits, with the ultimate aim of defining putative subtypes of pediatric irritability and developing targeted interventions (e.g., precision medicine).

The fourth and fifth sections cover Clinical Presentation and Treatment, respectively. The fourth section highlights the transdiagnostic nature of irritability, describing the clinical presentation of irritability within autism, disruptive behavior disorders (i.e., ODD, ADHD, conduct disorder [CD]), and mood disorders (i.e., DMDD, MDD, BD). The Treatment section provides a comprehensive overview of the psychotherapeutic and pharmacological interventions currently in use or being developed to address symptoms of pediatric irritability. What is clear from both of these sections is that pediatric irritability poses a significant clinical challenge in terms of appropriate diagnosis and treatment. Since most treatment studies have focused primarily on diagnostic groups, there is little known about the treatment of irritability transdiagnostically and whether the same treatments could be used for irritability across disorders. Furthermore, few pharmacological studies have examined irritability as an outcome variable, but instead have observed it as a side effect.

Conclusion and Future Directions

In sum, the past 20 years have witnessed significant empirical advances in the etiology, pathophysiology, diagnosis, and treatment of pediatric irritability. However, challenges remain when these children and adolescents present for clinical assessment and treatment: Is the irritability a symptom of a mood or a behavioral disorder, or both? Does it reflect a heightened response to frustration and/or deficient regulation of that response? What is the best psychosocial and/or pharmacological treatment for this child? Clearly, more work is needed to inform the prediction of clinical outcomes and the development of novel mechanism-based interventions. This work is likely to depend on advances in computational methods, such as bifactor models and other latent variable approaches, that allow us to take advantage of large extant datasets to better understand the irritability phenotype. These models will be even more effective when used with longitudinal datasets to predict outcomes. As we learn more about the basic neural, cognitive, and familial factors contributing to pediatric irritability, novel, targeted interventions can be developed. For example, initial trials of cognitive training aimed at deficits in social information processing in irritable youth are under way. Other psychosocial treatments are being developed that adapt existing cognitive behavioral and dialectical behavior therapies to meet the specific needs of pediatric irritability. It is our hope that this book will provide clinicians and clinical researchers a strong foundation in the current state of pediatric irritability research and thus serve as a launching point for important new discoveries.

References

Althoff, R. R., Crehan, E. T., He, J. P., Burstein, M., Hudziak, J. J., & Merikangas, K. R. (2016). Disruptive mood dysregulation disorder at ages 13–18: Results from the National Comorbidity Survey-Adolescent Supplement. *Journal of Child and Adolescent Psychopharmacology, 26*(2), 107–113. doi:10.1089/cap.2015.0038

American Psychiatric Association (APA). (2013). *Diagnostic and statistical manual of mental disorders* (5th edition). Washington, DC: American Psychiatric Publishing.

Axelson, D., Findling, R. L., Fristad, M. A., Kowatch, R. A., Youngstrom, E. A., Horwitz, S. M., . . . Birmaher, B. (2012). Examining the proposed disruptive mood dysregulation disorder diagnosis in children in the Longitudinal Assessment of Manic Symptoms study. *Journal of Clinical Psychiatry, 73*(10), 1342–1350. doi:10.4088/JCP.12m07674

Biederman, J., Faraone, S. V., Wozniak, J., Mick, E., Kwon, A., & Aleardi, M. (2004). Further evidence of unique developmental phenotypic correlates of pediatric bipolar disorder: Findings from a large sample of clinically referred preadolescent children assessed over the last 7 years. *Journal of Affective Disorders, 82 Suppl 1*, S45–S58. doi:10.1016/j.jad.2004.05.021

Blader, J. C., & Carlson, G. A. (2007). Increased rates of bipolar disorder diagnoses among U.S. child, adolescent, and adult inpatients, 1996–2004. *Biological Psychiatry, 62*(2), 107–114.

Brotman, M. A., Kircanski, K., Stringaris, A., Pine, D. S., & Leibenluft, E. (2017). Irritability in youths: A translational model. *American Journal of Psychiatry, 174*(6), 520–532. doi:10.1176/appi.ajp.2016.16070839

Collishaw, S., Maughan, B., Natarajan, L., & Pickles, A. (2010). Trends in adolescent emotional problems in England: A comparison of two national cohorts twenty years apart. *Journal of Child Psychology and Psychiatry, 51*(8), 885–894. doi:10.1111/j.1469-7610.2010.02252.x

Copeland, W. E., Angold, A., Costello, E. J., & Egger, H. (2013). Prevalence, comorbidity, and correlates of DSM-5 proposed disruptive mood dysregulation disorder. *American Journal of Psychiatry, 170*(2), 173–179. doi:10.1176/appi.ajp.2012.12010132

Copeland, W. E., Shanahan, L., Egger, H., Angold, A., & Costello, E. J. (2014). Adult diagnostic and functional outcomes of DSM-5 disruptive mood dysregulation disorder. *American Journal of Psychiatry, 171*(6), 668–674. doi:10.1176/appi.ajp.2014.13091213

Freeman, A. J., Youngstrom, E. A., Youngstrom, J. K., & Findling, R. L. (2016). Disruptive mood dysregulation disorder in a community mental health clinic: Prevalence, comorbidity and correlates. *Journal of Child and Adolescent Psychopharmacology, 26*(2), 123–130. doi:10.1089/cap.2015.0061

Fristad, M. A., Wolfson, H., Algorta, G. P., Youngstrom, E. A., Arnold, L. E., Birmaher, B., . . . Group, L. (2016). Disruptive mood dysregulation disorder and bipolar disorder not otherwise specified: Fraternal or identical twins? *Journal of Child and Adolescent Psychopharmacology, 26*(2), 138–146. doi:10.1089/cap.2015.0062

Geller, B., Tillman, R., Bolhofner, K., & Zimerman, B. (2008). Child bipolar I disorder: Prospective continuity with adult bipolar I disorder; characteristics of second and third episodes; predictors of 8-year outcome. *Archives of General Psychiatry, 65*(10), 1125–1133. doi:10.1001/archpsyc.65.10.1125

Kircanski, K., White, L. K., Tseng, W. L., Wiggins, J. L., Frank, H. R., Sequeira, S., . . . Brotman, M. A. (2018). A latent variable approach to differentiating neural mechanisms of irritability and anxiety in youth. *JAMA Psychiatry, 75*(6), 631–639. doi:10.1001/jamapsychiatry.2018.0468

Leibenluft, E. (2011). Severe mood dysregulation, irritability, and the diagnostic boundaries of bipolar disorder in youths. *American Journal of Psychiatry, 168*(2), 129–142. doi:10.1176/appi.ajp.2010.10050766

Leibenluft, E. (2017). Pediatric irritability: A systems neuroscience approach. *Trends in Cognitive Science, 21*(4), 277–289. doi:10.1016/j.tics.2017.02.002

Margulies, D. M., Weintraub, S., Basile, J., Grover, P. J., & Carlson, G. A. (2012). Will disruptive mood dysregulation disorder reduce false diagnosis of bipolar disorder in children? *Bipolar Disorder, 14*(5), 488–496. doi:10.1111/j.1399-5618.2012.01029.x

Mayes, S. D., Mathiowetz, C., Kokotovich, C., Waxmonsky, J., Baweja, R., Calhoun, S. L., & Bixler, E. O. (2015). Stability of disruptive mood dysregulation disorder symptoms (irritable-angry mood and temper outbursts) throughout childhood and adolescence in a general population sample. *Journal of Abnormal Child Psychology, 43*(8), 1543–1549. doi:10.1007/s10802-015-0033-8

Mayes, S. D., Waxmonsky, J. D., Calhoun, S. L., & Bixler, E. O. (2016). Disruptive mood dysregulation disorder symptoms and association with oppositional defiant and other disorders in a general population child sample. *Journal of Child and Adolescent Psychopharmacology, 26*(2), 101–106. doi:10.1089/cap.2015.0074

Mitchell, R. H., Timmins, V., Collins, J., Scavone, A., Iskric, A., & Goldstein, B. I. (2016). Prevalence and correlates of disruptive mood dysregulation disorder among adolescents with bipolar disorder. *Journal of Child and Adolescent Psychopharmacology, 26*(2), 147–153. doi:10.1089/cap.2015.0063

Moreno, C., Laje, G., Blanco, C., Jiang, H., Schmidt, A. B., & Olfson, M. (2007). National trends in the outpatient diagnosis and treatment of bipolar disorder in youth. *Archives of General Psychiatry, 64*(9), 1032–1039. doi:10.1001/archpsyc.64.9.1032

Orri, M., Galera, C., Turecki, G., Forte, A., Renaud, J., Boivin, M., . . . Geoffroy, M. C. (2018). Association of childhood irritability and depressive/anxious mood profiles with adolescent suicidal ideation and attempts. *JAMA Psychiatry, 75*(5), 465–473. doi:10.1001/jamapsychiatry.2018.0174

Perlman, S. B., Luna, B., Hein, T. C., & Huppert, T. J. (2014). fNIRS evidence of prefrontal regulation of frustration in early childhood. *NeuroImage, 85*(Pt 1), 326–334. doi:10.1016/j.neuroimage.2013.04.057

Peterson, B. S., Zhang, H., Santa Lucia, R., King, R. A., & Lewis, M. (1996). Risk factors for presenting problems in child psychiatric emergencies. *Journal of the American Academy of Child and Adolescent Psychiatry, 35*(9), 1162–1173.

Pickles, A., Aglan, A., Collishaw, S., Messer, J., Rutter, M., & Maughan, B. (2010). Predictors of suicidality across the life span: The Isle of Wight study. *Psychological Medicine, 40*(9), 1453–1466. doi:10.1017/S0033291709991905

Roy, A. K., Lopes, V., & Klein, R. G. (2014). Disruptive mood dysregulation disorder: A new diagnostic approach to chronic irritability in youth. *American Journal of Psychiatry, 171*(9), 918–924. doi:10.1176/appi.ajp.2014.13101301

Stringaris, A. (2011). Irritability in children and adolescents: A challenge for DSM-5. *European Child and Adolescent Psychiatry, 20*(2), 61–66. doi:10.1007/s00787-010-0150-4

Stringaris, A., Cohen, P., Pine, D. S., & Leibenluft, E. (2009). Adult outcomes of youth irritability: A 20-year prospective community-based study. *American Journal of Psychiatry, 166*(9), 1048–1054. doi:10.1176/appi.ajp.2009.08121849

Stringaris, A., & Goodman, R. (2009). Longitudinal outcome of youth oppositionality: Irritable, headstrong, and hurtful behaviors have distinctive predictions. *Journal of the American Academy of Child and Adolescent Psychiatry, 48*(4), 404–412. doi:10.1097/CHI.0b013e3181984f30

Stringaris, A., Goodman, R., Ferdinando, S., Razdan, V., Muhrer, E., Leibenluft, E., & Brotman, M. A. (2012). The Affective Reactivity Index: A concise irritability scale for clinical and research settings. *Journal of Child Psychology and Psychiatry, 53*(11), 1109–1117. doi:10.1111/j.1469-7610.2012.02561.x

Vidal-Ribas, P., Brotman, M. A., Valdivieso, I., Leibenluft, E., & Stringaris, A. (2016). The status of irritability in psychiatry: A conceptual and quantitative review. *Journal of the American Academy of Child and Adolescent Psychiatry, 55*(7), 556–570. doi:10.1016/j.jaac.2016.04.014

Wakschlag, L. S., Briggs-Gowan, M. J., Choi, S. W., Nichols, S. R., Kestler, J., Burns, J. L., . . . Henry, D. (2014). Advancing a multidimensional, developmental spectrum approach to preschool disruptive behavior. *Journal of the American Academy of Child and Adolescent Psychiatry, 53*(1), 82–96 e83. doi:10.1016/j.jaac.2013.10.011

Wakschlag, L. S., Briggs-Gowan, M. J., Hill, C., Danis, B., Leventhal, B. L., Keenan, K., . . . Carter, A. S. (2008). Observational assessment of preschool disruptive behavior, part II: Validity of the Disruptive Behavior Diagnostic Observation Schedule (DB-DOS). *Journal of the American Academy of Child and Adolescent Psychiatry, 47*(6), 632–641. doi:10.1097/CHI.0b013e31816c5c10

Wakschlag, L. S., Hill, C., Carter, A. S., Danis, B., Egger, H. L., Keenan, K., . . . Briggs-Gowan, M. J. (2008). Observational assessment of preschool disruptive behavior, part I: Reliability of the Disruptive Behavior Diagnostic Observation Schedule (DB-DOS). *Journal of the American Academy of Child and Adolescent Psychiatry, 47*(6), 622–631. doi:10.1097/CHI.0b013e31816c5bdb

Wakschlag, L. S., Perlman, S. B., Blair, R. J., Leibenluft, E., Briggs-Gowan, M. J., & Pine, D. S. (2018). The neurodevelopmental basis of early childhood disruptive behavior: Irritable and callous phenotypes as exemplars. *American Journal of Psychiatry, 175*(2), 114–130. doi:10.1176/appi.ajp.2017.17010045

Perspectives on Assessment and Measurement

Epidemiology of Pediatric Irritability

Giovanni Abrahão Salum

Introduction

Irritability, defined as proneness to anger relative to peers (Brotman, Kircanski, & Leibenluft, 2017; Brotman, Kircanski, Stringaris, Pine, & Leibenluft, 2017), is a common complaint in the clinical practice of a mental health professional (Peterson, Zhang, Santa Lucia, King, & Lewis, 1996). It is a trait, continuously distributed in the population, that can become pathological and require clinical attention (Vidal-Ribas, Brotman, Valdivieso, Leibenluft, & Stringaris, 2016). Irritability is common in both internalizing and externalizing disorders (Shaw, Stringaris, Nigg, & Leibenluft, 2014; Stoddard et al., 2014) and is also the core feature of disruptive mood dysregulation disorder (DMDD), a relatively new diagnosis introduced in the fifth edition of the *Diagnostic and Statistical Manual of Mental Disorders* (DSM-5) (American Psychiatric Association [APA], 2013). In this chapter, I first review the epidemiology of irritability as a dimension. Then I present the epidemiology of DMDD as the diagnostic category that most explicitly captures the clinical features of pathological irritability. In both sections, I summarize the available evidence and discuss the current challenges of epidemiological research in pediatric irritability. To illustrate some of the topics discussed here, I also present some unpublished data from the Brazilian High-Risk Cohort (HRC) Study for Psychiatric Disorders (Salum et al., 2015).

The Epidemiology of Irritability as a Dimension

Most of the current knowledge on pediatric irritability emerged from the study of irritability as a dimension in community samples (Leibenluft, Cohen, Gorrindo, Brook, & Pine, 2006; Salum et al., 2017; Stringaris, Cohen, Pine, & Leibenluft, 2009; Stringaris & Goodman, 2009a, 2009b). In these studies, irritability is commonly operationalized as a combination of temper outbursts, a low threshold for being annoyed, and angry mood. Using data from existing cohorts, items from questionnaires and interviews, such as the Diagnostic Interview Schedule for Children (DISC; Costello, Edelbrock, & Costello, 1985), Child and Adolescent Psychiatric Assessment (CAPA; Angold & Costello, 2000), and Development and Well-Being Behavior Assessment (DAWBA; Goodman, Ford, Richards, Gatward, & Meltzer, 2000), have been used to generate a composite of items indicating the presence of irritability in children and adolescents. Despite not using measures specifically designed to measure irritability, these early epidemiological studies helped to validate the irritability construct in multiple ways. First, they demonstrated that the oppositional defiant disorder (ODD) category was too heterogeneous and that irritability should have a place by itself as a significant trait in the field's nosology. Second, these studies separated chronic from episodic forms of irritability and contributed to the debate on how to fit chronic irritability into diagnostic frameworks (Leibenluft et al., 2006). Lastly, this work differentiated irritability from aggression, shifting attention from sole behavioral manifestations of irritability to the mood component of the trait (Leibenluft & Stoddard, 2013), as described in the next section.

The empirical distinction between irritability and oppositionality occurred within wider research demonstrating that oppositionality relates broadly to distinct behavioral and affective disorders (Rowe, Costello, Angold, Copeland, & Maughan, 2010; Stringaris et al., 2009), and, as a consequence of that, there could be value to studying irritability as a distinct construct. This research showed that ODD encompasses multidimensional traits that include at least three aspects: irritability (temper loss and easy annoyance), hurtfulness (spitefulness and vindictiveness), and headstrongness (argumentativeness, noncompliance, and rule-breaking behaviors; Stringaris & Goodman, 2009b). This line of research elucidated that these three dimensions are distinct in four ways: (1) in associations with other forms of psychopathology (Krieger et al., 2013; Stringaris & Goodman, 2009b), (2) in longitudinal predictions (Stringaris & Goodman, 2009a), (3) in associations with family history (Krieger et al., 2013), and (4) in etiological correlates (Stringaris, Zavos, Leibenluft, Maughan, & Eley, 2012). When integrated, these validators converge to demonstrate that, whereas the irritability dimension relates more strongly to anxiety and unipolar depression, the hurtful dimension more strongly relates to conduct problems, and the headstrong dimension is more strongly associated with attention deficit/hyperactivity disorder (ADHD). Thus, these findings highlight the distinction between irritability and other oppositional behaviors that was previously ignored by the field.

Epidemiological studies were also important to differentiate chronic from episodic presentations of irritability. Leibenluft and colleagues (Leibenluft et al., 2006) investigated a community sample of youths who had received structured diagnostic interviews at three time points (14, 16, and 22 years of age). They examined associations between separate composites of items about chronic and episodic irritability and the emergence of later psychiatric diagnosis. This study showed that chronic irritability predicted ADHD and major depression, while episodic irritability predicted simple phobias and hypo/mania. These findings highlighted the importance of differentiating these two distinct aspects of irritability and the importance for the field to begin studying chronic forms of irritable mood, and not only the episodic forms of irritability that characterize bipolar disorder (BD).

Last, the conceptual and empirical distinction between irritability and aggression was also an essential step toward establishing the value of irritability as a distinct construct for developmental psychopathology that was somewhat informed by epidemiological studies (Leibenluft & Stoddard, 2013). *Aggression* is defined as behavior intended to harm another (Berkowitz, 1983), and it is frequently divided into *proactive aggression* (i.e., a behavior designed to attain a goal) and *reactive aggression* (i.e., signs of anger that occur in response to frustrating events or perceived threats). The concept of reactive aggression is closely related to the behavioral aspects of irritability. However, reactive aggression does not necessarily capture the affective or mood component of irritability (i.e., the conscious feeling of annoyance and touchiness that does not inevitably result in aggression). Epidemiological research started to disentangle behavioral (i.e., reactive aggression) and affective (i.e., irritable mood) components of irritability in order to study if these constructs are indeed dissociable (Copeland, Brotman, & Costello, 2015). In that regard, Copeland and colleagues investigated two aspects of irritability in young children: phasic and tonic (Copeland et al., 2015). While the phasic component consists of acute times of anger or temper outbursts, the tonic aspect was characterized by a generalized angry or grumpy mood. Although the main distinction between phasic and tonic irritability in children relied on the duration of the manifestation (i.e., tonic lasting longer than phasic), operational ways of classifying tonic and phasic irritability relied a great deal on the mood and behavior distinction, with mood representing proneness to persistently experience anger as an emotion and behavior representing proneness to respond frequently with anger to frustration. The research so far shows that those components often overlap, with young children showing outbursts more often than irritable mood (Copeland et al., 2015). In any case, this conceptualization of the irritability construct brought attention to the possibility of conceptualizing irritability as a pathological mood and not solely as a behavior.

Tonic and phasic irritability are very common in community samples. The average prevalence of tantrums in the community, as estimated from meta-analyzed data from five community samples of 3- to 15-year-olds, is 46%, varying from 5% to 80% (Althoff et al., 2016; Copeland, Angold, Costello, & Egger, 2013; Dougherty et al., 2014). Age was a significant moderator of the prevalence of tantrums in a meta-regression analysis from these studies, decreasing by 4% each year and accounting for 54% of the variance in tantrum prevalence. The meta-analytic scatterplot in Figure 2.1 depicts the prevalence of tantrums according to age as predicted by the meta-regression model. Angry mood in those studies was less common

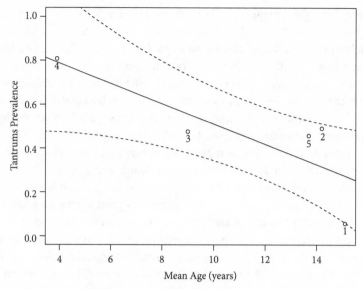

FIGURE 2.1 *Meta-analytic scatter plot of the prevalence of tantrums in community samples.*
Note: 1, Althoff (2016); 2, Dougherty (2016); 3, Copeland (2013, Duke Preschool); 4, Copeland (2013, Great Smoky Mountains); 5, Copeland (2013, Caring for Children).

than temper tantrums. The average prevalence of angry mood in the community estimated from meta-analyzed data from four community samples was 17%, varying from 8% to 27% (Althoff et al., 2016; Copeland et al., 2013; Dougherty et al., 2014).

How Common Is Irritability as a Trait, and How Is this Trait Distributed?

In addition to characterizing the prevalence of core features, the most common way to characterize irritability as a trait in community samples is by combining several items that capture behaviors, thoughts, and emotions from a rating scale that commonly quantifies frequency or duration. Given that there is a high amount of variability in the format of available rating scales, it is difficult to describe the frequency of irritability as a trait from available evidence. Also, prevalence of trait irritability is directly dependent on the instrument used to characterize frequency and duration of irritable mood and temper outbursts.

Figure 2.2 is an example of how irritability is distributed in the community using unpublished rating scale data from the Brazilian HRC. The Child Behavior Checklist (CBCL; Achenbach & Rescorla, 2001) Irritability Scale defines irritability as indicated by a child presenting with "temper tantrums or hot temper," who "sulks a lot," is "stubborn, sullen, or irritable," has "sudden changes in mood or feelings," and who "argues a lot." A scale quantifying those symptoms as "Not true (value of 0)," "Sometimes true (value of 1)," and "Often true (value of 2)"

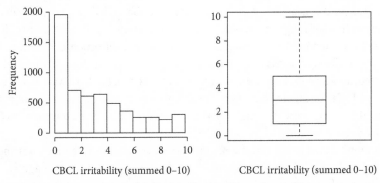

FIGURE 2.2 *Distribution of Child Behavior Checklist (CBCL) irritability in community samples.*

Unpublished data from the Brazilian High-Risk Cohort Study (*n* = 2,511, ages 6–14, baseline; *n* = 2,009, ages 9–17 in wave 2, CBCL Irritability Scale).

generates a score of 0 to 10. A histogram of this short scale shows that whereas there are several children in the community who do not present with any irritability symptoms, there are high variations in irritability levels among children and adolescents, with half of the participants having a score of 3 or more (Figure 2.2).

These data show that irritability is not normally distributed in the population, meaning that existing instruments might serve to characterize irritability more specifically in subjects with high levels of symptoms. Other brief instruments, such as the Affective Reactivity Index (ARI), also present similar issues with frequency of distributions (Stringaris, Goodman et al., 2012). More detailed instruments, such as the Temper Loss Scale from the Multidimensional Assessment of Preschool Disruptive Behavior (MAP-DB) (Wakschlag et al., 2015), are more sensitive to capture the nuance of normal and pathological irritability. Nevertheless, the MAP-DB still focuses its discriminative power on children with high levels of symptoms, which is consistent with the clinical purpose of the instrument.

Newly designed measures, such as the Disruptive Mood Dysregulation Disorder version of the Extended Strengths and Weaknesses of Normal Behavior (E-SWAN), are focused on characterizing children from the community with high and low ability to regulate emotions. Consistent with that purpose, the E-SWAN instrument has shown normal distributions and might be suitable to characterize variation in community samples (Alexander, Salum, Swanson, & Milham, 2017). The E-SWAN version for irritability traits can be found online (www.eswan.org). This type of approach holds promise in epidemiological studies that include both children with and without psychiatric disorders.

IRRITABILITY AS A TRAIT ACROSS DEVELOPMENT

Very few longitudinal studies have addressed the trajectories of irritability over time. In a cross-sectional community sample of preschoolers (3–8 years of age),

Wakschlag and colleagues (Wakschlag et al., 2015) found decreases in levels of irritability in this age range (0.2 standard deviation [SD] per year), with no sex effects or age-by-sex interactions. Leibenluft and colleagues (Leibenluft et al., 2006) also found age effects on levels of irritability in a community sample showing that, for children, adolescents, and young adults (9–21 years of age), there was an inverted-U shaped relationship for both sexes, peaking approximately at age 13 for boys and 15 for girls. Girls presented higher irritability scores than boys, but there was no age-by-sex interaction.

In unpublished data from the Brazilian HRC study spanning four assessments of the CBCL irritability subscale and including children 6–17 years of age, we observe a significant interaction between age and sex on levels of irritability over time. A stratified analysis of age effects by sex shows that whereas there is a substantial linear increase in levels of irritability symptoms over time for girls, the same does not occur for boys. Mean levels of irritability were nominally higher for boys before age 12 as compared to girls and nominally higher for girls as compared to boys from age 12 until age 17 (Figure 2.3).

Using the CBCL, Wiggins, Mitchell, Stringaris, and Leibenluft (2014) examined longitudinal data from 4,898 families when children were at ages 3, 5, and 9 years. Using latent growth analysis, which finds clusters of symptom trajectories over time, they found that irritability follows five specific trajectories. Most children had low (61%) and moderate (21%) levels of irritability at age 3, decreasing slightly until age 9. The other three trajectories presented with a high number of symptoms at age 3, with one group continuing to be steady-high (10%), another group decreasing dramatically (5%), and another continuing to increase (2%) in the number of symptoms until age 9. This highlights the diverse number of possible trajectories of irritability symptoms over time at the individual level.

CO-OCCURRENCE OF TRAIT IRRITABILITY WITH OTHER CLINICAL TRAITS

Irritability as a trait is common to both internalizing and externalizing disorders (Shaw et al., 2014; Stoddard et al., 2014). In unpublished data from the Brazilian HRC, the irritability scale relates strongly to all other domains of psychopathology, with stronger correlations with aggression, followed by anxiety/depression and attention domains (Figure 2.4). Also, a network analysis of all CBCL items showed that irritability items are at the midpoint between internalizing and externalizing symptoms, consistent with the high prevalence of those symptoms in both internalizing and externalizing disorders (Figure 2.4).

Moreover, levels of irritability are higher in children and adolescents with all types of mental disorders (phobias, major depression, generalized anxiety, ADHD, and disruptive behavior disorder) compared to children with typical development (Figure 2.5). This is consistent with the ubiquity of irritability as a symptom in the diagnostic manuals and the prominence of this symptom in clinical practice.

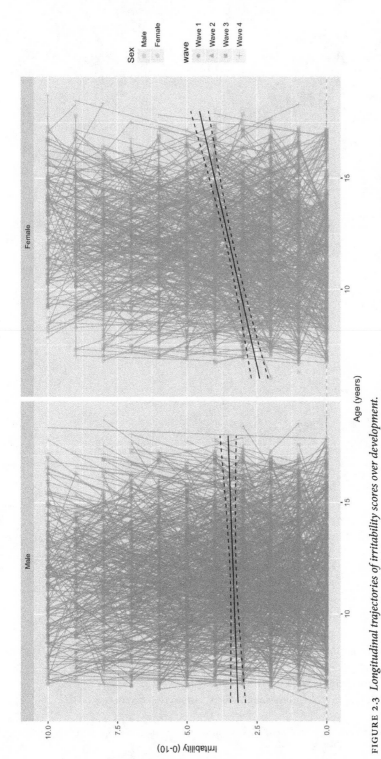

FIGURE 2.3 *Longitudinal trajectories of irritability scores over development.*

Unpublished data from the Brazilian High-Risk Cohort Study (wave 1 household assessment *n* = 771; wave 1 imaging assessment *n* = 2,511; wave 2 household assessment *n* = 2,009; wave 2 imaging assessment *n* = 484).

(a)

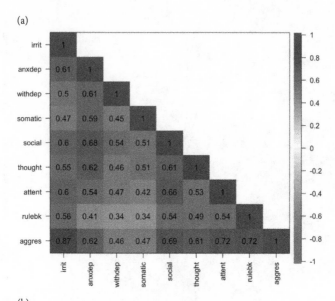

(b)

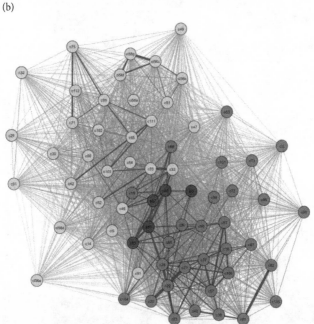

FIGURE 2.4 *Relationship between irritability symptoms and irritability dimensions with other symptoms and domains of psychopathology.*
Right panel: Irritability symptoms (darkest gray) are in the middle of internalizing (lightest gray) and externalizing (medium gray) symptoms as measured by the Child Behavior Checklist (CBCL). Left Panel: Correlation between Irritability and narrow band CBCL dimensions.

Unpublished data from the High-Risk Cohort Study (*n* = 2,511, ages 6–14, baseline assessment, CBCL Irritability Scale; Giovanni Abrahão Salum et al., 2015).

We can also see that in the Brazilian HRC, there are several children with typical development who have high levels of irritability. Given that these children do not meet criteria for any of the clinical diagnoses examined, this suggests there might be room for new diagnostic categories such as DMDD to clinically characterize irritability in the community.

Despite this, data from three community studies (Copeland, Shanahan, Egger, Angold, & Costello, 2014) suggest that the vast majority of children with DMDD using the current diagnostic thresholds (62–92%) present with comorbid internalizing and externalizing disorders, and that, therefore, DMDD currently does not capture most children with purer forms of irritability.

Longitudinal data also support a strong relationship with other mental disorders, showing a pattern of heterotypic continuity. Dougherty and colleagues (Dougherty et al., 2013), investigating the longitudinal predictors of trait irritability in preschoolers at 3 years of age, showed that a continuous measure of irritability derived from Preschool Age Psychiatric Assessment (PAPA) items predicted depression, ODD, and functional impairment at 6 years after adjusting for baseline disorders.

DEFINING CUTOFFS IN TRAIT IRRITABILITY FOR CLINICAL PRACTICE

Similar to other dimensions of negative affectivity, such as anxiety and depression, irritability, when assessed with measures with sufficient sensitivity, distributes continuously in the population (Wakschlag et al., 2015). Cutoffs defining normal from abnormal levels are likely to represent the necessity of dichotomous or stratified clinical decisions (e.g., to treat or not to treat) rather than "natural joints" in the trait distribution (Markon, Chmielewski, & Miller, 2011). Therefore, given that

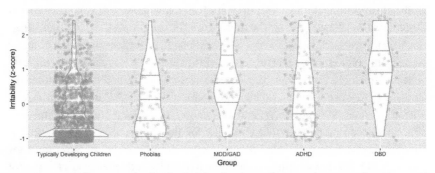

FIGURE 2.5 *Differences in levels of irritability between subjects with non-overlapping mental disorders.*

Abbreviations: MDD, major depressive disorder; GAD, generalized anxiety disorder; ADHD, attention deficit/ hyperactivity disorder; BDD, disruptive behavior disorders.

Unpublished data from the Brazilian High-Risk Cohort Study (n = 2,263, ages 6–14, baseline assessment, CBCL irritability scale; Giovanni Abrahão Salum et al., 2015).

we are not expected to have clear cutoffs, the next essential step is understanding how irritability distributes in the population, and epidemiological studies play a major role in this process.

Epidemiological studies now use modern psychometrics to separate normative misbehavior from clinically salient problems that require clinical attention (Wakschlag et al., 2015; Wiggins et al., 2018). Wakschlag and collaborators (2015) provide an example of using item response theory analysis to investigate which symptoms represent normative misbehavior and which symptoms indicate clinically significant problems. By investigating the patterns of responses from each item of a questionnaire, they showed that some behaviors, such as acting "aggressively when frustrated, angry, or upset," are typical and normative and only represent problems when their frequency is high or very high. Other responses, such as a child who "acts aggressively to try to get something he or she wanted," are only seen in children already presenting with several other symptoms, and these are called *problem indicators* (i.e., their mere presence already indicates the presence of a significant problem that requires clinical attention) (Wakschlag et al., 2014). This strategy holds promise to both refine diagnostic manuals to improve the validity of current categories and also as a way to integrate dimensional assessments into clinical practice and inform clinicians when to worry and when not to worry about children's moods and behaviors (Wakschlag et al., 2017). A psychometric approach applied to epidemiological studies is necessary to move the field forward and help define boundaries that combine clinical experience with data-driven methods.

The Epidemiology of Irritability as a Category

As discussed earlier, DMDD is a diagnostic category that captures the two core clinical features of pathological irritability (i.e., tonic and phasic). As discussed in more detail in other chapters, the motivation for the proposition of a new diagnostic category to classify children with severe and chronic expressions of anger came from epidemiological assessments of the rates of BD in children using data collected from 1990 and 2006. Those studies detected a fivefold increase in the diagnosis of BD in children in inpatient populations (Blader & Carlson, 2007; Case, Olfson, Marcus, & Siegel, 2007) and as much as a 40-fold increase in outpatient clinics (Moreno et al., 2007). The reasons for that increase were debatable, but some researchers proposed that it was a result of broadening the symptoms for pediatric BD by incorporating nonepisodic irritability and hyperarousal as part of the criteria and ignoring the requirements of clearly demarcated episodes of hypomania and mania (Brotman, Kircanski, & Leibenluft, 2017).

To empirically test the formulation of severe and chronic irritability as a distinct form of pediatric BD, Leibenluft and colleagues (Leibenluft, 2011; Leibenluft, Charney, Towbin, Bhangoo, & Pine, 2003) operationalized criteria for a syndrome called *severe mood dysregulation* (SMD) and conducted a series of studies to investigate commonalities and differences between SMD and BD in children. Those studies converged to demonstrate that there was little evidence to support SMD as an early presentation of BD based on accumulated evidence from epidemiology, family history, clinical description, and a series of laboratory studies (Leibenluft, 2011). The understanding that these children suffered significant impairments (Dougherty et al., 2014) that led to frequent hospitalization and the preliminary validity of SMD syndrome served as the basis for the DMDD diagnosis proposed in DSM-5.

HOW COMMON IS DMDD IN THE COMMUNITY?

Multiple studies have estimated DMDD prevalence in community-ascertained samples. Because the diagnosis is new, most studies (with one exception: Munhoz et al., 2017) needed to use secondary data from instruments not directly designed to diagnose DMDD. While this is a limitation, these studies are still informative for future research.

Copeland and collaborators (Copeland et al., 2013) used data from three regionally representative samples: the Duke Preschool Anxiety Study (Study 1: n = 918, ages 2–6 years recruited from primary care pediatric clinics), the Great Smoky Mountains Study (Study 2: n = 1,420, ages 9–17 recruited from 11 rural counties from North Carolina), and the Caring for Children in the Community Study (Study 3: n = 920, ages 9–17 recruited from four rural counties from North Carolina). They investigated the prevalence of DMDD using questions from the PAPA (Study 1) and the Child and Adolescent Psychiatric Assessment (CAPA; Studies 2 and 3), which have the required domains to generate a DMDD diagnosis. Using the full criteria, they found a prevalence of DMDD of 3.3%, 1.1%, and 0.8% for studies 1, 2, and 3, respectively.

Dougherty and collaborators (Dougherty et al., 2014) used data from 462 families living within 20 miles of Stony Brook University as identified by a commercial mailing list. They assessed children at 3 years of age and reassessed them at 6 years of age using adapted questions from the PAPA; these questions were not specifically designed to assess DMDD but did assess the required domains of temper tantrums and irritable mood necessary to generate a DMDD diagnosis. The 3-month prevalence rate of DMDD at 6 years of age in this sample was 8.2%.

Althoff and collaborators (Althoff et al., 2016) used data from the Adolescent Supplement from the National Comorbidity Survey (NCS-A) to generate proxies for the DMDD diagnosis using this nationally representative sample of 6,483 adolescents 12–18 years of age. By using questions from several modules of the Composite International Diagnostic Interview (CIDI), they showed that the prevalence of a narrow definition of DMDD in this sample was 0.12%. When excluding the frequency criterion (Criterion C) and ignoring the exclusion of subjects with elevated/expansive mood (Criterion I), the prevalence rate of DMDD was 5.26%.

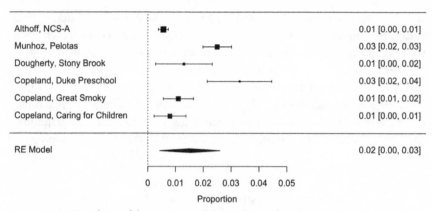

FIGURE 2.6 *Prevalence of disruptive mood dysregulation disorder in community samples.*

Finally, Munhoz and collaborators (Munhoz et al., 2017) used data from the 2004 Pelotas Birth Cohort using a regionally representative sample of 3,563 participants 11 years of age. They used an instrument constructed to assess DMDD from the DAWBA. The DAWBA consists of open and closed questions quantifying the occurrence of symptoms based on the diagnostic manuals. The open questions allow qualitative description of the symptoms, frequency, and other characteristics of the disorders assessed, which are then rated by psychiatrists. Using this method, the authors showed that the prevalence of DMDD in this population was 2.5%.

As seen in Figure 2.6, there are wide variations in the estimated prevalence of DMDD in each specific study; these are represented by squares in the forest plot and the precision of each study to provide prevalence estimates is represented by the whiskers of those squares. The diamond at the end of the plot represents the weighted overall prevalence for all the studies. A meta-analysis investigating the overall prevalence of DMDD from the available data resulted in a prevalence of 2%.

RELIABILITY AND VALIDITY OF DMDD

It is important to note that the prevalence of DMDD, or any disorder, is directly related to the reliability and validity of that diagnosis. *Reliability* refers the degree to which two clinicians could independently agree on the presence or absence of a DMDD diagnosis when the same patient was interviewed on separate occasions. Results from DSM-5 field trials showed that reliability for DMDD was good for the site that included the largest number of patients and where the patients were predominantly from inpatient services (kappa = 0.49) (Regier et al., 2013). The two other sites that included participants obtained primarily from outpatient settings produced unacceptable kappa levels of between 0.06 and 0.11. These results denote that, consistent with the origins of the "severe mood dysregulation" diagnosis, the DMDD category performs best for differentiating patients with a severe presentation of irritability and that further research on providing an empirical basis for DMDD diagnosis is still needed.

The *validity* of a diagnosis indicates the percentage of person-to-person variability within that diagnosis, which relates to the variance of the disease for which the diagnosis is meant (Kraemer, 2007). That is, validity is the work the diagnosis does in the world; that is, by knowing that a patient is in a diagnostic class, we learn something important about the patient (First, Kendler, & Parnas, 2012). The validity of DMDD has been partially supported by studies investigating the clinical description, laboratory studies, delimitation from other disorders, longitudinal courses, and family studies (Robins & Guze, 1970). The clinical description has been demonstrated in the frequent co-occurrence of the two main clinical features—severe and recurrent temper outbursts and persistent angry mood between outbursts (Copeland et al., 2015)—which significantly impacts children's functioning (Copeland et al., 2013; Dougherty et al., 2014). Laboratory studies show some neurocognitive and brain alterations when comparing those with DMDD with children with other disorders (Brotman, Kircanski, Stringaris, et al., 2017; Leibenluft, 2017); however, as in other mental disorders, effect sizes for those differences so far are low and have little impact on the DMDD diagnosis (Kapur, Phillips, & Insel, 2012). The validity of DMDD as a distinct disorder is also challenged by the fact that boundaries between normal and abnormal levels of irritability are still being delineated, and high rates of comorbidity denote the importance of reconsidering the placement of irritability as a symptom in other DSM-5 syndromes. Follow-up studies indicate the long-term prognosis of children with DMDD is marked by impaired functioning (Copeland et al., 2014). Family studies indicate that there is a significant association between DMDD and maternal depression (Munhoz et al., 2017) and parental anxiety (Dougherty et al., 2014).

THE BUILDING BLOCKS OF THE DMDD DIAGNOSIS

Given that the specific diagnostic criteria for DMDD is still a topic of empirical study, it is important to understand the building blocks that define this phenotype. As outlined earlier in this chapter, the presence of severe tantrums is extremely common in communities and particularly in preschool children, reaching 80% of all children in some studies (Figure 2.7). The diagnostic constraints imposed by frequency of the tantrums, the presence of negative mood between tantrums, duration, the necessity of behaviors occurring in multiple settings, and the application of the full criteria with "and" rules defines the lower prevalence of DMDD we see in the five studies described in Figure 2.7 (Althoff et al., 2016; Copeland et al., 2013; Dougherty et al., 2014).

However, the extent to which those criteria are valid from a clinical standpoint and the degree to which the diagnostic label captures most children with a severe irritability that require clinical attention still merits further research. For example, an empirical way of determining groups with distinct severity levels of irritability is by the use of latent methods such as latent class analysis (LCA). This method investigates the pattern of response to several items to find classes of subjects with distinct levels of severity. This analysis in the Brazilian HRC demonstrated the existence of three groups: a low symptoms group (53%), a sometimes irritable group

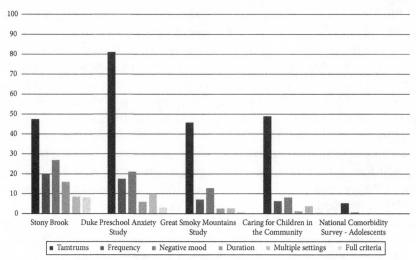

FIGURE 2.7 *The building blocks of the disruptive mood dysregulation disorder diagnostic definition.*

(32%), and an often irritable group (15%) (Salum et al., 2017). These results suggest that current DMDD criteria might be overly strict in capturing the phenomena in the population, given that only around 2% would meet diagnostic criteria. Moreover, given the prominence of age effects on both severity and frequency of irritability symptoms in the community, neurodevelopmentally appropriate criteria will be required to separate normal from abnormal levels of irritability for diagnostic manuals (Wakschlag et al., 2017; Wiggins et al., 2018).

PATTERNS OF CO-OCCURRENCE OF DMDD

Comorbidity with other disorders is substantial as DMDD co-occurs with all common mental disorders in children and adolescents. In the Duke Preschool Anxiety, Great Smoky Mountains, and Caring for Children in the Community Studies, DMDD occurred with another disorder 62–92% of the time and occurred with both an emotional and behavioral disorder 32–68% of the time (Copeland et al., 2013). Without applying exclusionary criteria, co-occurrence with ODD reaches an odds ratio (OR) from 52.9 to 103.0 (Copeland et al., 2013).

In preschool children (Copeland et al., 2013; Dougherty et al., 2014), the highest levels of co-occurrence were with depressive disorder (OR between 3.4 and 9.9), conduct disorder (OR 3.8), ADHD (OR between 1.5 and 12.6), and anxiety disorders (OR between 1.47 and 6.1). In children and adolescents (Althoff et al., 2016; Copeland et al., 2013), co-occurrence was again higher for depressive disorders (OR between 5 and 23), conduct disorder (OR between 4.4 and 11.9), ADHD (OR between 1.95 and 7.6), and anxiety disorders (OR between 1.13 and 5.2). Significant levels of co-occurrence were also found for substance abuse in one study (OR 2.36) (Althoff et al., 2016).

DMDD AND DEMOGRAPHIC CHARACTERISTICS

The prevalence of DMDD appears to be equally distributed across sexes (Althoff et al., 2016; Copeland et al., 2013; Dougherty et al., 2014; Munhoz et al., 2017). There were no prevalence differences of DMDD between ethnicities as assessed by four studies (Althoff et al., 2016; Copeland et al., 2013; Dougherty et al., 2014; Munhoz et al., 2017). All studies showed that DMDD is more common in impoverished families (Althoff et al., 2016; Copeland et al., 2013; Dougherty et al., 2014; Munhoz et al., 2017). The association with lower parental education is mixed, with some studies reporting significant associations with this factor (Althoff et al., 2016; Munhoz et al., 2017), while other failed to report such associations (Copeland et al., 2013; Dougherty et al., 2014).

Conclusion

I reviewed here evidence related to the epidemiology of irritability both dimensionally and related to the DMDD syndrome. The following conclusions can be drawn. First, whereas irritability as a trait is tremendously common, DMDD as a categorical syndrome affects around 2% of the population. Second, there are developmental effects on levels of irritability over time, with epidemiological data suggesting profound age-related differences in how irritability manifests. This also affects prevalence rates of DMDD and denotes the importance to adapt diagnostic criteria for the nuance of developmental presentations of both temper tantrums and irritable mood. Third, work is still needed to bring reliability and validity to measuring irritability as a dimension with scales that are sensitive to detect the normal–abnormal spectrum of irritability. Also, research must address the extent to which DMDD is a representative category of severe irritability given the low-reliability estimates and still modest evidence for validity according to classical parameters. Last, despite preliminary evidence of discriminability, the extent to which irritability differs from other psychiatry-relevant traits and to which DMDD differs from other common mental disorders still needs to be further assessed and conceptualized to separate common from dissociable aspects of psychopathology.

References

Achenbach, T.M., & Rescorla, L.A. (2001). Manual for the ASEBA School-Age Forms & Profiles. Burlington, VT: University of Vermont, Research Center for Children, Youth, & Families.

Alexander, L. M., Salum, G., Swanson, J. M., & Milham, M. P. (2017). Balancing strengths and weaknesses in dimensional psychiatry. *bioRxiv*, http://dx.doi.org/10.1101/207019.

Althoff, R. R., Crehan, E. T., He, J. P., Burstein, M., Hudziak, J. J., & Merikangas, K. R. (2016). Disruptive mood dysregulation disorder at ages 13–18: Results from the National

Comorbidity Survey—Adolescent Supplement. *Journal of Child and Adolescent Psychopharmacology*, 26(2), 107–113.

American Psychiatric Association (APA). (2013). *Diagnostic and statistical manual of mental disorders (DSM-5)*. Washington, DC: American Psychiatric Pub.

Angold, A., & Costello, E. J. (2000). The Child and Adolescent Psychiatric Assessment (CAPA). *Journal of the American Academy of Child and Adolescent Psychiatry*, 39(1), 39–48.

Berkowitz, L. (1983). Aversively stimulated aggression: Some parallels and differences in research with animals and humans. *American Psychologist*, 38(11), 1135.

Blader, J. C., & Carlson, G. A. (2007). Increased rates of bipolar disorder | diagnoses among US child, adolescent, and adult inpatients, 1996–2004. *Biological Psychiatry*, 62(2), 107–114.

Brotman, M. A., Kircanski, K., & Leibenluft, E. (2017). Irritability in children and adolescents. *Annual Review of Clinical Psychology*, 13, 317–341.

Brotman, M. A., Kircanski, K., Stringaris, A., Pine, D. S., & Leibenluft, E. (2017). Irritability in youths: A translational model. *American Journal of Psychiatry*, 174(6), 520–532.

Case, B. G., Olfson, M., Marcus, S. C., & Siegel, C. (2007). Trends in the inpatient mental health treatment of children and adolescents in US community hospitals between 1990 and 2000. *Archives of General Psychiatry*, 64(1), 89–96.

Copeland, W. E., Angold, A., Costello, E. J., & Egger, H. (2013). Prevalence, comorbidity, and correlates of DSM-5 proposed disruptive mood dysregulation disorder. *American Journal of Psychiatry*, 170(2), 173–179.

Copeland, W. E., Brotman, M. A., & Costello, E. J. (2015). Normative irritability in youth: Developmental findings from the Great Smoky Mountains Study. *Journal of the American Academy of Child & Adolescent Psychiatry*, 54(8), 635–642.

Copeland, W. E., Shanahan, L., Egger, H., Angold, A., & Costello, E. J. (2014). Adult diagnostic and functional outcomes of DSM-5 disruptive mood dysregulation disorder. *American Journal of Psychiatry*, 171(6), 668–674.

Costello, E. J., Edelbrock, C. S., & Costello, A. J. (1985). Validity of the NIMH Diagnostic Interview Schedule for Children: a comparison between psychiatric and pediatric referrals. *Journal of Abnormal Child Psychology*, 13(4), 579–595.

Dougherty, L. R., Smith, V. C., Bufferd, S. J., Carlson, G. A., Stringaris, A., Leibenluft, E., & Klein, D. N. (2014). DSM-5 disruptive mood dysregulation disorder: Correlates and predictors in young children. *Psychological Medicine*, 44(11), 2339–2350.

Dougherty, L. R., Smith, V. C., Bufferd, S. J., Stringaris, A., Leibenluft, E., Carlson, G. A., & Klein, D. N. (2013). Preschool irritability: longitudinal associations with psychiatric disorders at age 6 and parental psychopathology. *Journal of the American Academy of Child & Adolescent Psychiatry*, 52(12), 1304–1313. doi:10.1016/j.jaac.2013.09.007. Epub 2013 Sep 26.

First, M. B., Kendler, K. S., & Parnas, J. (2012). Philosophical issues in psychiatry II: Nosology.

Goodman, R., Ford, T., Richards, H., Gatward, R., & Meltzer, H. (2000). The Development and Well-Being Assessment: description and initial validation of an integrated assessment of child and adolescent psychopathology. *Journal of Child Psychology and Psychiatry*, 41(5), 645–655.

Kapur, S., Phillips, A. G., & Insel, T. R. (2012). Why has it taken so long for biological psychiatry to develop clinical tests and what to do about it?. *Molecular Psychiatry*, *17*(12), 1174.

Kraemer, H. C. (2007). DSM categories and dimensions in clinical and research contexts. *International Journal of Methods in Psychiatric Research*, *16*(S1) , S8–S15.

Krieger, F. V., Polanczyk, G. V., Goodman, R., Rohde, L. A., Graeff-Martins, A. S., Salum, G., . . . Stringaris, A. (2013). Dimensions of oppositionality in a Brazilian community sample: Testing the DSM-5 proposal and etiological links. *Journal of the American Academy of Child & Adolescent Psychiatry*, *52*(4), 389–400.

Leibenluft, E. (2011). Severe mood dysregulation, irritability, and the diagnostic boundaries of bipolar disorder in youths. *American Journal of Psychiatry*, *168*(2), 129–142.

Leibenluft, E. (2017). Pediatric irritability: A systems neuroscience approach. *Trends in Cognitive Sciences*, *21*(4), 277–289.

Leibenluft, E., Charney, D. S., Towbin, K. E., Bhangoo, R. K., & Pine, D. S. (2003). Defining clinical phenotypes of juvenile mania. *American Journal of Psychiatry*, *160*(3), 430–437.

Leibenluft, E., Cohen, P., Gorrindo, T., Brook, J. S., & Pine, D. S. (2006). Chronic versus episodic irritability in youth: A community-based, longitudinal study of clinical and diagnostic associations. *Journal of Child & Adolescent Psychopharmacology*, *16*(4), 456–466.

Leibenluft, E., & Stoddard, J. (2013). The developmental psychopathology of irritability. *Development and Psychopathology*, *25*(4pt2), 1473–1487.

Markon, K. E., Chmielewski, M., & Miller, C. J. (2011). The reliability and validity of discrete and continuous measures of psychopathology: A quantitative review. *Psychological Bulletin*, *137*(5), 856.

Moreno, C., Laje, G., Blanco, C., Jiang, H., Schmidt, A. B., & Olfson, M. (2007). National trends in the outpatient diagnosis and treatment of bipolar disorder in youth. *Archives of General Psychiatry*, *64*(9), 1032–1039.

Munhoz, T. N., Santos, I. S., Barros, A. J., Anselmi, L., Barros, F. C., & Matijasevich, A. (2017). Perinatal and postnatal risk factors for disruptive mood dysregulation disorder at age 11: 2004 Pelotas Birth Cohort Study. *Journal of Affective Disorders*, *215*, 263–268.

Peterson, B. S., Zhang, H., Santa Lucia, R., King, R. A., & Lewis, M. (1996). Risk factors for presenting problems in child psychiatric emergencies. *Journal of the American Academy of Child & Adolescent Psychiatry*, *35*(9), 1162–1173.

Regier, D. A., Narrow, W. E., Clarke, D. E., Kraemer, H. C., Kuramoto, S. J., Kuhl, E. A., & Kupfer, D. J. (2013). DSM-5 field trials in the United States and Canada, Part II: Test-retest reliability of selected categorical diagnoses. *American Journal of Psychiatry*, *170*(1), 59–70.

Robins, E., & Guze, S. B. (1970). Establishment of diagnostic validity in psychiatric illness: Its application to schizophrenia. *American Journal of Psychiatry*, *126*(7), 983–987.

Rowe, R., Costello, E. J., Angold, A., Copeland, W. E., & Maughan, B. (2010). Developmental pathways in oppositional defiant disorder and conduct disorder. *Journal of Abnormal Child Psychology*, *119*(4), 726–738. doi:10.1037/a0020798

Salum, G. A., Gadelha, A., Pan, P. M., Moriyama, T. S., Graeff-Martins, A. S., Tamanaha, A. C., . . . Sato, J. R. (2015). High risk cohort study for psychiatric disorders in childhood: Rationale, design, methods and preliminary results. *International Journal of Methods in Psychiatric Research*, *24*(1), 58–73.

Salum, G. A., Mogg, K., Bradley, B. P., Stringaris, A., Gadelha, A., Pan, P. M., . . . Leibenluft, E. (2017). Association between irritability and bias in attention orienting to threat in children and adolescents. *Journal of Child Psychology and Psychiatry, 58*(5), 595–602.

Shaw, P., Stringaris, A., Nigg, J., & Leibenluft, E. (2014). Emotion dysregulation in attention deficit hyperactivity disorder. *American Journal of Psychiatry, 171*(3), 276–293.

Stoddard, J., Stringaris, A., Brotman, M. A., Montville, D., Pine, D. S., & Leibenluft, E. (2014). Irritability in child and adolescent anxiety disorders. *Depression and Anxiety, 31*(7), 566–573.

Stringaris, A., Cohen, P., Pine, D. S., & Leibenluft, E. (2009). Adult outcomes of youth irritability: A 20-year prospective community-based study. *American Journal of Psychiatry, 166*(9), 1048–1054.

Stringaris, A., & Goodman, R. (2009a). Longitudinal outcome of youth oppositionality: Irritable, headstrong, and hurtful behaviors have distinctive predictions. *Journal of the American Academy of Child & Adolescent Psychiatry, 48*(4), 404–412.

Stringaris, A., & Goodman, R. (2009b). Three dimensions of oppositionality in youth. *Journal of Child Psychology and Psychiatry, 50*(3), 216–223.

Stringaris, A., Goodman, R., Ferdinando, S., Razdan, V., Muhrer, E., Leibenluft, E., & Brotman, M. A. (2012). The Affective Reactivity Index: A concise irritability scale for clinical and research settings. *Journal of Child Psychology and Psychiatry, 53*(11), 1109–1117.

Stringaris, A., Zavos, H., Leibenluft, E., Maughan, B., & Eley, T. C. (2012). Adolescent irritability: Phenotypic associations and genetic links with depressed mood. *American Journal of Psychiatry, 169*(1), 47–54.

Vidal-Ribas, P., Brotman, M. A., Valdivieso, I., Leibenluft, E., & Stringaris, A. (2016). The status of irritability in psychiatry: A conceptual and quantitative review. *Journal of the American Academy of Child & Adolescent Psychiatry, 55*(7), 556–570.

Wakschlag, L. S., Briggs-Gowan, M. J., Choi, S. W., Nichols, S. R., Kestler, J., Burns, J. L., Carter, A. S., & Henry, D. (2014). Advancing a multidimensional, developmental spectrum approach to preschool disruptive behavior. *Journal of the American Academy of Child & Adolescent Psychiatry, 53*(1), 82–96.e3. doi:10.1016/j.jaac.2013.10.011. Epub 2013 Nov 7.

Wakschlag, L. S., Estabrook, R., Petitclerc, A., Henry, D., Burns, J. L., Perlman, S. B., . . . Briggs-Gowan, M. L. (2015). Clinical implications of a dimensional approach: The normal-abnormal spectrum of early irritability. *Journal of the American Academy of Child & Adolescent Psychiatry, 54*(8), 626–634.

Wakschlag, L. S., Perlman, S. B., Blair, R. J., Leibenluft, E., Briggs-Gowan, M. J., & Pine, D. S. (2017). The neurodevelopmental basis of early childhood disruptive behavior: Irritable and callous phenotypes as exemplars. *American Journal of Psychiatry, 175*, 114–130.

Wiggins, J. L., Briggs-Gowan, M. J., Estabrook, R., Brotman, M. A., Pine, D. S., Leibenluft, E., & Wakschlag, L. S. (2018). Identifying Clinically Significant Irritability in Early Childhood. *Journal of the American Academy of Child & Adolescent Psychiatry, 57*(3), 191–199.e2. doi:10.1016/j.jaac.2017.12.008. Epub 2017 Dec 28.

Wiggins, J. L., Mitchell, C., Stringaris, A., & Leibenluft, E. (2014). Developmental trajectories of irritability and bidirectional associations with maternal depression. *Journal of the American Academy of Child & Adolescent Psychiatry, 53*(11), 1191–205, 1205. e1–4. doi:10.1016/j.jaac.2014.08.005. Epub 2014 Sep 3.

3

Measurement of Irritability in Children and Adolescents

Merelise Ametti and Robert R. Althoff

Background

Irritability has been part of the official psychiatric nomenclature since it was used to describe episodes of mania in the first edition of the *Diagnostic Statistical Manual* (DSM) published in 1952 (Safer, 2009). Since then, it has been incorporated into the diagnostic criteria for 15 psychiatric illnesses, including mood, anxiety, behavioral, substance use, and personality disorders (American Psychiatric Association [APA], 2013; Toohey & DiGiuseppe, 2017). Yet, despite longevity and ubiquity, irritability has remained an ill-defined and underresearched phenomenon until relatively recently.

The need for further conceptual development and phenotypic refinement was brought into sharp relief during the late 1990s and early 2000s by an upsurge in the rates of juvenile bipolar disorder (J-BPD) diagnoses, particularly in the United States (Blader & Carlson, 2007). There was a suggestion in the literature and in consensus panels that J-BPD rates were being inflated by the misinterpretation of chronic irritability as a symptom of (hypo)mania. Further, it was postulated that impairing, nonepisodic irritability during childhood may constitute a distinct clinical phenotype with unique trajectories and treatment needs (Leibenluft, Charney, Towbin, Bhangoo, & Pine, 2003). In order to test this hypothesis, valid and reliable methods of isolating and measuring nonepisodic irritability were imperative. Unfortunately, the few extant measures of clinical irritability at the time had been only minimally validated and were primarily intended for use in adult populations (Burns, Folstein, Brandt, & Folstein, 1990; Caprara, Renzi, Alcini, Imperio, & Travaglia, 1983; Snaith, Constantopoulos, Jardine, & McGuffin, 1978).

Since that time, there have been multiple attempts made to measure irritability in childhood and adolescence. There have been changes in both the diagnostic system and the measurement landscape (APA, 2013). The purpose of the current chapter is to provide an overview of the various approaches that have been used in the measurement and empirical study of pediatric irritability. However, it would be remiss to do so without first addressing the ontological and definitional challenges that beset the construct of irritability and inevitably complicate its measurement. In general, most scientists agree that irritability describes a psychological experience in which one's propensity toward anger and/or sadness is elevated and which may become pathological when its frequency and/or intensity is incommensurate with developmental level and/or situational triggers (Toohey & DiGiuseppe, 2017). Nevertheless, there is no explicit operational definition of irritability, and many essential features of the construct continue to be debated. For instance, it remains unclear whether irritability is most appropriately conceptualized as an affective or a behavioral symptom. This confusion is highlighted by the inconsistency and ambiguity in the psychiatric vernacular related to the term. In the DSM-5, *irritability, irritable mood*, and *irritable behavior* are all used in the criteria of various diagnoses with little rationale or clinical guidance for their differentiation. Recently, the National Institute of Mental Health (NIMH) expert group proposed the division of the construct into two distinct, but related components: (1) a "tonic" component, which describes affective symptoms of irritability, such as anger and touchiness, and (2) a "phasic" component which includes behavioral manifestations, namely temper loss and tantrums (National Institute of Mental Health, 2014). Although taxonomically useful, further study is required to determine whether the distinction between tonic and phasic irritability is phenomenologically valid (Avenevoli, Blader, & Leibenluft, 2015).

Another area of uncertainty concerns the establishment of normative levels and developmental course of irritability (Copeland, Shanahan, Egger, Angold, & Costello, 2014; Wiggins, Mitchell, Stringaris, & Leibenluft, 2014). During childhood, levels of irritability are inherently higher than during other periods of development, making it clinically challenging to discern early pathological presentations from developmentally appropriate fluctuations (Wakschlag et al., 2012). This is further complicated by inconsistent findings regarding the homotypic continuity of irritability and uncertainty regarding whether irritability should be regarded as a temporary mood state or a more stable characterological trait (Leadbeater & Homel, 2015; Roberson-Nay et al., 2015; Whelan, Stringaris, Maughan, & Barker, 2013).

A final challenge in the measurement of irritability is its conceptual boundaries with associated emotional-behavioral problems, such as anger and aggression. By some perspectives, irritability can be distinguished from anger based on the level of intensity and is equated to a mild form of anger. Others have posited that irritability represents anger in the absence of a clear cause or provocation. Most definitions, however, do not attempt to delineate between these two perspectives (Toohey & DiGiuseppe, 2017). This lack of clarity and face validity

TABLE 3.1 Overview of methods for measuring pediatric irritability

Methods for Measuring Pediatric Irritability

STANDARDIZED DIAGNOSTIC INTERVIEWS

- Kiddie Schedule for Affective Disorders and Schizophrenia (K-SADS)
- Developmental and Well-Being Assessment (DAWBA)
- Diagnostic Interview Schedule for Children (DISC)
- Computerized Diagnostic Interview Schedule for Children (C-DISC)
- Child and Adolescent Psychiatric Assessment (CAPA)

BEHAVIOR RATING SCALES

- Youth Self-Report (YSR)
- Child Behavior Checklist (CBCL)
- Child Symptom Inventory (CSI)
- Emory Diagnostic Rating Scale (EDRS)
- Child and Adolescent Psychopathology Scale (CAPS)
- Hypomania Checklist-32 (HCL-32)
- Connor's Parent Rating Scale (CPRS)
- Affective Reactivity Index (ARI)
- Multidimensional Assessment of Preschool Disruptive Behavior (MAP-DB)

DIRECT OBSERVATION

- Disruptive Behavior Diagnostic Observation Schedule (DB-DOS)

DIAGNOSTIC CRITERIA

- Disruptive Mood Dysregulation Disorder (DMDD)
- Severe Mood Dysregulation (SMD; provisional)

threatens to affect the ratings of both patients and clinicians on standardized diagnostic interviews and questionnaires and to compromise the accuracy of data on irritability.

Despite these limitations, the existing methods of measuring pediatric irritability have yielded important information that continues to inform an iterative process of construct reification and measurement refinement. Here, we describe the early attempts at measuring irritability with standardized diagnostic interviews (SDIs), then discuss how statistical models have shaped these earliest measures, and end with models and measures that are emerging (see Table 3.1).

Early Measurement: Standardized Diagnostic Interviews

As attention shifted toward the role of irritability in developmental psychopathology, most early research relied on secondary analyses of symptoms extracted from SDIs primarily for DSM-IV disorders to measure irritability. Mick et al. (2005) were among the first to utilize this approach by identifying three subtypes of irritability symptoms within the Kiddie Schedule for Affective Disorders and Schizophrenia (K-SADS; Kaufman et al., 1997). Specifically, they defined (1) a "mad/cranky" type measured by the major depression (MDD) criteria of *feeling mad or cranky most of the time for 2 weeks or longer,* (2) a "super-angry/grouchy/ cranky" type based on the mania symptom of *feeling super angry, grouchy, cranky (or irritable) all of the time for a week or longer,* and (3) an "oppositional defiant disorder (ODD)-type" which was measured by the questions *loses temper frequently, feels angry or resentful,* and *is easily annoyed* from the ODD module. The authors demonstrated in a sample of school-aged children with attention deficit/ hyperactivity disorder that these three types of irritability were differentially associated with DSM-IV mood disorders and level of impairment. In particular, only endorsement of "super-angry/grouchy/cranky" irritability was associated with a J-BPD diagnosis, whereas all three types of irritability were common in children with unipolar depression, thus highlighting both the heterogeneity of the construct as well as its insufficiency as a hallmark symptom of bipolar disorder in children (Mick, Spencer, Wozniak, & Biederman, 2005).

Stringaris and Goodman (2009a, 2009b) used the Developmental and Well-Being Assessment (DAWBA), another SDI, to examine the role of irritability within the context of ODD. They parsed the diagnostic criteria for ODD into three a priori dimensions: irritable, hurtful, and headstrong. The irritable dimension, which was measured by the symptoms *often loses temper, often angry and resentful,* and *often touchy or easily annoyed by others* (during the past 6 months), was strongly related to emotional disorders, both at baseline and at 3-year follow-up (Stringaris & Goodman, 2009a, 2009b). In another study using a different method for measuring irritability, Stringaris, Cohen, Pine, and Liebenluft (2009) reported similar associations between adolescent irritability and adult mood and anxiety disorders at 20-year follow-up. Here, irritability was measured by the summation of frequency scores on items from the Diagnostic Interview Schedule for Children for DSM-III disorders (DISC-III) and the Disorganized Poverty Index (DIPOV). The specific items that comprised the scale were (1) *Does child tantrum when parent makes him/her do things?* (2) *Does child tantrum when teacher makes him/her do things?* (3) *How often is child angry on an average day?* Parents responded either "no," "sometimes," or "yes" for questions 1 and 2 and either "never," "once in a while," "often," or "constantly" for question 3. For each question, more frequent symptoms were indicative of more severe irritability.

Brotman et al. (2006) used existing data on DSM-IV diagnoses obtained from the Child and Adolescent Psychiatric Assessment (CAPA) to approximate severe mood dysregulation (SMD) diagnoses, a provisional set of diagnostic criteria for persistent and severe childhood irritability. Notably, to assess the SMD criterion of abnormal mood (anger or sadness) that is present at least half of the time most days and noticeable to others, the items *touchy or easily annoyed, angry or resentful,* and *depressed mood* were extracted from the Depression module of the CAPA. Similarly, the ODD symptoms of *loses temper* and *temper tantrums* as well as the Depression symptom of *irritability or easily precipitated irritable mood* were used to capture the SMD symptom of "markedly increased reactivity to negative emotional stimuli." Additionally, this study was novel in that it included a criterion related to the pervasiveness of symptoms, specifying that they must be severe in at least one setting (e.g., home, school, with peers) and at least mild in another. This study found that SMD was prevalent in childhood (3.3%) and predicted depressive disorders in adulthood, although this work was limited by the common problem with studies of diagnostic interviews to date—that the interview was not designed to examine SMD specifically and so diagnoses were applied post-hoc.

The secondary use of SDI data was an important advance in the empirical refinement and evaluation of pediatric irritability. Taken together, the findings of these studies support both the reliability and validity of the construct as measured by DSM symptoms. That is, irritability was a robust predictor of negative outcomes, especially emotional disorders in child and adulthood, across different interviews and study samples. Additionally, SDIs supported the theoretical convergence of irritability with affective and behavioral symptoms such as headstrongness and aggression while also reifying the divergence of irritability from mania and J-BPD. Nevertheless, there are substantial limitations to the measurement approaches described in these studies. First, irritability scales were constructed based on a priori definitions used for items taken from other constructs. This introduces the risk that the variables selected to measure irritability may have been poor indicators of the construct or that other, important indicators had been omitted. Furthermore, SDIs most typically identify irritability using categorical measures (e.g., Yes/No decisions) which may truncate the variance of symptoms and conceal phenotypic nuances.

Statistical Models of Irritability

In response to the methodological issues of SDI symptom counts, many researchers have begun to utilize more empirically rigorous methods of examining the structure and organization of irritability symptoms in children and adolescents. Broadly, this has taken two analytical forms: variable-centered and person-centered approaches.

VARIABLE-CENTERED METHODS

Factor analysis is the most common variable-centered method that has been applied to the study of pediatric irritability. Both exploratory (EFA) and confirmatory factor analysis (CFA) are statistical techniques used to measure the strength of associations between observed variables and hypothesized underlying dimension(s). Typically, EFA is appropriate when there is limited theoretical precedent for a model, as the number of dimensions and their associations with observed variables are determined based on the data. In CFA, on the other hand, models are theory-driven, and the researcher must specify the hypothesized number of dimensions and variables associated with each (Brown, 2014).

To date, the most empirical support exists for defining irritability as a distinct dimension within ODD. In particular, Stringaris et al. (2009; Stringaris & Goodman, 2009a) aforementioned a priori irritable-headstrong-hurtful dimensions have been widely tested using factor analytic methods. Although some studies have not found statistical justification for the inclusion of the hurtful dimension, irritability has been consistently supported as a distinct dimension of ODD. In a later study, Stringaris et al. (2012) performed an EFA of oppositionality items (i.e., *argue a lot, mean to others, destroy others' things, disobey parents, disobey at school, have a hot temper, tease others a lot, stubborn sullen or irritable, mood/feelings change suddenly*) from the Youth Self-Report (YSR) and Adult Self Report (ASR). In their model, the items *have a hot temper, stubborn sullen or irritable,* and *mood/feelings change suddenly* loaded clearly onto an irritability dimension, whereas *argue a lot* loaded onto both the irritability and headstrong/hurtful dimensions. The structure of irritability was consistent across adolescence and predicted depressed mood. Similarly, Aebi, Plattner, Metzke, Bessler, and Steinhausen (2013) identified a similar irritability dimension defined by the items *have a hot temper, stubborn sullen or irritable,* and *mood/feelings change suddenly* in a CFA using the same oppositionality items from the YSR and Child Behavior Checklist (CBCL). It is worth noting the complexity of the item *stubborn sullen or irritable* in these models. Because both behavioral and affective features of irritability are aggregated in this single item, it is not possible to examine the unique relationships of these components to irritability (Burke, 2017).

Burke et al. (Burke, Hipwell, & Loeber, 2010) have proposed a competing model of ODD symptoms in which irritability symptoms are subsumed within a broader negative affect dimension. In separate EFA studies of boys and girls, the authors identified negative affect as a dimension of oppositionality, which included the symptoms *angry, touchy,* and *spiteful* from the Child Symptom Inventory (CSI-IV). Interestingly, in girls, two additional dimensions (i.e., oppositional behavior and antagonistic behavior) were identified, whereas in boys, oppositional behavior was the only other dimension of ODD symptoms identified.

Several studies have performed direct comparisons of Stringaris's and Burke's models. Krieger et al. (2013) found that in a sample of Brazilian youth, Stringaris's irritable-headstrong-hurtful model demonstrated the best fit to the data. Additionally, the irritability dimension was associated with childhood emotional disorders and maternal history of depression and suicidality. By contrast, Herzhoff and Tackett (2016) found evidence for Burke et al.'s (2010) two-factor (negative affect and oppositional behavior) model in two large community samples. Burke et al. also compared his own to model to other competing models of ODD in five samples using different assessments of ODD symptoms (i.e., DISC-IV, CSI-IV, DAWBA, Emory Diagnostic Rating Scale, and Child and Adolescent Psychopathology Scale). In general, Stringaris' irritability dimension demonstrated better fit to the observed symptoms than did Burke's own negative affect dimension; however, the fit of Stringaris' irritability dimension was further improved by the use of a different statistical approach, known as *bifactor modeling*. Bifactor models are comprised of both a general factor, which accounts for covariance in observed symptoms, as well as specific factors, which account for the unique variance in symptoms over and above the general factor (Brown, 2014). Burke et al. specified a bifactor model consisting of a general ODD factor and oppositional behavior and irritability as correlated specific factors, and this best represented the structure of ODD symptoms across all five samples. The emergence of irritability as a significant specific factor, even after partialing out the general ODD factor, demonstrates the importance of irritability as a specific domain of ODD.

A substantially smaller body of research has used variable-centered approaches to evaluate pediatric irritability within the context of bipolar disorder. For example, a validation study of the Hypomania Checklist-32 (HCL-32) conducted in a school-based sample of German adolescents identified an "irritable-erratic" dimension of hypomania using factor analysis. In particular, this dimension was defined by the following items: *engage in a lot of new things, more easily distracted, more impatient/get irritable more easily, spend more/too much money, drive faster/ take more risks when driving, get into more quarrels, thoughts jump from topic to topic, exhausting/irritating for others, want/do travel more, plan more activities/ projects, take more risks in daily life,* and *need less sleep.* However, this dimension did not significantly predict self-reported hypomania, but rather was associated with conduct, hyperactivity-inattention, and peer problems (Holtmann et al., 2009). In an alternative model of youth mania symptoms developed by Stringaris et al. (Stringaris, Stahl, Santosh, & Goodman, 2011; Stringaris et al., 2014), irritability was conceptualized as an indicator of a broader construct of episodic undercontrol, which included other symptoms such as *invades space, overconfident, risk-taking, distractible, less self-control, poor concentration,* and *flight of ideas* taken from the Mania section of the DAWBA. Another study by Pan et al. (2014), which examined dimensions of manic symptoms in a community sample of Brazilian youth aged 6–12, found that the episodic undercontrol dimension was uniquely associated with psychiatric morbidity, psychosocial impairment, and a family history of mania, depression, or suicide attempts.

PERSON-CENTERED METHODS

Support for irritability as an important dimension of ODD has been corroborated by studies using person-centered analytic approaches. Unlike variable-centered approaches that model variance and covariance among items or symptoms, person-centered approaches identify groups of individuals with similar patterns of responding across items or symptoms. With regard to irritability research, latent class analysis (LCA) has been the most common technique for conducting person-centered research (Laursen & Hoff, 2006).

In a community sample of 9- to 10-year-old children, Herzoff and Tackett (2016) performed an LCA of ODD symptoms from the Computerized Diagnostic Interview Schedule for Children (C-DISC) and identified three classes of individuals: (1) oppositional, (2) irritable, and (3) low symptoms. More specifically, the oppositional class was characterized by high probability of endorsement of symptoms of *loses temper, argues,* and *defies.* The irritable class, on the other hand, had high probabilities of being *touchy, angry,* and *spiteful.* The authors confirmed the validity of this three-class solution in a replication sample and also examined personality traits as external validators of class membership. Of note, a personality profile of low Agreeableness, Conscientiousness, and Extraversion and high Neuroticism seemed to be a risk factor for membership in both the oppositional and irritable classes; however, at 2-year follow-up, the irritable class had higher levels of internalizing symptoms as compared with the oppositional class.

Other studies using LCA of ODD symptoms have found support for four distinct classes of symptoms. In a large general population sample of Dutch twins, Kuny et al. (2013) identified four classes based on the ODD subscale of the Connor's Parent Rating Scale: (1) no symptoms, (2) defiant, (3) irritable, and (4) high symptoms. The defiant class had high probabilities of endorsing *actively defies and refuses to comply with adults' request, deliberately does things that annoy other people,* and *argues with adults*; the irritable class was characterized by high probabilities for *lose temper, irritable,* and *angry.* The high symptoms class had high item endorsement probabilities on all items. The defiant, irritable, and high symptoms classes exhibited higher levels of externalizing problems than did the no symptom class. In addition, the high symptoms class also had higher levels of internalizing problems, and the irritable class had elevated mood symptoms. These four classes were also identified by Althoff et al. (2014) using the CBCL in three large samples of children from the United States and Holland. In this study, only membership in the irritable and high-symptoms classes was associated with psychiatric disorders during childhood, particularly ODD. Membership in the defiant or high symptom classes during childhood predicted later adult violent criminal behavior, whereas membership in the irritable class predicted later adult mood disorders.

Taken together, both variable- and person-centered statistical models of pediatric irritability have yielded relatively robust evidence for the conceptualization of irritability as a core dimension of ODD that comprises both affective and behavioral symptoms. This dimension has been consistent across samples, measures, and statistical techniques and has been shown to predict psychiatric disorders both in childhood and adulthood. In particular, these symptoms seem to represent a pathway by which behavioral disorders during childhood may lead to future mood disorders.

By contrast, in the limited available research on the symptom structure of pediatric mania, irritability has not emerged as a unique dimension, but rather as a symptom of a broader construct of episodic undercontrol. Although more research is needed, this calls into question the applicability of irritability as a hall-mark symptom of bipolar disorder in youth.

Emerging Measures of Irritability for Clinical Settings

While statistical models have yielded valuable insight into the symptoms, presentations, and trajectories of pediatric irritability, these methods have limited direct clinical utility, and further work is required to translate this empirical knowledge into useful tools for clinicians. While empirically based assessments of pediatric irritability are still in their nascent stages, this section provides an overview of some of the currently available tools.

DISRUPTIVE MOOD DYSREGULATION DISORDER

The addition of disruptive mood dysregulation disorder (DMDD) as a mood disorder in the DSM-5 represented an important step in the integration of research and clinical conceptualizations of pediatric irritability (APA, 2013). DMDD has established a standardized set of symptoms and criteria for evaluating pathological irritability which, as described in Chapter 11, requires symptoms of both chronic irritable mood and temper outbursts that are severe and present in more than one setting (APA, 2013). While the diagnosis has served to address concerns related the misdiagnosis of J-BPD, further research is required to evaluate the validity of DMDD as a distinct diagnosis. This has been hindered by the lack of widely available clinical interviews for explicitly assessing DMDD criteria (Baweja, Mayes, Hameed, & Waxmonsky, 2016).

AFFECTIVE REACTIVITY INDEX

Developed by Stringaris et al. in 2012, the Affective Reactivity Index (ARI) is a seven-item questionnaire with analogous parent and self-report versions intended to capture symptoms and impairment associated with chronic irritable mood. More specifically, six symptoms of irritability (i.e., *easily annoyed by others, often lose temper, stay angry for a long time, angry most of the time, get angry frequently,* and *lose temper easily*) are rated as 0 (*not true*), 1 (*somewhat true*), and 2 (*certainly true*) to yield a total irritability score ranging from 0 to 12. Preliminary psychometric analyses have demonstrated promising results, with items loading closely onto a single irritability factor and high internal consistency among items. Additionally, the ARI has been shown to converge with measures of anxiety and depression, as well as to discriminate between J-BPD, SMD, and healthy controls (Mulraney, Melvin, & Tonge, 2014; Stringaris et al., 2012). Due to its brevity and linguistic simplicity, the ARI is appropriate for assessing irritability in clinical as well as research settings. However, given the emphasis on chronic irritability, it is important to note that the ARI may be less appropriate for use in more acute and hospital settings (Mathews, Carlson, Pang, & Klein, 2017).

MULTIDIMENSIONAL ASSESSMENT OF PRESCHOOL DISRUPTIVE BEHAVIOR

The Multidimensional Assessment of Preschool Disruptive Behavior (MAP-DB) is a comprehensive 111-item parent report measure of disruptive behaviors in pre-school children. In particular, the MAP-DB is intended to capture variations in symptoms across different interactions (e.g., with parents/teachers/other children) and different contexts (e.g., when tired/hungry/sick). All items are rated in terms for frequency on a 6-point Likert scale (0 = Never; 1 = Rarely [less than once per week]; 2 = Some [1–3] days of the week; 3 = Most [4–6] days of the week; 4 = Every day of the week; 5 = Many times each day). In particular, the MAP-DB contains a 22-item Temper Loss subscale with empirically derived severity cutoffs useful for distinguishing normative and pathological manifestations of temper loss. In general, temper loss symptoms present more than 4–6 days of the week were considered pathological (Wakschlag et al., 2012, 2014). The MAP-DB provides valuable information about the context and frequency of phasic irritability symptoms that are not captured by the ARI. However, its applicability to only preschool-aged children and lack of multi-informant reports are major limitations of the measure (Mick, Biederman, Pandina, & Faraone, 2003).

DISRUPTIVE BEHAVIOR DIAGNOSTIC OBSERVATION SCHEDULE

The Disruptive Behavior Diagnostic Observation Schedule (DB-DOS) is a complementary, observational assessment tool to the MAP-DB for measuring irritability in preschool children. The DB-DOS is designed to assess for a wide range of disruptive behaviors through different tasks (Galanter et al., 2003) and conditions (i.e., with parent, with examiner, alone) and has been demonstrated to have good psychometric properties (Wakschlag, Briggs-Gowan et al., 2008; Wakschlag, Hill et al., 2008).

In particular, the DB-DOS assesses 21 behaviors, each of which is categorized as 0 = normative behavior, 1 = normative misbehavior, 2 = of concern, or 3 = atypical. These items are divided into two broad domains of disruptive behavior: Behavioral Regulation and Anger Modulation. The latter domain is particularly relevant to the assessment of irritability as it captures *intensity of irritable/angry behavior, predominance of irritable/angry behavior, ease of elicitation of irritable/angry behavior, rapid escalation of irritable/angry behavior,* and *difficulty recovering from irritable/angry episode* (Wakschlag, Hill et al., 2008). The DB-DOS may be a useful tool for clinicians to understand child functioning without relying solely on potentially biased parental reports (Bunte et al., 2013). As with the MAP-DB, the DB-DOS is limited insofar as it is only appropriate to the assessment of preschool children. There are several additional noteworthy limitations. First, the DB-DOS is both time- and resource-intensive, requiring approximately 50 minutes to administer and additional time to review and code behaviors. Second, the behavioral coding criteria of the DB-DOS does not differentiate between irritable and anger behaviors, thus hindering the clinician/researcher's ability to isolate irritability.

CHILD BEHAVIOR CHECKLIST DYSREGULATION PROFILE

A set of constructs based on the CBCL have gained increasing use as measures of broad emotional self-regulation in relation to irritability. Initially envisioned as a way to compare children with bipolar disorder across sites, the CBCL-Dysregulation Profile (CBCL-DP) consists of elevated scores on the attention problems, aggressive behavior, and anxious-depressed scales (Mick et al., 2003). It was studied initially under the name of the CBCL-Juvenile Bipolar Disorder or CBCL-Mania profile (Galanter et al., 2003; Hudziak, Althoff, Derks, Faraone, & Boomsma, 2005). As studies began to examine this profile, however, it became evident that high scores on the CBCL-DP did not necessarily predict concurrent or subsequent bipolar disorder (Youngstrom et al., 2005) but rather predicted a host of other outcomes, including substance use disorders, anxiety and depression, and personality disorders (Althoff, Verhulst, Rettew, Hudziak, & van der Ende, 2010; Meyer et al., 2009). This profile was subsequently renamed the CBCL-Dysregulation Profile (Althoff et al., 2010), and it has been used to examine the role of emotion regulation in studies of children with other disorders (Frazier et al., 2015; Surman et al., 2013). The precise manner in which the profile is calculated has varied from a variable-centered summed score in genetic studies (Boomsma et al., 2006) to a person-centered profile approach using latent class analysis (Althoff, Rettew, Faraone, Boomsma, & Hudziak, 2006; Althoff et al., 2010) and, most recently, to using the statistical technique of bivariate modeling to parse the specific and unique predictive power associated with each individual scale as compared to the total scale (Deutz, Geeraerts, van Baar, Deković, & Prinzie, 2016). The profile has been useful as a transdiagnostic construct that can be used to examine biological markers (Poustka et al., 2015), cognitive function (Basten et al., 2014), and clinical outcomes (Masi, Muratori, Manfredi, Pisano, & Milone, 2015), among others. Because of the ease of administration of the CBCL and the nearly ubiquitous collection of this instrument in studies of developmental psychopathology, the CBCL has immense potential to allow for the study of broad dysregulation and irritability.

Conclusion

The past decade has witnessed substantial progress in the definition, measurement, and assessment of irritability in children and adolescents. Various approaches have been taken to the study of pediatric irritability, including the use of SDI, questionnaires, advanced statistical modeling, and direct behavioral observation. Taken together, these methods have helped shaped our definitions of irritability, differentiate between normative and pathological manifestations, and predict long-term trajectories for irritable children. However, much work remains to adequately serve the children and families affected by these impairing psychiatric symptoms. In particular, to date, the vast majority of research related to irritability has been conducted within the context of ODD. Given the transdiagnostic nature of irritability, efforts should be made to understand the relationship of irritability to various forms of developmental psychopathology. For this to occur, specific measurement of the component of irritability in relation to other diagnoses (bipolar disorder, posttraumatic stress disorder, ADHD, etc.) needs to be prioritized. Additionally, more research is needed to clarify the connection between irritability and broader constructs and processes, such as emotion regulation, mood lability, and frustrative nonreward. Finally, the use of psychophysiological measures as well as ecological momentary assessment represents promising novel avenues for future research to gain insight into pediatric irritability.

References

Aebi, M., Plattner, B., Metzke, C. W., Bessler, C., & Steinhausen, H. C. (2013). Parent- and self-reported dimensions of oppositionality in youth: Construct validity, concurrent validity, and the prediction of criminal outcomes in adulthood. *Journal of Child Psychology and Psychiatry, 54*(9), 941–949.

Althoff, R. R., Kuny-Slock, A. V., Verhulst, F. C., Hudziak, J. J., & van der Ende, J. (2014). Classes of oppositional-defiant behavior: Concurrent and predictive validity. *Journal of Child Psychology and Psychiatry, 55*(10), 1162–1171.

Althoff, R. R., Rettew, D. C., Faraone, S. V., Boomsma, D. I., & Hudziak, J. J. (2006). Latent class analysis shows strong heritability of the child behavior checklist–juvenile bipolar phenotype. *Biological Psychiatry, 60*(9), 903–911.

Althoff, R. R., Verhulst, F. C., Rettew, D. C., Hudziak, J. J., & van der Ende, J. (2010). Adult outcomes of childhood dysregulation: A 14-year follow-up study. *Journal of the American Academy of Child and Adolescent Psychiatry, 49*(11), 1105–1116.

American Psychiatric Association (APA). (2013). *Diagnostic and statistical manual of mental disorders* (5th edition). Arlington, VA: American Psychiatric Publishing.

Avenevoli, S., Blader, J. C., & Leibenluft, E. (2015). Irritability in youth: An update. *Journal of the American Academy of Child & Adolescent Psychiatry, 54*(11), 881–883.

Basten, M., van der Ende, J., Tiemeier, H., Althoff, R. R., Rijlaarsdam, J., Jaddoe, V. W., . . . White, T. (2014). Nonverbal intelligence in young children with dysregulation: The Generation R Study. *European Child and Adolescent Psychiatry, 23*(11), 1061–1070.

Baweja, R., Mayes, S. D., Hameed, U., & Waxmonsky, J. G. (2016). Disruptive mood dysregulation disorder: Current insights. *Neuropsychiatric Disease and Treatment, 12*, 2115–2124.

Blader, J. C., & Carlson, G. A. (2007). Increased rates of bipolar disorder diagnoses among US child, adolescent, and adult inpatients, 1996–2004. *Biological Psychiatry, 62*(2), 107–114.

Boomsma, D. I., Rebollo, I., Derks, E. M., Van Beijsterveldt, T. C., Althoff, R. R., Rettew, D. C., & Hudziak, J. J. (2006). Longitudinal stability of the CBCL-juvenile bipolar disorder phenotype: A study in Dutch twins. *Biological Psychiatry, 60*(9), 912–920.

Brotman, M. A., Schmajuk, M., Rich, B. A., Dickstein, D. P., Guyer, A. E., Costello, E. J., . . . Leibenluft, E. (2006). Prevalence, clinical correlates, and longitudinal course of severe mood dysregulation in children. *Biological Psychiatry, 60*(9), 991–997.

Brown, T. A. (2014). *Confirmatory factor analysis for applied research.* New York: Guilford.

Bunte, T. L., Laschen, S., Schoemaker, K., Hessen, D. J., van der Heijden, P. G., & Matthys, W. (2013). Clinical usefulness of observational assessment in the diagnosis of DBD and ADHD in preschoolers. *Journal of Clinical Child and Adolescent Psychology, 42*(6), 749–761.

Burke, J. (2017). *Panel on measurement and definition.* Paper presented at the 2nd Congress on Pediatric Irritability and Dysregulation, Burlington, VT.

Burke, J. D., Hipwell, A. E., & Loeber, R. (2010). Dimensions of oppositional defiant disorder as predictors of depression and conduct disorder in preadolescent girls. *Journal of the American Academy of Child and Adolescent Psychiatry, 49*(5), 484–492.

Burns, A., Folstein, S., Brandt, J., & Folstein, M. (1990). Clinical assessment of irritability, aggression, and apathy in Huntington and Alzheimer disease. *Journal of Nervous and Mental Disease, 178*(1), 20–26.

Caprara, G. V., Renzi, P., Alcini, P., Imperio, G., & Travaglia, G. (1983). Instigation to aggress and escalation of aggression examined from a personological perspective: The role of irritability and of emotional susceptibility. *Aggressive Behavior, 9*(4), 345–351.

Copeland, W. E., Shanahan, L., Egger, H., Angold, A., & Costello, E. J. (2014). Adult diagnostic and functional outcomes of DSM-5 disruptive mood dysregulation disorder. *American Journal of Psychiatry, 171*(6), 668–674.

Deutz, M. H., Geeraerts, S. B., van Baar, A. L., Deković, M., & Prinzie, P. (2016). The Dysregulation Profile in middle childhood and adolescence across reporters: Factor structure, measurement invariance, and links with self-harm and suicidal ideation. *European Child and Adolescent Psychiatry, 25*(4), 431–442.

Frazier, J. A., Wood, M. E., Ware, J., Joseph, R. M., Kuban, K. C., O'Shea, M., . . . Leviton, A. (2015). Antecedents of the child behavior checklist–dysregulation profile in children born extremely preterm. *Journal of the American Academy of Child and Adolescent Psychiatry, 54*(10), 816–823.

Galanter, C. A., Carlson, G. A., Jensen, P. S., Greenhill, L. L., Davies, M., Li, W., . . . March, J. S. (2003). Response to methylphenidate in children with attention deficit hyperactivity disorder and manic symptoms in the multimodal treatment study of children with attention deficit hyperactivity disorder titration trial. *Journal of Child and Adolescent Psychopharmacology, 13*(2), 123–136.

Herzhoff, K., & Tackett, J. L. (2016). Subfactors of oppositional defiant disorder: Converging evidence from structural and latent class analyses. *Journal of Child Psychology and Psychiatry, 57*(1), 18–29.

Holtmann, M., Portner, F., Duketis, E., Flechtner, H. H., Angst, J., & Lehmkuhl, G. (2009). Validation of the Hypomania Checklist (HCL-32) in a nonclinical sample of German adolescents. *Journal of Adolescence, 32*(5), 1075–1088.

Hudziak, J. J., Althoff, R. R., Derks, E. M., Faraone, S. V., & Boomsma, D. I. (2005). Prevalence and genetic architecture of Child Behavior Checklist–juvenile bipolar disorder. *Biological Psychiatry, 58*(7), 562–568.

Kaufman, J., Birmaher, B., Brent, D., Rao, U., Flynn, C., Moreci, P., . . . Ryan N. (1997). Schedule for Affective Disorders and Schizophrenia for School-Age Children-Present and Lifetime Version (K-SADS-PL): Initial reliability and validity data. *Journal of the American Academy of Child and Adolescent Psychiatry, 36*(7), 980–988.

Krieger, F. V., Polanczyk, V. G., Goodman, R., Rohde, L. A., Graeff-Martins, A. S., Salum, G., . . . Stringaris, A. (2013). Dimensions of oppositionality in a Brazilian community sample: Testing the DSM-5 proposal and etiological links. *Journal of the American Academy of Childand Adolescent Psychiatry, 52*(4), 389–400.e381.

Kuny, A. V., Althoff, R. R., Copeland, W., Bartels, M., Beijsterveldt, V., Baer, J., & Hudziak, J. J. (2013). Separating the domains of oppositional behavior: Comparing latent models of the Conners' oppositional subscale. *Journal of the American Academy of Child and Adolescent Psychiatry, 52*(2), 172–183.

Laursen, B. P., & Hoff, E. (2006). Person-centered and variable-centered approaches to longitudinal data. *Merrill-Palmer Quarterly, 52*(3), 377–389.

Leadbeater, B. J., & Homel, J. (2015). Irritable and defiant sub-dimensions of ODD: Their stability and prediction of internalizing symptoms and conduct problems from adolescence to young adulthood. *Journal of Abnormal Child Psychology, 43*(3), 407–421.

Leibenluft, E., Charney, D. S., Towbin, K. E., Bhangoo, R. K., & Pine, D. S. (2003). Defining clinical phenotypes of juvenile mania. *American Journal of Psychiatry, 160*(3), 430–437.

Masi, G., Muratori, P., Manfredi, A., Pisano, S., & Milone, A. (2015). Child behaviour checklist emotional dysregulation profiles in youth with disruptive behaviour disorders: Clinical correlates and treatment implications. *Psychiatry Research, 225*(1), 191–196.

Mathews, B., Carlson, G. A., Pang, P., & Klein, D. (2017). *The Irritability Inventory: Assessing the phasic aspect of irritability to better predict behavior in the hospital.* Paper presented at the American Academy of Child and Adolescent Psychiatry, Washington DC.

Meyer, S. E., Carlson, G. A., Youngstrom, E., Ronsaville, D. S., Martinez, P. E., Gold, P. W., . . . Radke-Yarrow, M. (2009). Long-term outcomes of youth who manifested the CBCL-Pediatric Bipolar Disorder phenotype during childhood and/or adolescence. *Journal of Affective Disorders, 113*(3), 227–235.

Mick, E., Biederman, J., Pandina, G., & Faraone, S. V. (2003). A preliminary meta-analysis of the child behavior checklist in pediatric bipolar disorder. *Biological Psychiatry, 53*(11), 1021–1027.

Mick, E., Spencer, T., Wozniak, J., & Biederman, J. (2005). Heterogeneity of irritability in attention-deficit/hyperactivity disorder subjects with and without mood disorders. *Biological Psychiatry, 58*(7), 576–582.

Mulraney, M. A., Melvin, G. A., & Tonge, B. J. (2014). Psychometric properties of the Affective Reactivity Index in Australian adults and adolescents. *Psychological Assessment, 26*(1), 148.

National Institute of Mental Health (NIMH). (2014). *Childhood irritability and the pathophysiology of mental illness.* Rockville, MD: NIMH.

Pan, P. M., Salum, G. A., Gadelha, A., Moriyama, T., Cogo-Moreira, H., Graeff-Martins, A. S., . . . Bressan, R. A. (2014). Manic symptoms in youth: Dimensions, latent classes, and associations with parental psychopathology. *Journal of the American Academy of Child and Adolescent Psychiatry, 53*(6), 625–634.

Poustka, L., Zohsel, K., Blomeyer, D., Jennen-Steinmetz, C., Schmid, B., Trautmann-Villalba, P., . . . Schmidt, M. H. (2015). Interacting effects of maternal responsiveness, infant regulatory problems and dopamine D4 receptor gene in the development of dysregulation during childhood: A longitudinal analysis. *Journal of Psychiatric Research, 70*, 83–90.

Roberson-Nay, R., Leibenluft, E., Brotman, M. A., Myers, J., Larsson, H., Lichtenstein, P., & Kendler, K. S. (2015). Longitudinal stability of genetic and environmental influences on irritability: From childhood to young adulthood. *American Journal of Psychiatry, 172*(7), 657–664.

Safer, D. J. (2009). Irritable mood and the Diagnostic and Statistical Manual of Mental Disorders. *Child and Adolescent Psychiatry and Mental Health, 3*(1), 35.

Snaith, R. P., Constantopoulos, A. A., Jardine, M. Y., & McGuffin, P. (1978). A clinical scale for the self-assessment of irritability. *The British Journal of Psychiatry, 132*(2), 164–171.

Stringaris, A., Castellanos-Ryan, N., Banaschewski, T., Barker, G. J., Bokde, A. L., Bromberg, U., . . . Frouin, V. (2014). Dimensions of manic symptoms in youth: Psychosocial impairment and cognitive performance in the IMAGEN sample. *Journal of Child Psychology and Psychiatry, 55*(12), 1380–1389.

Stringaris, A., Cohen, P., Pine, D. S., & Leibenluft, E. (2009). Adult outcomes of youth irritability: A 20-year prospective community-based study. *American Journal of Psychiatry, 166*(9), 1048–1054.

Stringaris, A., & Goodman, R. (2009a). Longitudinal outcome of youth oppositionality: Irritable, headstrong, and hurtful behaviors have distinctive predictions. *Journal of the American Academy of Child and Adolescent Psychiatry, 48*(4), 404–412.

Stringaris, A., & Goodman, R. (2009b). Three dimensions of oppositionality in youth. *Journal of Child Psychology and Psychiatry, 50*(3), 216–223.

Stringaris, A., Goodman, R., Ferdinando, S., Razdan, V., Muhrer, E., Leibenluft, E., & Brotman, M. A. (2012). The Affective Reactivity Index: A concise irritability scale for clinical and research settings. *Journal of Child Psychology and Psychiatry, 53*(11), 1109–1117.

Stringaris, A., Stahl, D., Santosh, P., & Goodman, R. (2011). Dimensions and latent classes of episodic mania-like symptoms in youth: An empirical enquiry. *Journal of Abnormal Child Psychology, 39*(7), 925–937.

Stringaris, A., Zavos, H., Leibenluft, E., Maughan, B., & Eley, T. C. (2012). Adolescent irritability: Phenotypic associations and genetic links with depressed mood. *American Journal of Psychiatry, 169*(1), 47–54.

Surman, C. B., Biederman, J., Spencer, T., Miller, C. A., McDermott, K. M., & Faraone, S. V. (2013). Understanding deficient emotional self-regulation in adults with attention deficit hyperactivity disorder: A controlled study. *ADHD Attention Deficit and Hyperactivity Disorders, 5*(3), 273–281.

Toohey, M. J., & DiGiuseppe, R. (2017). Defining and measuring irritability: Construct clarification and differentiation. *Clinical Psychology Review, 53*, 93–108.

Wakschlag, L. S., Briggs-Gowan, M. J., Choi, S. W., Nichols, S. R., Kestler, J., Burns, J. L., . . . Henry, D. (2014). Advancing a multidimensional, developmental spectrum approach to preschool disruptive behavior. *Journal of the American Academy of Child and Adolescent Psychiatry, 53*(1), 82–96.

Wakschlag, L. S., Briggs-Gowan, M. J., Hill, C., Danis, B., Leventhal, B. L., Keenan, K., . . . Carter, A. S. (2008). Observational assessment of preschool disruptive behavior, part II: Validity of the Disruptive Behavior Diagnostic Observation Schedule (DB-DOS). *Journal of the American Academy of Child and Adolescent Psychiatry, 47*(6), 632–641.

Wakschlag, L. S., Choi, S. W., Carter, A. S., Hullsiek, H., Burns, J., McCarthy, K., . . . Briggs-Gowan, M. J. (2012). Defining the developmental parameters of temper loss in early childhood: Implications for developmental psychopathology. *Journal of Child Psychology and Psychiatry, 53*(11), 1099–1108.

Wakschlag, L. S., Hill, C., Carter, A. S., Danis, B., Egger, H. L., Keenan, K., . . . Briggs-Gowan, M. J. (2008). Observational assessment of preschool disruptive behavior, part I: Reliability of the Disruptive Behavior Diagnostic Observation Schedule (DB-DOS). *Journal of the American Academy of Child and Adolescent Psychiatry, 47*(6), 622–631.

Whelan, Y. M., Stringaris, A., Maughan, B., & Barker, E. D. (2013). Developmental continuity of oppositional defiant disorder subdimensions at ages 8, 10, and 13 years and their distinct psychiatric outcomes at age 16 years. *Journal of the American Academy of Child and Adolescent Psychiatry, 52*(9), 961–969.

Wiggins, J. L., Mitchell, C., Stringaris, A., & Leibenluft, E. (2014). Developmental trajectories of irritability and bidirectional associations with maternal depression. *Journal of the American Academy of Child and Adolescent Psychiatry, 53*(11), 1191–1205.

Youngstrom, E., Meyers, O., Demeter, C., Youngstrom, J., Morello, L., Piiparinen, R., . . . Findling, R. L. (2005). Comparing diagnostic checklists for pediatric bipolar disorder in academic and community mental health settings. *Bipolar Disorders, 7*(6), 507–517.

4

Behavioral and Psychophysiological Investigations of Irritability

Mariah DeSerisy and Christen M. Deveney

Clinically significant irritability is typically defined as excessive anger and/or a low threshold for frustration that manifests in temper outbursts/rages that are frequent, severe, and disproportionate to the child's developmental stage (Carlson, Potegal, Margulies, Gutkovich, & Basile, 2009; Leibenluft, 2017; Roy et al., 2013). Irritability is associated with marked impairment in both treatment-seeking and community samples. Children referred for severe temper outbursts experience higher rates of inpatient hospitalization, diagnostic comorbidity, and greater deficits in emotional and behavioral control when compared to children referred for nonirritable symptoms (Carlson et al., 2009; Roy et al., 2013). In community settings, children with irritability experience greater disruptions in peer and parent relationships, greater deficits in school performance, and are more likely to be involved with the legal system than are children without temper outbursts or children without psychopathology (Copeland, Angold, Costello, & Egger, 2013; Girard, Pingault, Doyle, Falissard, & Tremblay, 2016). Early childhood irritability also predicts poorer outcomes in adulthood (Copeland, Shanahan, Egger, Angold, & Costello, 2014). Thus, there is a critical need to improve our understanding of the neurocognitive basis of irritability in order to inform treatments and improve quality of life for these children.

Despite the clinical relevance of this symptom, research into the mechanisms of irritability is in its nascent stages. The focus of this chapter is on behavioral and psychophysiological investigations of irritability-related mechanisms in children and adolescents. Behavioral measures include assessments of performance (e.g., accuracy and response time) during cognitive tasks as well as self-reported emotional responses and judgments about emotional stimuli. Psychophysiological measures include heart rate, startle response, skin sweating response, respiration rates, and electrical measures of neural activity (Andreassi, 1995). The majority of psychophysiological studies of irritability have relied on brain-based event-related potentials (ERPs). These are time-locked averages of electroencephalographic (EEG) signals reflecting the synchronous activity of hundreds to thousands of neurons (Andreassi, 1995). ERPs are calculated in response to specific trial events (e.g., correct and incorrect responses; negative and positive images) and index specific cognitive processes including response inhibition, error monitoring, and emotional responsivity (Luck, 2014).

Both behavioral and psychophysiological methods are uniquely positioned to provide insights into potential mechanisms underlying irritability in youth. They provide real-time and noninvasive monitoring of physiological functioning that is easily tolerated and, relative to other neuroimaging techniques, is afford-able and accessible (Andreassi, 1995; Huettel, Song, & McCarthy, 2009; Nelson & McCleery, 2008). The greater temporal specificity of these methods (Luck, 2014) also allow more temporally precise measures of irritability-related deficits than can be probed using magnetic resonance imaging (MRI). ERPs also allow researchers to measure baseline functioning as well as changes in response to specific task demands and/or task conditions (Woodman, 2010). In combina-tion with data from cognitive neuroscience and neuroimaging investigations of irritability, behavioral and psychophysiological investigations may identify key neurophysiological deficits that can be targeted in treatment and prevention efforts.

The existing behavioral and psychophysiological literature on irritability has investigated three primary domains: (1) executive functioning, (2) reward pro-cessing, and (3) responses to emotional stimuli. As is typical of the pediatric irrita-bility literature, these studies characterize irritability using categorical (i.e., severe mood dysregulation [SMD] (Leibenluft, Charney, Towbin, Bhangoo, & Pine, 2003); disruptive mood dysregulation disorder [DMDD]) and/or transdiagnostic dimensional approaches. This chapter summarizes this research and proposes areas for future study.

Executive Functioning

The symptoms of severe and persistent irritability suggest potential under-lying deficits in several executive functioning domains. For example, emo-tion dysregulation and temper outbursts in response to frustration may stem from difficulties inhibiting motor responses and shifting behavior in response to feedback. To date, executive functioning among children with severe irrita-bility has been studied in three primary domains: (1) inhibitory control, (2) error monitoring, and (3) attention. In the following sections, we review evidence for associations between childhood irritability and altered executive functioning in each of these domains.

RESPONSE INHIBITION

Response inhibition, and more broadly inhibitory control, is a measure of one's ability to inhibit automatic responses that interfere with goal achievement (Logan, Cowan, & Davis, 1984; Logan, Schachar, & Tannock, 1997). Core deficits in the ability to inhibit emotional and behavioral responses may underlie the emotional reactivity and aggressive responses characteristic of youth with clinically significant irritability. One early study by Gagne and Goldsmith (2011) examined the relationship between laboratory-induced anger and inhibitory control in 735 young children (aged 12 and 36 months) using the Laboratory Temperament Assessment Battery (Lab-TAB), an assessment battery designed to assess temperament in early childhood (Gagne & Goldsmith, 2011). Higher levels of laboratory anger at 12 months of age predicted poorer inhibitory control at 36 months (Gagne & Goldsmith, 2011). Further analyses suggested that this relationship was particularly strong for male infants, and the correlations were stronger for monozygotic versus dizygotic twins, suggestive of a genetic contribution (Gagne & Goldsmith, 2011).

In older children, the gold standard for measuring response inhibition is the Stop Signal Task (Logan et al., 1984, 1997). The Stop Signal Task requires participants to execute a motor response following each target stimulus unless a "stop" signal appears shortly after target onset. Among 30 healthy preadolescents, greater variability in anger over a 3- to 4-day period was associated with poorer response inhibition on the Stop Signal task, suggesting that response inhibition difficulties may impair anger regulation (Hoeksma, Oosterlaan, & Schipper, 2004). In contrast, a later study of school-age children and adolescents did not detect behavioral impairments on a Stop Signal Task in those with SMD ($n = 26$) relative to typically developing comparisons ($n = 21$) (Deveney, Connolly, Jenkins, Kim, Fromm, Brotman et al., 2012). During this study, the behavioral task was completed during a functional MRI (fMRI) scan. The novelty of the scanning environment may have obscured group differences, as has been observed in studies of youth with bipolar disorder and those with attention deficit/hyperactivity disorder (ADHD)—populations which have demonstrated robust impairments on response inhibition tasks administered in non-scanning settings (McClure et al., 2005; Rubia, Oosterlaan, Sergeant, Brandeis, & v Leeuwen, 1998; Schachar, Mota, Logan, Tannock, & Klim, 2000).

Response inhibition can also be measured using go/no-go tasks. During these tasks, participants press a button in response to one frequent stimulus ("go"), but withhold a response to a less frequent stimulus ("no-go"). A recent study of 50 preschoolers with high or low levels of disruptive behaviors—of which irritability is common—provides some evidence for response inhibition deficits in irritability (Grabell, Olson, Tardif, Thompson, & Gehring, 2017). Traditional behavioral measures (e.g., accuracy and response time) did not differ between groups. However, children with disruptive behavior took longer to complete the task than did children in the low disruptive behavior group, suggesting that the go and no-go stimuli needed to be presented for longer durations in order to ensure successful response inhibition within this population. Only one study has used the go no-go task to examine response inhibition as a function of irritability symptoms, specifically (Deveney et al., 2018). In that ERP study, higher levels of irritability among 4–7 year-olds ($n = 46$) was associated with reduced accuracy and increased conflict monitoring (i.e., larger N2 amplitudes) during no-go trials during frustration.

Other studies have explored whether irritability is associated with difficulty in generating appropriate alternative responses. Such deficits may manifest as a child being able to stop him- or herself from yelling but having difficulty substituting a more adaptive response to frustration. The Change Task—a modified Stop Signal Task developed to study inhibitory control and response flexibility—has been used to study this possibility. During change trials, children inhibit the prepotent response and substitute a unique third response. Relative to healthy comparison children ($n = 43$), those with SMD ($n = 44$) were less accurate and slower to respond on change trials. However, the more precise measure of how well individuals can execute a flexible response—the change signal reaction time—did not differ between groups (Dickstein et al., 2007). Studies of associated cognitive flexibility, measured using the Wisconsin Card Sorting Task and the Trail Making Task, do not show poorer performance in youth with SMD ($n = 24$; Uran & Kılıç, 2015).

ERROR MONITORING

Difficulties identifying errors and subsequently adjusting behavior may contribute to behavioral and emotional self-regulation impairments in youth with clinically significant irritability. Indeed, atypical error monitoring processes have been linked to depression, anxiety, and externalizing symptoms in healthy children and adults (Hajcak, McDonald, & Simons, 2004; Luu, Collins, & Tucker, 2000; Santesso, Segalowitz, & Schmidt, 2005). Furthermore, error monitoring processes are aberrant among individuals with irritability-related psychopathology including unipolar depression and anxiety (Chiu & Deldin, 2007; Holmes & Pizzagalli, 2008; Ladouceur, Dahl, Birmaher, Axelson, & Ryan, 2006; Olvet & Hajcak, 2008; Schachar et al., 2004). Given these prior associations, error monitoring deficits may exist in youth with chronic and severe irritability.

There are two ERP components that are typically associated with error monitoring, error-related negativity (ERN) and error positivity (Pe). The ERN is thought to reflect error or conflict detection (Carter et al., 1998; Coles, Scheffers, & Holroyd, 2001; Gehring, Goss, Coles, Meyer, & Donchin, 1993), learning or performance modification (Holroyd & Coles, 2002), or the negative affect triggered by making an error (Luu, Tucker, Derryberry, Reed, & Poulsen, 2003). Enhanced ERN amplitudes have been associated with internalizing disorders including anxiety and depression (Gorka, Burkhouse, Afshar, & Phan, 2017). In a longitudinal investigation, Kessel, Meyer, and colleagues (2016) found that children with persistent irritability at age 3 who also displayed enhanced ERN amplitudes during a go/no-go task at age 6 exhibited higher internalizing symptoms at age 9. In contrast, children with early persistent irritability at age 3 but decreased ERN amplitudes at age 6 displayed higher externalizing symptoms at age 9. This study suggests that while irritability alone is not predictive of specific ERN patterns, interactions between irritability and such error-monitoring processes may predict longitudinal clinical outcome in these youth (Kessel, Meyer et al., 2016). Such studies may help clarify how early childhood irritability leads to the development of unipolar mood and anxiety disorders in adulthood (Stringaris, Cohen, Pine, & Leibenluft, 2009).

The Pe component occurs slightly later and over more posterior scalp regions than the ERN and is thought to reflect the conscious processing or evaluation of errors after they have occurred (Nieuwenhuis, Yeung, van den Wildenberg, & Ridderinkhof, 2003), greater autonomic nervous system response to error (Hajcak, Simons, Nieuwenhuis, & Ridderinkhof, 2003; Wessel, Danielmeier, & Ullsperger, 2011), and processing of post-error negative affect (Falkenstein, Hoormann, & Hohnsbein, 1999; Overbeek, Nieuwenhuis, & Ridderinkhof, 2005; Tops, Koole, & Wijers, 2013). No studies have examined the relationship between irritability and Pe amplitude. However, in a recent study, youth with elevated disruptive behavior symptoms did not display the expected enhancement of the Pe component on error relative to correct trials, even though ERN patterns were intact (Grabell, Olson, et al., 2017). This finding raises the possibility that youth with irritability will display deficits during the evaluative stage of error processing. This is consistent with a recent study noting Pe deficits in adults with high trait anger (Lievaart et al., 2016).

ATTENTION

The ability to control one's attention is essential for successful emotion regulation, particularly in early childhood (Mischel, Shoda, & Rodriguez, 1989). Among typically developing children, poor attentional control is associated with increased negative affect and more frequent aggressive behaviors (Morasch & Bell, 2012; Morris et al., 2011; Reijntjes, Stegge, Terwogt, Kamphuis, & Telch, 2006; Rothbart, Ahadi, Hershey, & Fisher, 2001). Despite the clinical relevance of attention, only a handful of studies have examined whether youth with irritability have impairments on attention tasks.

Uran & Kılıç (2015)) compared performance on standard attention tasks (the Color Word Stroop and the Trail Making Tests) in children with SMD ($n = 24$), ADHD ($n = 67$), and a typically developing population ($n = 21$). Youth with SMD did not differ from the typically developing children on either task. In contrast, youth with ADHD performed more poorly relative to the typically developing control participants (Uran & Kılıç, 2015).

Attention has also been measured using the Affective Posner Task—a cued attention task that is completed under non-frustration and frustration conditions

(Pérez-Edgar & Fox, 2005). During the non-frustration ("baseline") condition, youth with SMD (n = 21) exhibited poorer accuracy and reduced early (i.e., N1 and P1), but not later (i.e., P3), ERP measures of attention relative to healthy comparison children (n = 26) (Rich et al., 2007). However, three subsequent studies using this paradigm did not replicate these behavioral effects (Deveney, Connolly, Jenkins, Kim, Fromm, Pine et al., 2012; Rich et al., 2011; Tseng et al., 2018). Rather, the results from these studies pointed to attention deficits that were specific to the frustration condition or related to participant age. These studies are discussed in the later frustrative non-reward section.

SUMMARY OF EXECUTIVE FUNCTIONING AND IRRITABILITY

Although preliminary evidence provides some support for irritability-related deficits in the domains of response inhibition, error monitoring, and attention, current behavioral and psychophysiological investigations are limited, sample sizes are small, and the findings are mixed. Much work remains to be done examining the relationship between irritability and executive functioning in order to better understand the directionality of this relationship and its ability to predict later psychopathology. In addition, many studies have relied on behavioral indices of executive function. These may not be sensitive to the presence of subtle differences that could result in deficits during more challenging conditions. For example, response inhibition may be intact when inhibition is the primary task demand but may be impaired when the child is managing strong negative emotions or engaged in a complex cognitive task in school. Indeed, a recent study of 4–7 year-olds (n = 46) indicated that associations between irritability and response inhibition were specific to a frustration condition (Deveney et al., 2018). Future research should capitalize on the temporal sensitivity of ERPs and assess response inhibition under different task demands before definitive conclusions about irritability and executive functioning are drawn.

Reward Responsivity, Frustrative Non-Reward, and Reward Learning

Early definitions of irritability conceptualized this symptom as a low tolerance for frustration—the negative affect experienced when an expected reward is not received (Brotman, Kircanski, Stringaris, Pine, & Leibenluft, 2017; Leibenluft, Blair, Charney, & Pine, 2003)—indicating that dysfunctional reward processes may be key underlying mechanisms of irritability (Brotman et al., 2017). There are several theoretical reasons to link developmental irritability with atypical reward processing. As an approach emotion, state anger has been associated with increased behavioral and ERP indices of reward-seeking and hedonic responses to rewards (i.e., reward responsivity) in adults (Angus, Kemkes, Schutter, & Harmon-Jones,

2015; Carver & Harmon-Jones, 2009; Ford et al., 2010; Ford, Tamir, Gagnon, Taylor, & Brunyé, 2012) For example, anger manipulations increase attention to rewarding stimuli and may increase the reward positivity (RewP), an ERP measure of hedonic responses to rewards (Angus et al., 2015; Ford et al., 2010, 2012; Proudfit, 2015). However, childhood irritability increases risk for unipolar depression (Stringaris et al., 2009), a disorder in which reduced reward responsivity is consistently observed using behavioral, ERP, and neuroimaging measures (Eshel & Roiser, 2010; Pizzagalli, 2014; Zisner & Beauchaine, 2016). Therefore, while irritability may be associated with altered reward responsivity, the directionality of this effect is unclear. In addition, a recent review by Zisner and Beauchaine (2016) suggests that reduced dopaminergic activity during reward anticipation and associative learning may be a shared feature of internalizing and externalizing symptoms, including irritability.

It is important to note that reward processing is a broad construct encompassing several subprocesses including reward anticipation, hedonic response to reward receipt, reactions to the omission of expected rewards, the ability to associate cues with positive or negative outcomes, and the ability to use feedback to alter behavior. While each of these subprocesses involves dopaminergic systems and interacts with one another, they are frequently distinguished in the empirical literature (Zisner & Beauchaine, 2016). To date, the research on reward processing in irritability has focused on three primary domains that will be reviewed in the subsequent paragraphs: (1) reward responsivity, (2) frustrative non-reward, and (3) reward learning.

REWARD RESPONSIVITY AND SENSITIVITY

Reward responsivity refers to the hedonic response to received rewards that is mediated by mesolimbic dopaminergic systems and measured via self-report as well as frontocentral ERPs and striatal activation in response to rewarding stimuli (Zisner & Beauchaine, 2016). Since anger is an approach emotion (Carver & Harmon-Jones, 2009), youth with irritability may be more sensitive to rewarding stimuli. Alternatively, links between irritability and depression suggest reduced hedonic responses to naturally occurring rewards. A small literature has examined whether irritability is associated with altered experiences during the consumption of rewards.

Reward responsivity is probed using ERPs elicited by rewarding feedback (i.e., "You Win 50¢!") compared to the ERPs elicited by loss feedback (i.e., "You Lost 50¢!") to generate a component called *reward positivity* (RewP; Proudfit, 2015). Greater reward responsivity is associated with higher RewP amplitudes. A recent physiological study examined the relationship between early childhood irritability and RewP amplitude using a gambling task that has been used extensively to probe reward responsivity in adults with depression. In a community sample of 373 children, severe irritability at age 3 predicted enhanced RewP amplitudes at age 9, reflecting greater reward responsivity (Kessel, Dougherty et al., 2016). Findings from this initial study suggest that children with irritability may be more responsive to rewards and may have a greater tendency to seek them out. However, irritability at age 9 did not predict reward responsivity at the same age, so further research is needed to interpret these results.

A related but distinct process of reward sensitivity was explored by Rau and colleagues (2008) using a behavioral task that measures how well participants discriminate between stimuli associated with varying degrees of reward and punishment (Blair, Peschardt, Budhani, Mitchell, & Pine, 2006). Relative to healthy comparison children (n = 31), youth with severe irritability (SMD, n = 37) did not demonstrate impairments on this task, suggesting no difference in the experience of rewards between children who struggle with irritability and those who do not (Rau et al., 2008).

FRUSTRATIVE NON-REWARD

The frequent and developmentally inappropriate temper tantrums characteristic of youth with irritability often occur when the child is frustrated (i.e., when being asked to stop doing something or when they do not get an expected reward). Accordingly, research has examined whether youth with irritability have exaggerated responses on frustrative non-reward tasks. *Frustrative non-reward* is an RDoC construct that describes the reaction elicited when an individual is prevented from receiving an expected reward despite sustained or persistent efforts (Insel et al., 2010). The majority of behavioral and psychophysiological research on frustrative non-reward in irritability has used the Affective Posner task. As mentioned earlier, this is a cued attention task designed to test attentional shifts under non-frustration and frustration conditions (Pérez-Edgar & Fox, 2005). Frustration is induced via rigged performance feedback that informs participants that they responded too slowly and have lost money.

Consistent with clinical reports of exaggerated emotional responses to frustration, youth with severe irritability (operationalized as either SMD or DMDD) self-report greater unpleasant arousal or frustration in response to the frustration manipulation in the Affective Posner task than do typically developing children (Deveney et al. 2013; Rich et al., 2007, 2011). Although one study of youth with SMD (n = 21) documented accuracy and early attention-related ERP deficits during non-frustration that were not exacerbated by the frustration manipulation (Rich et al., 2007), two subsequent neuroimaging studies indicate that youth with SMD are characterized by frustration-specific attentional impairments (Deveney, Connolly, Jenkins, Kim, Fromm, Pine et al., 2012; Rich et al., 2011). Relative to healthy comparison children, youth with SMD displayed poorer accuracy (n_{HC} = 20; n_{SMD} = 20) (Rich et al., 2011) and slower response times (n_{HC} = 23; n_{SMD} = 19) (Deveney et al., 2013) during frustration. Groups did not differ during the non-frustration condition in these studies. These studies also revealed atypical neural activation patterns during frustration among youth with SMD as well as among children with greater irritability symptoms that are detailed in Chapter 8 (Deveney et al., 2013; Rich et al. 2011). Interestingly, a recent neuroimaging study of children with DMDD ($n = 52$), ADHD ($n = 52$), anxiety disorders ($n = 40$), or no psychiatric history ($n = 61$) detected neural, but not behavioral, associations with dimensional measures of irritability across the entire participant sample (Tseng et al., 2018).

A similar paradigm (FETCH) has been used to explore frustrative non-reward in preschool children with irritability and irritability-related symptoms (Grabell, Li, et al., 2017; Perlman, Luna, Hein, & Huppert, 2013; Perlman et al., 2015). The neural findings from these studies are discussed in Chapter 8. A modified go/no-go task that includes a negative, frustrating mood induction block has been used to examine cognitive control in youth with internalizing and externalizing symptoms and/or disruptive behavior symptoms (Lewis, Lamm, Segalowitz, Stieben, & Zelazo, 2006; Stieben et al., 2007). In these studies, researchers measure an early frontocentral ERP component elicited by no-go stimuli ($N2_{no-go}$), which is a measure of conflict detection and response inhibition (Falkenstein, Hoormann, & Hohnsbein, 2002; Huster, Enriquez-Geppert, Lavallee, Falkenstein, & Herrmann, 2013). Relative to typically developing school-age youth ($n = 15$), those with externalizing symptoms only ($n = 8$) displayed reduced N2 amplitudes in both non-frustration and frustration conditions. This suggested impaired response inhibition ability irrespective of the affective demands of the task. In contrast, youth with externalizing and internalizing symptoms demonstrated an augmentation of N2 amplitudes during frustration. The latter finding was interpreted as a sign that these youth needed to mobilize cognitive resources in order to successfully inhibit responses during the frustration block. To date, no published work has examined whether irritability correlates with performance on this task.

REWARD LEARNING

Research has also examined how well youth with irritability adapt to changing reward contingencies and use performance feedback to guide future behavior. Difficulties adapting to changing reward contingencies has been associated with increased frustration and negative affect, which may in turn underlie the development of clinical irritability in youth (Blair, 2004; Blair & Cipolotti, 2000). Responses to changing learning contingencies is measured using reversal learning tasks (Cools, Clark, & Robbins, 2004; Stemme, Deco, Busch, & Schneider, 2005). During these tasks, participants learn a reward contingency and then adjust their behavior upon receiving feedback that the contingency has changed (i.e., the prior choice is no longer correct) (Budhani, Marsh, Pine, & Blair, 2007; Finger et al., 2008). While error monitoring reflects responses to the actual error, reversal learning tasks explore how individuals use feedback to adjust behavior. Failures in behavioral adjustments following errors may signal deficits in reward processing regions like the orbitofrontal cortex and the ventral striatum (Blair, Colledge, & Mitchell, 2001; Budhani et al., 2007; Clark, Cools, & Robbins, 2004; Cools et al., 2004; Dickstein et al., 2010; Knutson, Westdorp, Kaiser, & Hommer, 2000; O'Doherty et al., 2004).

Deficits in reversal learning among youth with irritability have been explored in three studies. In the first study, Dickstein and colleagues (2007) compared reversal learning across youth with bipolar disorder ($n = 50$), SMD ($n = 44$), and no psychiatric history ($n = 43$). The task consisted of two phases—a simple reversal during which a previously incorrect stimulus became the correct response and a compound reversal phase during which a previously irrelevant stimulus became the correct response. While youth with bipolar disorder were impaired during both phases of the task, youth with SMD were only impaired during the compound response reversal phases, suggesting that reward learning deficits were specific to more challenging task demands and were intact on simpler tasks in the latter population (Dickstein et al., 2007).

Two subsequent studies did not detect reversal learning deficits among youth with SMD ($n = 22$; 35) (Adleman et al., 2011; Dickstein et al., 2010). While this suggests that irritability may not be associated with reversal learning deficits, two important caveats should be noted. First, neither of these tasks included the compound reversal phase that may be more sensitive to irritability-related deficits. As noted in Dickstein et al. (2007), youth with SMD may be characterized by impairments on more challenging reversals but have intact performance on simple reversals. Second, although Adleman et al. (2011) did not detect behavioral differences, neural activation patterns differed between youth with SMD and healthy comparison children, providing some evidence for reversal learning deficits in youth with irritability (see Chapter 8).

SUMMARY OF REWARD PROCESSING STUDIES OF IRRITABILITY

The behavioral and psychophysiological evidence provides partial support for atypical reward processes in youth with irritability. The present findings suggest that irritability may be related to enhanced hedonic responses to reward at a later age, atypical responses to frustrative non-reward, and difficulty using feedback to make complex, but not simple, behavioral changes. However, only a few studies have been conducted, sample sizes are small, and studies are limited to a narrow set of reward processes. Other domains of reward processing represent important avenues for future research. For example, Zisner and Beauchaine (2016) highlight dysfunctional reward encoding ability and reward anticipation as potential common features of internalizing and externalizing disorders. To date, these processes have not been explored as a function of irritability specifically. Careful attention to the specific reward subprocesses that are linked to irritability may help identify domain-specific deficits in irritability and their associated neurophysiological correlates.

Emotional Stimulus Processing

Finally, researchers have examined links between irritability and atypical responses to emotional stimuli. Atypical emotion processing and emotion recognition are commonly found in psychiatric populations and are implicated in poor social relationships, low perceived social support, and altered executive functioning when faced with emotionally salient stimuli (Bediou et al., 2012; Dalgleish, 2004; Kohler, Turner, Gur, & Gur, 2004; Phillips, 2003). Among children with irritability, studies of emotional stimulus processing fall into four primary domains: (1) identification of emotion from facial expressions and auditory cues, (2) hostile interpretation biases, (3) threat biases, and (4) responses to emotional images.

FACE EMOTION IDENTIFICATION

Numerous studies have explored face emotion identification in children with severe irritability. In part, this reflects the early literature's focus on examining whether severe and persistent irritability is a developmental form of bipolar disorder (for review, see Leibenluft, 2011); emotion identification deficits are observed in youth with bipolar disorder (Guyer et al., 2007; Kim et al., 2013; McClure et al., 2005; Rocca, Heuvel, Caetano, & Lafer, 2009). However, such studies also provide important information about potential underlying mechanisms of irritability and may improve the field's understanding of the social impairments displayed by this population (Greene et al., 2002; Rich et al., 2008).

The ability to recognize emotions from facial expressions has been probed using two primary paradigms: static emotional face identification tasks and dynamic face morphing tasks. During *static* emotion identification tasks, participants view images of facial expressions which vary in terms of the type (e.g., happy, sad) and, in some tasks, the intensity (e.g., 50% angry/50% neutral) of the emotion displayed. Participants identify the emotion displayed by each stimulus, typically from a limited set of choices. Higher task accuracy reflects better face emotion identification ability. During *dynamic* face morphing tasks, participants view neutral images that slowly morph into a 100% prototypical emotional expression in a movie-like format. Participants are instructed to stop the video when they first detect the emotional expression displayed. The earlier a video is stopped, the less intensity that was required to identify the emotional expression and the better the participant's emotion identification ability.

Youth with severe irritability demonstrate impaired face emotion identification in both static and dynamic tasks. Across several studies, relative to healthy comparison children, those with SMD were less accurate when identifying all emotions during a static face emotion identification task ($n = 67$ across two studies) (Guyer et al., 2007; Kim et al., 2013) and required more emotional intensity to identify a face emotion correctly in a dynamic morphing task ($n = 31$) (Rich et al., 2008). The emotion identification deficits displayed by youth with

SMD are similar to those with bipolar disorder, but greater than youth with mood and/or anxiety disorders (Guyer et al., 2007; Kim et al., 2013). In addition, one study suggests that youth with SMD ($n = 67$) performed more poorly on a task requiring them to recognize the emotional tone (prosody) of brief sentences than did their typically developing peers ($n = 57$) (Deveney, Brotman, Decker, Pine, & Leibenluft, 2012). Together, these results suggest that emotion labeling may represent a general problem for youth with chronic irritability. However, a recent study indicates that future work examining associations between irritability and face emotion identification deficits should account for co-occurring depression symptoms (Vidal-Ribas et al., 2018).

Existing studies have only assessed the ability of youth to identify the six basic emotions (anger, fear, happiness, sadness, disgust, and surprise). Whether similar deficits exist in tasks requiring participants to identify more complex emotional expressions is unknown. Future face emotion identification research should also directly assess social skills or interpersonal functioning in youth with irritability. To date, only one study has done so, and, while it links deficits on the face emotion task with poorer interpersonal functioning (Rich et al., 2008), future research is necessary to replicate these findings in larger samples. Finally, while neuroimaging studies have probed face emotion processing (see Chapter 8), we are unaware of any psychophysiological (i.e., ERP) studies in youth with irritability. Such information may contribute to our understanding of subprocesses involved in face emotion identification deficits associated with irritability.

HOSTILE INTERPRETATION BIASES

Recent studies have probed associations between irritability and a tendency to perceive threat/hostility from ambiguous social information (i.e., hostile interpretation biases) (Leibenluft, 2017). This area of research builds on prior work on trait anger and disruptive behavior disorders that relate aggression and anger to hostile interpretation biases (Crick & Dodge, 1994, 1996). A tendency to perceive hostile intent may contribute to the temper outbursts exhibited by youth with irritability. An early fMRI study provided initial evidence for hostile interpretation biases in youth with irritability. Neutral faces, which are ambiguous, were rated as more threatening by youth with SMD ($n = 29$), than by the healthy comparison children ($n = 37$) (Brotman et al., 2010).

Recent behavioral work has provided a more fine-grained assessment of hostile interpretation biases in this population. In these paradigms, prototypical angry and happy faces are morphed together at different intensity levels (e.g., 20% angry/80% happy or 60% angry/40% happy) to generate ambiguous facial expressions. Participants are asked to identify each face morph as being happy or angry. Researchers plot the frequency with which participants rate each face as being angry and measure the point at which participants shift from identifying faces as happy to interpreting them as being angry. Relative to healthy comparison youth, the shifting point of those with DMDD occurs at lower anger intensity levels, suggesting a hostile interpretation bias in this population (Stoddard et al., 2016).

THREAT BIAS

Threat biases refer to preferential attention to threatening stimuli (Leibenluft, 2017). These are typically defined as bias toward (selectively attending to) or bias away from (selectively attending away) threat. Numerous studies in adults document increased attention to threatening stimuli among individuals with high trait anger and/or aggression (Smith & Waterman, 2003; van Honk, Tuiten, de Haan, van den Hout, & Stam, 2001). Studies of threat bias in irritability have used the *dot probe paradigm*—a task that has been used extensively to research threat biases in anxiety (Bar-Haim, Lamy, Pergamin, Bakermans-Kranenburg, & van, 2007; Ehrenreich & Gross, 2002; Shechner et al., 2012). During this task, participants briefly view emotional (i.e., threatening) and neutral stimuli in two locations on a computer screen. One of the stimuli is quickly replaced by a target probe (i.e., a letter or an arrow). If a participant preferentially attends to the threatening stimulus, she or he will identify the probe that appears in that location (congruent trials) more quickly than a probe appearing behind the neutral stimulus (incongruent trials). The degree to which individuals are faster to respond on threat-congruent relative to -incongruent trials is a measure of threat bias (Shechner et al., 2012).

Two behavioral studies have examined threat in populations characterized by severe irritability and/or externalizing behaviors. In one study, children and adolescents with SMD ($n = 74$) displayed greater threat biases than healthy comparison children ($n = 42$) (Hommer et al., 2014). This finding was replicated in a large community sample of children ($n = 1,872$), oversampled for individuals experiencing current psychiatric symptoms or who had family histories of psychiatric disorders (Salum et al., 2017). Children in a high-irritability group ($n = 73$) (operationalized using the CBCL Irritability subscale) displayed greater attention biases toward angry faces than children in the low-irritability group ($n = 73$). In addition, dimensional analyses linked higher CBCL Irritability scores with greater threat biases across the entire sample. Importantly, irritability was unrelated to biases toward happy faces in both studies, suggesting that irritability is not associated with heightened attention to all emotional stimuli. Rather, it is specific to threatening faces and remains significant even after accounting for potential confounds such as anxiety (Hommer et al., 2014; Salum et al., 2016).

Although the findings from these studies are consistent and a robust literature uses the dot probe paradigm to explore threat biases in anxiety, significant questions exist about the reliability and validity of this paradigm. Test-retest reliability for threat biases in those with anxiety is poor (Kappenman, Farrens, Luck, & Proudfit, 2014), and it is unclear whether the task measures initial attention/

orienting or difficulty disengaging attention (Grafton & MacLeod, 2014; Koster, Crombez, Verschuere, & De Houwer, 2004; Rudaizky, Basanovic, & MacLeod, 2014). The developing literature on irritability and threat biases would benefit from being aware of these limitations and the existence of paradigms/techniques that may help parse the specific attentional mechanisms associated with irritability. For example, Grafton and MacLeod (2014) developed a variant of the dot probe that disentangles selective attention from attention disengagement. Using this paradigm, the researchers were able to link social anxiety symptoms in adults with selective attention to negative information, specifically (Grafton & MacLeod, 2014). In conjunction with eye tracking techniques like the one used by Kim et al. (2013), paradigms that clarify the specific attentional processes underlying threat biases will help identify the relevant neural circuits and potential interventions for irritability. Finally, this field may benefit from combining behavioral and neural measures of threat bias. Several studies have capitalized on the temporal sensitivity of ERPs to investigate threat biases in populations characterized by elevated anxiety symptoms or risk factors for anxiety, yet we are unaware of any such studies examining threat biases in irritability.

RESPONSIVITY TO EMOTIONAL, NONFACIAL IMAGES

As reviewed earlier, much of the research on atypical emotional processing in irritability focuses on responses to emotional faces. However, researchers have also explored whether irritability is related to atypical responses to other types of emotional stimuli, including emotionally evocative images like those contained in the International Affective Picture System (Hajcak & Dennis, 2009; Lang, Bradley, & Cuthbert, 2005). Atypical responses to emotional images in addition to emotional faces may suggest broader deficits in limbic regions and/or deficits in the prefrontal regulatory regions.

Only a few studies have explored the relationship between irritability and emotional images and the findings are mixed. In an early behavioral study using the Emotional Interrupt task, a task designed to explore sensitivity to emotional stimuli and cognitive task performance, Rich and colleagues (2010) found that youth with SMD ($n = 41$) were less impacted by the emotional stimuli as compared to children with bipolar disorder ($n= 57$) and healthy volunteers ($n = 33$) (Rich et al., 2010). In contrast, a recent physiological study linked high levels of irritability in early childhood (age 3) with greater responsivity to emotional stimuli in later childhood in a sample of 338 youth (Kessel et al., 2017). Specifically, youth with early levels of irritability and a maternal history of depression demonstrated a larger late positive potential (LPP) ERP component to both positively and negatively valenced images, suggesting greater responsivity to emotional stimuli. Heightened irritability in early childhood in the absence of maternal history of depression was unrelated to LPP amplitudes to emotional images. Similar to the RewP and ERN studies reviewed earlier (Kessel, Meyer, et al., 2016; Kessel, Dougherty et al., 2016), interactions between irritability and ERP components are important to evaluate. The relationship between irritability and atypical responses to emotional stimuli remains underexplored in behavioral and psychophysiological paradigms and represents a promising avenue for future investigations.

SUMMARY OF EMOTIONAL STIMULI STUDIES

Atypical responses to emotional stimuli represent one of the most robust findings in studies of severe irritability. Youth with severe irritability are characterized by impaired face emotion identification abilities, a tendency to interpret ambiguous images as threatening, and biased attention toward threatening stimuli. Deficits in these domains may underlie both the social deficits and frustration that characterize clinically significant irritability. Although additional work is necessary to replicate these findings, the early work on hostile interpretation and threat biases suggests potential interventions for irritability. Attention bias modification (ABM) treatment has been shown to reduce anxiety symptoms in populations with anxiety (Bar-Haim, 2010; Lowther & Newman, 2014). ABM may reduce threat biases and irritability symptoms in youth characterized by problematic irritability as well, although this remains to be tested. Early pilot work also suggests that a computerized intervention designed to reduce hostile interpretation biases called Interpretation Bias Training (IBT) reduces irritability symptoms and alters neural activation to threatening faces among youth with DMDD (Stoddard et al., 2016) and among older populations with anger/aggression (Penton-Voak et al., 2013). Should future research replicate these findings, ABM and IBT may be promising, low-cost, and easy-to-disseminate interventions for children with severe irritability.

Conclusion and Future Directions

Behavioral and psychophysiological investigations of childhood irritability have focused on executive functioning, reward processing, and responses to emotional stimuli. First, while some evidence links irritability with impaired executive functioning as evidenced by response inhibition, error monitoring, and early attention, findings are somewhat mixed. Second, irritability may be characterized by atypical reward processing, including enhanced hedonic responses to reward, atypical responses to frustrative non-reward, and difficulty using feedback to adjust behavior. And, third, irritability is related to clear deficits in responses to emotional stimuli including impaired face emotion identification ability, hostile interpretation biases, and greater attention toward threatening stimuli. It is important to note that research into each of these domains is limited, samples sizes are small, and additional research using temporally sensitive tools is necessary to gain a comprehensive understanding of the mechanisms underlying irritability and to resolve existing discrepancies in the literature.

A consistent theme emerging from this literature is that emotion-cognition interactions may be critical for understanding the mechanisms underlying irritability. Irritability-related deficits were robust in studies of frustrative non-reward and of attentional control during frustration manipulations. Such findings raise the possibility that baseline executive functioning and reward processing is intact in youth with irritability but becomes impaired during conditions of marked negative affect. This parallels research on populations with externalizing symptoms (Lewis et al., 2006; Stieben et al., 2007) and some research on adults with high trait anger (Eckhardt & Cohen, 1997). Future research focusing on emotion-cognition interactions may benefit the field's understanding of irritability. Such research should also explore whether deficits are specific to frustration manipulations or whether they extend to other affective conditions including sadness, anxiety, and stress, as well as to overall cognitive resource depletion.

Future behavioral and psychophysiological research would also benefit from adopting a dimensional approach when measuring irritability. Much of the existing behavioral and psychophysiological literature on irritability has utilized a categorical approach. In part, this reflects the lack of developmentally appropriate measures of irritability at the time many of these studies were conducted. The recent availability of dimensional assessment tools such as the ARI (Stringaris et al., 2012) and the MAP-DB (Wakschlag et al., 2014) should facilitate future dimensional research into irritability in children and adolescents. Such studies would facilitate transdiagnostic investigations of irritability, would be consistent with National Institute of Mental Health's (NIMH) Research Domain Criteria approach (Insel et al., 2010; Insel, 2013), and may address concerns that current diagnostic criteria for DMDD may not adequately capture all youth with impairing irritability (Deveney et al., 2015; Roy, Lopes, & Klein, 2014).

Finally, irritability is a transdiagnostic symptom that is present in numerous disorders that have also been associated with atypical neuropsychological, reward, and emotional processing deficits. Therefore, an important avenue for future research is whether deficits are specific to irritability or whether they are driven by co-occurring mood, anxiety, attention, and externalizing symptoms. Studies of threat biases carefully controlled for anxiety symptoms to reveal irritability-related deficits on these tasks (Hommer et al., 2014; Salum et al., 2016). Similar efforts are necessary for studies in other domains for which there are known behavioral and physiological dysfunction.

Irritability is associated with significant impairment in functioning and a high mental health burden on children and their families (Carlson et al., 2009; Raine, 1996; Roy et al., 2013). Behavioral and psychophysiological investigations play a valuable role in elucidating the underlying mechanisms of irritability and have translated to potential treatments for this impairing symptom (Stoddard et al., 2016). However, the field of irritability research is young and much work is necessary to fully understand this impairing symptom and its impact on children and their families.

References

Adleman, N. E., Kayser, R., Dickstein, D., Blair, R. J. R., Pine, D., & Leibenluft, E. (2011). Neural correlates of reversal learning in severe mood dysregulation and pediatric bipolar disorder. *Journal of the American Academy of Child & Adolescent Psychiatry, 50*, 1173–1185.e1172. Retrieved from https://doi.org/10.1016/j.jaac.2011.07.011

Andreassi, J. L. (1995). *Psychophysiology: Human behavior and psychophysiological response* (3rd ed.). Hillsdale, NJ: Erlbaum.

Angus, D. J., Kemkes, K., Schutter, D. J., & Harmon-Jones, E. (2015). Anger is associated with reward-related electrocortical activity: Evidence from the reward positivity. *Psychophysiology, 52*, 1271–1280. doi:10.1111/psyp.12460

Bar-Haim, Y. (2010). Research review: Attention bias modification (ABM): A novel treatment for anxiety disorders. *Journal of Child Psychology and Psychiatry, 51*, 859–870. doi:10.1111/j.1469-7610.2010.02251.x

Bar-Haim, Y., Lamy, D., Pergamin, L., Bakermans-Kranenburg, M. J., & van, I. M. H. (2007). Threat-related attentional bias in anxious and nonanxious individuals: A meta-analytic study. *Psychological Bulletin, 133*, 1–24. doi:10.1037/0033-2909.133.1.1

Bediou, B., Brunelin, J., d'Amato, T., Fecteau, S., Saoud, M., Hénaff, M.-A., & Krolak-Salmon, P. (2012). A comparison of facial emotion processing in neurological and psychiatric conditions. *Frontiers in Psychology, 3*, 98. doi:10.3389/fpsyg.2012.00098

Blair, R. J. (2004). The roles of orbital frontal cortex in the modulation of antisocial behavior. *Brain and Cognition, 55*, 198–208. doi:10.1016/s0278-2626(03)00276-8

Blair, R. J., & Cipolotti, L. (2000). Impaired social response reversal. A case of "acquired sociopathy." *Brain, 123 (Pt 6)*, 1122–1141.

Blair, R. J., Colledge, E., & Mitchell, D. G. (2001). Somatic markers and response reversal: Is there orbitofrontal cortex dysfunction in boys with psychopathic tendencies? *Journal of Abnormal Child Psychology, 29*, 499–511.

Blair, R. J., Peschardt, K. S., Budhani, S., Mitchell, D. G. V., & Pine, D. S. (2006). The development of psychopathy. *Journal of Child Psychology and Psychiatry, 47*, 262–276. doi:10.1111/j.1469-7610.2006.01596.x

Brotman, M. A., Kircanski, K., Stringaris, A., Pine, D. S., & Leibenluft, E. (2017). Irritability in youths: A translational model. *American Journal of Psychiatry*, appiajp201616070839. doi:10.1176/appi.ajp.2016.16070839

Brotman, M. A., Rich, B. A., Guyer, A. E., Lunsford, J. R., Horsey, S. E., Reising, M. M., . . . Leibenluft, E. (2010). Amygdala activation during emotion processing of neutral faces in children with severe mood dysregulation versus ADHD or bipolar disorder. *American Journal of Psychiatry, 167*, 61–69. doi:10.1176/appi.ajp.2009.09010043

Budhani, S., Marsh, A. A., Pine, D. S., & Blair, R. J. R. (2007). Neural correlates of response reversal: Considering acquisition. *NeuroImage, 34*, 1754–1765. doi:10.1016/j.neuroimage.2006.08.060

Carlson, G. A., Potegal, M., Margulies, D., Gutkovich, Z., & Basile, J. (2009). Rages: What are they and who has them? *Journal of Child and Adolescent Psychopharmacology, 19*, 281–288. doi:10.1089/cap.2008.0108

Carter, C. S., Braver, T. S., Barch, D. M., Botvinick, M. M., Noll, D., & Cohen, J. D. (1998). Anterior cingulate cortex, error detection, and the online monitoring of performance. *Science, 280*, 747–749.

Carver, C. S., & Harmon-Jones, E. (2009). Anger is an approach-related affect: Evidence and implications. *Psychological Bulletin, 135,* 183–204. doi:10.1037/a0013965

Chiu, P. H., & Deldin, P. J. (2007). Neural evidence for enhanced error detection in major depressive disorder. *American Journal of Psychiatry, 164,* 608–616. doi:10.1176/ajp.2007.164.4.608

Clark, L., Cools, R., & Robbins, T. W. (2004). The neuropsychology of ventral prefrontal cortex: Decision-making and reversal learning. *Brain and Cognition, 55,* 41–53. doi:10.1016/S0278-2626(03)00284-7

Coles, M. G., Scheffers, M. K., & Holroyd, C. B. (2001). Why is there an ERN/Ne on correct trials? Response representations, stimulus-related components, and the theory of error-processing. *Biological Psychology, 56,* 173–189.

Cools, R., Clark, L., & Robbins, T. W. (2004). Differential responses in human striatum and prefrontal cortex to changes in object and rule relevance. *Journal of Neuroscience, 24,* 1129–1135. doi:10.1523/JNEUROSCI.4312-03.2004

Copeland, W. E., Angold, A., Costello, E. J., & Egger, H. (2013). Prevalence, comorbidity, and correlates of DSM-5 proposed disruptive mood dysregulation disorder. *American Journal of Psychiatry, 170,* 173–179. doi:10.1176/appi.ajp.2012.12010132

Copeland, W. E., Shanahan, L., Egger, H., Angold, A., & Costello, E. J. (2014). Adult diagnostic and functional outcomes of DSM-5 disruptive mood dysregulation disorder. *American Journal of Psychiatry, 171,* 668–674. doi:10.1176/appi.ajp.2014.13091213

Crick, N. R., & Dodge, K. A. (1994). A review and reformulation of social information-processing mechanisms in children's social-adjustment. *Psychological Bulletin, 115,* 74–101. doi:10.1037/0033-2909.115.1.74

Crick, N. R., & Dodge, K. A. (1996). Social information-processing mechanisms in reactive and proactive aggression. *Child Development, 67,* 993–1002.

Dalgleish, T. (2004). Timeline: The emotional brain. *Nature Reviews Neuroscience, 5,* 583–589. doi:10.1038/nrn1432

Deveney, C. M., Briggs-Gowan, M. J., Pagliaccio, D., Estabrook, C.R., Zobel, E., Burns, J. L., . . . Wakschlag, L. S. (2018). Temporally sensitive neural measures of inhibition in preschool children across a spectrum of irritability. *Developmental Psychobiology.* doi:10.1002/dev.21792. [Epub ahead of print]

Deveney, C. M., Brotman, M. A., Decker, A. M., Pine, D. S., & Leibenluft, E. (2012). Affective prosody labeling in youths with bipolar disorder or severe mood dysregulation. *Journal of Child Psychology and Psychiatry, 53,* 262–270. doi:10.1111/j.1469-7610.2011.02482.x

Deveney, C. M., Connolly, M. E., Haring, C. T., Bones, B. L., Reynolds, R. C., Kim, P., . . . Leibenluft, E. (2013). Neural mechanisms of frustration in chronically irritable children. *American Journal of Psychiatry, 170,* 1186–1194. doi:10.1176/appi.ajp.2013.12070917 1695222 [pii]

Deveney, C. M., Connolly, M. E., Jenkins, S. E., Kim, P., Fromm, S. J., Brotman, M. A., . . . Leibenluft, E. (2012). Striatal dysfunction during failed motor inhibition in children at risk for bipolar disorder. *Progress in Neuropsychopharmacology and Biological Psychiatry, 38,* 127–133. doi:S0278-5846(12)00046-2 [pii] 10.1016/j.pnpbp.2012.02.014

Deveney, C. M., Connolly, M. E., Jenkins, S. E., Kim, P., Fromm, S. J., Pine, D. S., & Leibenluft, E. (2012). Neural recruitment during failed motor inhibition differentiates youths with bipolar disorder and severe mood dysregulation. *Biological Psychology, 89,* 148–155. doi:10.1016/j.biopsycho.2011.10.003

Deveney, C. M., Hommer, R. E., Reeves, E., Stringaris, A., Hinton, K. E., Haring, C. T., . . . Leibenluft, E. (2015). A prospective study of severe irritability in youths: 2- and 4-year follow-up. *Depression and Anxiety, 32*, 364–372. doi:10.1002/da.22336

Dickstein, D. P., Finger, E. C., Brotman, M. A., Rich, B. A., Pine, D. S., Blair, J. R., & Leibenluft, E. (2010). Impaired probabilistic reversal learning in youths with mood and anxiety disorders. *Psychological Medicine, 40*, 1089–1100. doi:10.1017/S0033291709991462

Dickstein, D. P., Nelson, E. E., McClure, E. B., Grimley, M. E., Knopf, L., Brotman, M. A., . . . Leibenluft, E. (2007). Cognitive flexibility in phenotypes of pediatric bipolar disorder. *Journal of the American Academy of Child and Adolescent Psychiatry, 46*, 341–355. doi:10.1097/chi.0b013e31802d0b3d S0890-8567(09)61678-6 [pii]

Eckhardt, C. I., & Cohen, D. J. (1997). Attention to anger-relevant and irrelevant stimuli following naturalistic insult. *Personality and Individual Differences, 23*, 619–629. doi:10.1016/S0191-8869(97)00074-3

Ehrenreich, J. T., & Gross, A. M. (2002). Biased attentional behavior in childhood anxiety. A review of theory and current empirical investigation. *Clinical Psychology Review, 22*, 991–1008.

Eshel, N., & Roiser, J. P. (2010). Reward and punishment processing in depression. *Biological Psychiatry, 68*, 118–124. doi:10.1016/j.biopsych.2010.01.027

Falkenstein, M., Hoormann, J., & Hohnsbein, J. (1999). ERP components in Go/Nogo tasks and their relation to inhibition. *Acta Psychology (Amst), 101*, 267–291.

Falkenstein, M., Hoormann, J., & Hohnsbein, J. (2002). Inhibition-related ERP components: Variation with modality, age, and time-on-task. *Journal of Psychophysiology, 16*, 167–175. doi:10.1027//0269-8803.16.3.167

Finger, E. C., Marsh, A. A., Mitchell, D. G., Reid, M. E., Sims, C., Budhani, S., . . . Blair, J. R. (2008). Abnormal ventromedial prefrontal cortex function in children with psychopathic traits during reversal learning. *Archives of General Psychiatry, 65*, 586–594. doi:10.1001/archpsyc.65.5.586

Ford, B. Q., Tamir, M., Brunyé, T. T., Shirer, W. R., Mahoney, C. R., & Taylor, H. A. (2010). Keeping your eyes on the prize: Anger and visual attention to threats and rewards. *Psychological Science, 21*, 1098–1105. doi:10.1177/0956797610375450

Ford, B. Q., Tamir, M., Gagnon, S. A., Taylor, H. A., & Brunyé, T. T. (2012). The angry spotlight: Trait anger and selective visual attention to rewards. *European Journal of Personality, 26*, 90–98. doi:10.1002/per.1840

Gagne, J. R., & Goldsmith, H. H. (2011). A longitudinal analysis of anger and inhibitory control in twins from 12 to 36 months of age. *Developmental Science, 14*, 112–124. doi:10.1111/j.1467-7687.2010.00969.x

Gehring, W. J., Goss, B., Coles, M. G., Meyer, D. E., & Donchin, E. (1993). A neural system for error detection and compensation. *Psychological Science, 4*, 385–390.

Girard, L.-C., Pingault, J.-B., Doyle, O., Falissard, B., & Tremblay, R. E. (2016). Developmental associations between conduct problems and expressive language in early childhood: A population-based study. *Journal of Abnormal Child Psychology, 44*, 1033–1043. doi:10.1007/s10802-015-0094-8

Gorka, S. M., Burkhouse, K. L., Afshar, K., & Phan, K. L. (2017). Error-related brain activity and internalizing disorder symptom dimensions in depression and anxiety. *Depression and Anxiety, 34*, 985–995. doi:10.1002/da.22648

Grabell, A. S., Li, Y., Barker, J. W., Wakschlag, L. S., Huppert, T. J., & Perlman, S. B. (2017). Evidence of non-linear associations between frustration-related prefrontal cortex activation and the normal:abnormal spectrum of irritability in young children. *Journal of Abnormal Child Psychology*. doi:10.1007/s10802-017-0286-5

Grabell, A. S., Olson, S. L., Tardif, T., Thompson, M. C., & Gehring, W. J. (2017). Comparing self-regulation-associated event related potentials in preschool children with and without high levels of disruptive behavior. *Journal of Abnormal Child Psychology*, 45, 1119–1132. doi:10.1007/s10802-016-0228-7

Grafton, B., & MacLeod, C. (2014). Enhanced probing of attentional bias: The independence of anxiety-linked selectivity in attentional engagement with and disengagement from negative information. *Cognition and Emotion*, 28, 1287–1302. doi:10.1080/02699931.2014.881326

Greene, R. W., Biederman, J., Zerwas, S., Monuteaux, M. C., Goring, J. C., & Faraone, S. V. (2002). Psychiatric comorbidity, family dysfunction, and social impairment in referred youth with oppositional defiant disorder. *The American Journal of Psychiatry*, 159, 1214–1224. doi:10.1176/appi.ajp.159.7.1214

Guyer, A. E., McClure, E. B., Adler, A. D., Brotman, M. A., Rich, B. A., Kimes, A. S., . . . Leibenluft, E. (2007). Specificity of facial expression labeling deficits in childhood psychopathology. *Journal of Child Psychology and Psychiatry*, 48, 863–871. doi:10.1111/j.1469-7610.2007.01758.x

Hajcak, G., & Dennis, T. A. (2009). Brain potentials during affective picture processing in children. *Biological Psychology*, 80, 333–338. doi:10.1016/j.biopsycho.2008.11.006

Hajcak, G., McDonald, N., & Simons, R. F. (2004). Error-related psychophysiology and negative affect. *Brain and Cognition*, 56, 189–197.

Hajcak, G., Simons, R. F., Nieuwenhuis, S., & Ridderinkhof, K. R. (2003). Error-preceding brain activity: A further investigation. *Psychophysiology*, 40, S45–S45.

Hoeksma, J. B., Oosterlaan, J., & Schipper, E. M. (2004). Emotion regulation and the dynamics of feelings: A conceptual and methodological framework. *Child Development*, 75, 354–360.

Holmes, A. J., & Pizzagalli, D. A. (2008). Spatiotemporal dynamics of error processing dysfunctions in major depressive disorder. *Archives of General Psychiatry*, 65, 179–188. doi:10.1001/archgenpsychiatry.2007.19

Holroyd, C. B., & Coles, M. G. H. (2002). The neural basis of human error processing: Reinforcement learning, dopamine, and the error-related negativity. *Psychological Review*, 109, 679–709. doi:10.1037/0033-295X.109.4.679

Hommer, R. E., Meyer, A., Stoddard, J., Connolly, M. E., Mogg, K., Bradley, B. P., . . . Brotman, M. A. (2014). Attention bias to threat faces in severe mood dysregulation. *Depression and Anxiety*, 31, 559–565. doi:10.1002/da.22145

Huettel, S. A., Song, A. W., & McCarthy, G. (2009). *Functional magnetic resonance imaging* (2nd ed.). Sunderland, MA: Sinauer.

Huster, R. J., Enriquez-Geppert, S., Lavallee, C. F., Falkenstein, M., & Herrmann, C. S. (2013). Electroencephalography of response inhibition tasks: Functional networks and cognitive contributions. *International Journal of Psychophysiology*, 87, 217–233. doi:https://doi.org/10.1016/j.ijpsycho.2012.08.001

Insel, T., Cuthbert, B., Garvey, M., Heinssen, R., Pine, D. S., Quinn, K., . . . Wang, P. (2010). Research Domain Criteria (RDoC): Toward a new classification framework for research on mental disorders. *American Journal of Psychiatry, 167,* 748–751. doi:10.1176/appi. ajp.2010.09091379

Insel, T. R. (2013). Mental disorders as brain disorders. *Tedx Caltech: The Brain.* Retrieved from http://tedxcaltech.caltech.edu/content/tom-insel. Accessed May 14, 2013.

Kappenman, E. S., Farrens, J. L., Luck, S. J., & Proudfit, G. H. (2014). Behavioral and ERP measures of attentional bias to threat in the dot-probe task: Poor reliability and lack of correlation with anxiety. *Frontiers in Psychology, 5,* 1368. doi:10.3389/fpsyg.2014.01368

Kessel, E. M., Dougherty, L. R., Kujawa, A., Hajcak, G., Carlson, G. A., & Klein, D. N. (2016b). Longitudinal associations between preschool disruptive mood dysregulation disorder symptoms and neural reactivity to monetary reward during preadolescence. *Journal of Child and Adolescent Psychopharmacology, 26,* 131–137. doi:10.1089/cap.2015.0071

Kessel, E. M., Kujawa, A., Dougherty, L. R., Hajcak, G., Carlson, G. A., & Klein, D. N. (2017). Neurophysiological processing of emotion in children of mothers with a history of depression: The moderating role of preschool persistent irritability. *Journal of Abnormal Child Psychology, 45,* 1599–1608. doi:10.1007/s10802-017-0272-y

Kessel, E. M., Meyer, A., Hajcak, G., Dougherty, L. R., Torpey-Newman, D. C., Carlson, G. A., & Klein, D. N. (2016a). Transdiagnostic factors and pathways to multifinality: The error-related negativity predicts whether preschool irritability is associated with internalizing versus externalizing symptoms at age 9. *Development and Psychopathology, 28,* 913–926. doi:10.1017/S0954579416000626

Kim, P., Arizpe, J., Rosen, B. H., Razdan, V., Haring, C. T., Jenkins, S. E., . . . Leibenluft, E. (2013). Impaired fixation to eyes during facial emotion labelling in children with bipolar disorder or severe mood dysregulation. *Journal of Psychiatry & Neuroscience, 38,* 407. doi:10.1503/jpn.120232

Knutson, B., Westdorp, A., Kaiser, E., & Hommer, D. (2000). FMRI visualization of brain activity during a monetary incentive delay task. *NeuroImage, 12,* 20–27. doi:10.1006/nimg.2000.0593

Kohler, C. G., Turner, T. H., Gur, R. E., & Gur, R. C. (2004). Recognition of facial emotions in neuropsychiatric disorders. *CNS Spectrums, 9,* 267–274. doi:10.1017/s1092852900009202

Koster, E. H. W., Crombez, G., Verschuere, B., & De Houwer, J. (2004). Selective attention to threat in the dot probe paradigm: Differentiating vigilance and difficulty to disengage. *Behaviour Research and Therapy, 42,* 1183–1192. doi:10.1016/j.brat.2003.08.001

Ladouceur, C. D., Dahl, R. E., Birmaher, B., Axelson, D. A., & Ryan, N. D. (2006). Increased error-related negativity (ERN) in childhood anxiety disorders: ERP and source localization. *Journal of Child Psychology and Psychiatry, 47,* 1073–1082.

Lang, P. J., Bradley, M. M., & Cuthbert, B. N. (2005). *International affective picture system (IAPS): Affective ratings of pictures and instruction manual.* Gainesville: University of Florida.

Leibenluft, E. (2011). Severe mood dysregulation, irritability, and the diagnostic boundaries of bipolar disorder in youths. *American Journal of Psychiatry, 168*(2), 129–142.

Leibenluft, E. (2017). Pediatric irritability: A systems neuroscience approach. *Trends in Cognitive Sciences.* 21, 277–289. doi:10.1016/j.tics.2017.02.002

Leibenluft, E., Blair, R. J., Charney, D. S., & Pine, D. S. (2003). Irritability in pediatric mania and other childhood psychopathology. *Annual New York Academy of Sciences, 1008,* 201–218.

Leibenluft, E., Charney, D. S., Towbin, K. E., Bhangoo, R. K., & Pine, D. S. (2003). Defining clinical phenotypes of juvenile mania. *American Journal of Psychiatry, 160*, 430–437.

Lewis, M. D., Lamm, C., Segalowitz, S. J., Stieben, J., & Zelazo, P. D. (2006). Neurophysiological correlates of emotion regulation in children and adolescents. *Journal of Cognitive Neuroscience, 18*, 430–443. doi:10.1162/089892906775990633

Lievaart, M., van der Veen, F. M., Huijding, J., Naeije, L., Hovens, J. E., & Franken, I. H. (2016). Trait anger in relation to neural and behavioral correlates of response inhibition and error-processing. *International Journal of Psychophysiology, 99*, 40–47. doi:10.1016/j.ijpsycho.2015.12.001

Logan, G. D., Cowan, W. B., & Davis, K. A. (1984). On the ability to inhibit simple and choice reaction-time responses: A model and a method. *Journal of Experimental Psychology-Human Perception and Performance, 10*, 276–291. doi:10.1037/0096-1523.10.2.276

Logan, G. D., Schachar, R. J., & Tannock, R. (1997). Impulsivity and inhibitory control. *Psychological Science, 8*, 60–64. doi:10.1111/j.1467-9280.1997.tb00545.x

Lowther, H., & Newman, E. (2014). Attention bias modification (ABM) as a treatment for child and adolescent anxiety: A systematic review. *Journal of Affective Disorders, 168*, 125–135. doi:10.1016/j.jad.2014.06.051

Luck, S. J. (2014). *An introduction to the event-related potential technique* (Second edition. ed.). Cambridge, MA: MIT Press.

Luu, P., Collins, P., & Tucker, D. M. (2000). Mood, personality, and self-monitoring: Negative affect and emotionality in relation to frontal lobe mechanisms of error monitoring. *Journal of Experimental Psychology: General, 129*, 43.

Luu, P., Tucker, D. M., Derryberry, D., Reed, M., & Poulsen, C. (2003). Electrophysiological responses to errors and feedback in the process of action regulation. *Psychological Science, 14*, 47–53.

McClure, E. B., Treland, J. E., Snow, J., Schmajuk, M., Dickstein, D. P., Towbin, K. E., . . . Leibenluft, E. (2005). Deficits in social cognition and response flexibility in pediatric bipolar disorder. *American Journal of Psychiatry, 162*, 1644–1651. doi:162/9/1644 [pii]10.1176/appi.ajp.162.9.1644

Mischel, W., Shoda, Y., & Rodriguez, M. I. (1989). Delay of gratification in children. *Science, 244*, 933–938.

Morasch, K. C., & Bell, M. A. (2012). Self-regulation of negative affect at 5 and 10 months. *Developmental Psychobiology, 54*, 215–221. doi:10.1002/dev.20584

Morris, A. S., Silk, J. S., Morris, M. D., Steinberg, L., Aucoin, K. J., & Keyes, A. W. (2011). The influence of mother-child emotion regulation strategies on children's expression of anger and sadness. *Developmental Psychology, 47*, 213–225. doi:2011-00627-014 [pii] 10.1037/a0021021

Nelson, C. A., & McCleery, J. P. (2008). Use of event-related potentials in the study of typical and atypical development. *Journal of American Academy of Child and Adolescent Psychiatry, 47*, 1252–1261. doi:10.1097/CHI.0b013e318185a6d8

Nieuwenhuis, S., Yeung, N., van den Wildenberg, W., & Ridderinkhof, K. R. (2003). Electrophysiological correlates of anterior cingulate function in a go/no-go task: Effects of response conflict and trial type frequency. *Cognitive, Affective, and Behavioral Neuroscience, 3*, 17–26.

O'Doherty, J., Dayan, P., Schultz, J., Deichmann, R., Friston, K., & Dolan, R. J. (2004). Dissociable roles of ventral and dorsal striatum in instrumental conditioning. *Science, 304*, 452–454. doi:10.1126/science.1094285

Olvet, D. M., & Hajcak, G. (2008). The error-related negativity (ERN) and psychopathology: Toward an endophenotype. *Clinical Psychology Review, 28*, 1343–1354.

Overbeek, T. J., Nieuwenhuis, S., & Ridderinkhof, K. R. (2005). Dissociable components of error processing: On the functional significance of the Pe vis-à-vis the ERN/Ne. *Journal of Psychophysiology, 19*, 319–329.

Penton-Voak, I. S., Thomas, J., Gage, S. H., McMurran, M., McDonald, S., & Munafò, M. R. (2013). Increasing recognition of happiness in ambiguous facial expressions reduces anger and aggressive behavior. *Psychological Science, 24*, 688–697. doi:10.1177/0956797612459657

Pérez-Edgar, K., & Fox, N. A. (2005). A behavioral and electrophysiological study of children's selective attention under neutral and affective conditions. *Journal of Cognition and Development, 6*(1), 89–118.

Perlman, S. B., Jones, B. M., Wakschlag, L. S., Axelson, D., Birmaher, B., & Phillips, M. L. (2015). Neural substrates of child irritability in typically developing and psychiatric populations. *Developmental Cognitive Neuroscience, 14*, 71–80. doi:10.1016/j.dcn.2015.07.003

Perlman, S. B., Luna, B., Hein, T. C., & Huppert, T. J. (2013). fNIRS evidence of prefrontal regulation of frustration in early childhood. *Neuroimage, 85*, 326–334. doi:10.1016/j.neuroimage.2013.04.057

Phillips, M. L. (2003). Understanding the neurobiology of emotion perception: Implications for psychiatry. *British Journal of Psychiatry, 182*, 190–192.

Pizzagalli, D. A. (2014). Depression, stress, and anhedonia: Toward a synthesis and integrated model. *Annual Reviews in Clinical Psychology, 10*, 393–423. doi:10.1146/annurev-clinpsy-050212-185606

Proudfit, G. H. (2015). The reward positivity: From basic research on reward to a biomarker for depression. *Psychophysiology, 52*, 449–459. doi:10.1111/psyp.12370

Raine, A. (1996). Autonomic nervous system factors underlying disinhibited, antisocial, and violent behavior. Biosocial perspectives and treatment implications. *Annals of the New York Academy of Sciences, 794*, 46–59.

Rau, G., Blair, K. S., Berghorst, L., Knopf, L., Skup, M., Luckenbaugh, D. A., . . . Leibenluft, E. (2008). Processing of differentially valued rewards and punishments in youths with bipolar disorder or severe mood dysregulation. *Journal of Child and Adolescent Psychopharmacology, 18*, 185–196. doi:10.1089/cap.2007.0053

Reijntjes, A., Stegge, H., Terwogt, M. M., Kamphuis, J. H., & Telch, M. J. (2006). Emotion regulation and its effects on mood improvement in response to an in vivo peer rejection challenge. *Emotion, 6*, 543–552. doi:2006-21788-001 [pii] 10.1037/1528-3542.6.4.543

Rich, B. A., Brotman, M. A., Dickstein, D. P., Mitchell, D. G. V., Blair, R. J. R., & Leibenluft, E. (2010). Deficits in attention to emotional stimuli distinguish youth with severe mood dysregulation from youth with bipolar disorder. *Journal of Abnormal Child Psychology, 38*, 695–706. doi:10.1007/s10802-010-9395-0

Rich, B. A., Carver, F. W., Holroyd, T., Rosen, H. R., Mendoza, J. K., Cornwell, B. R., . . . Leibenluft, E. (2011). Different neural pathways to negative affect in youth with pediatric bipolar disorder and severe mood dysregulation. *Journal of Psychiatric Research, 45,* 1283–1294. doi:10.1016/j.jpsychires.2011.04.006

Rich, B. A., Grimley, M. E., Schmajuk, M., Blair, K. S., Blair, R. J. R., & Leibenluft, E. (2008). Face emotion labeling deficits in children with bipolar disorder and severe mood dysregulation. *Development and Psychopathology, 20,* 529–546. doi:10.1017/S0954579408000266

Rich, B. A., Schmajuk, M., Perez-Edgar, K. E., Fox, N. A., Pine, D. S., & Leibenluft, E. (2007). Different psychophysiological and behavioral responses elicited by frustration in pediatric bipolar disorder and severe mood dysregulation. *American Journal of Psychiatry, 164*(2), 309–317.

Rocca, C. C. d. A., Heuvel, E. v. d., Caetano, S. C., & Lafer, B. (2009). Facial emotion recognition in bipolar disorder: A critical review. *Revista Brasileira de Psiquiatria, 31,* 171–180.

Rothbart, M. K., Ahadi, S. A., Hershey, K. L., & Fisher, P. (2001). Investigations of temperament at three to seven years: The Children's Behavior Questionnaire. *Child Development, 72,* 1394–1408.

Roy, A. K., Klein, R. G., Angelosante, A., Bar-Haim, Y., Leibenluft, E., Hulvershorn, L., . . . Spindel, C. (2013). Clinical features of young children referred for impairing temper outbursts. *Journal of Child and Adolescent Psychopharmacology, 23,* 588–596. doi:10.1089/cap.2013.0005

Roy, A. K., Lopes, V., & Klein, R. G. (2014). Disruptive mood dysregulation disorder: A new diagnostic approach to chronic irritability in youth. *American Journal of Psychiatry, 171,* 918–924. doi:10.1176/appi.ajp.2014.13101301 1901582 [pii]

Rubia, K., Oosterlaan, J., Sergeant, J. A., Brandeis, D., & v Leeuwen, T. (1998). Inhibitory dysfunction in hyperactive boys. *Behavioral Brain Research, 94,* 25–32. doi:S0166-4328(97)00166-6 [pii]

Rudaizky, D., Basanovic, J., & MacLeod, C. (2014). Biased attentional engagement with, and disengagement from, negative information: Independent cognitive pathways to anxiety vulnerability? *Cognition and Emotion, 28,* 245–259. doi:10.1080/02699931.2013.815154

Salum, G. A., Mogg, K., Bradley, B. P., Stringaris, A., Gadelha, A., Pan, P. M., . . . Leibenluft, E. (2016). Association between irritability and bias in attention orienting to threat in children and adolescents. *Journal of Child Psychology and Psychiatry, 58, 595- 602.* doi:10.1111/jcpp.12659

Salum, G. A., Mogg, K., Bradley, B. P., Stringaris, A., Gadelha, A., Pan, P. M., . . . Leibenluft, E. (2017). Association between irritability and bias in attention orienting to threat in children and adolescents. *Journal of Child Psychology and Psychiatry, 58,* 595–602. doi:10.1111/jcpp.12659

Santesso, D. L., Segalowitz, S. J., & Schmidt, L. A. (2005). ERP correlates of error monitoring in 10-year olds are related to socialization. *Biological Psychology, 70,* 79–87.

Schachar, R. J., Chen, S., Logan, G. D., Ornstein, T. J., Crosbie, J., Ickowicz, A., & Pakulak, A. (2004). Evidence for an error monitoring deficit in attention deficit hyperactivity disorder. *Journal of Abnormal Child Psychology, 32,* 285–293.

Schachar, R., Mota, V. L., Logan, G. D., Tannock, R., & Klim, P. (2000). Confirmation of an inhibitory control deficit in attention-deficit/hyperactivity disorder. *Journal of Abnormal Child Psychology, 28,* 227–235.

Shechner, T., Britton, J. C., Perez-Edgar, K., Bar-Haim, Y., Ernst, M., Fox, N. A., . . . Pine, D. S. (2012). Attention biases, anxiety, and development: Toward or away from threats or rewards? *Depression and Anxiety, 29*, 282–294. doi:10.1002/da.20914

Smith, P., & Waterman, M. (2003). Processing bias for aggression words in forensic and nonforensic samples. *Cognition & Emotion, 17*, 681–701. doi:10.1080/02699930244000192

Stemme, A., Deco, G., Busch, A., & Schneider, W. X. (2005). Neurons and the synaptic basis of the fMRI signal associated with cognitive flexibility. *NeuroImage, 26*, 454–470. doi:10.1016/j.neuroimage.2005.01.044

Stieben, J., Lewis, M. D., Granic, I., Zelazo, P. D., Segalowitz, S., & Pepler, D. (2007). Neurophysiological mechanisms of emotion regulation for subtypes of externalizing children. *Developmental Psychopathology, 19*, 455–480. doi:10.1017/S0954579407070228

Stoddard, J., Sharif-Askary, B., Harkins, E. A., Frank, H. R., Brotman, M. A., Penton-Voak, I. S., . . . Leibenluft, E. (2016). An open pilot study of training hostile interpretation bias to treat disruptive mood dysregulation disorder. *Journal of Child and Adolescent Psychopharmacology, 26*, 49–57. doi:10.1089/cap.2015.0100

Stringaris, A., Cohen, P., Pine, D. S., & Leibenluft, E. (2009). Adult outcomes of youth irritability: A 20-year prospective community-based study. *Am J Psychiatry, 166*, 1048–1054. doi:appi.ajp.2009.08121849 [pii] 10.1176/appi.ajp.2009.08121849

Stringaris, A., Goodman, R., Ferdinando, S., Razdan, V., Muhrer, E., Leibenluft, E., & Brotman, M. A. (2012). The Affective Reactivity Index: A concise irritability scale for clinical and research settings. *Journal of Child Psychology and Psychiatry, 53*, 1109–1117. doi:10.1111/j.1469-7610.2012.02561.x

Tops, M., Koole, S. L., & Wijers, A. A. (2013). The Pe of perfectionism. *Journal of Psychophysiology, 27*, 84–94. doi:10.1027/0269-8803/a000090

Tseng, W. L., Deveney, C. M., Stoddard, J., Kircanski, K., Frackman, A. E., Yi, J. Y., . . . Roule, A. (2018). Brain Mechanisms of Attention Orienting Following Frustration: Associations With Irritability and Age in Youths. *American Journal of Psychiatry, 176*, 67–76. https://doi.org/10.1176/appi.ajp.2018.18040491

Uran, P., & Kılıç, B. (2015). Comparison of neuropsychological performances and behavioral patterns of children with attention deficit hyperactivity disorder and severe mood dysregulation. *European Child & Adolescent Psychiatry, 24*, 21–30. doi:10.1007/s00787-014-0529-8

van Honk, J., Tuiten, A., de Haan, E., van den Hout, M., & Stam, H. (2001). Attentional biases for angry faces: Relationships to trait anger and anxiety. *Cognition & Emotion, 15*, 279–297. doi:10.1080/0269993004200222

Vidal-Ribas, P., Brotman, M. A., Salum, G. A., Kaiser, A., Meffert, L., Pine, D. S., . . . Stringaris, A. (2018). Deficits in emotion recognition are associated with depressive symptoms in youth with disruptive mood dysregulation disorder. *Depression and Anxiety, 35*(12), 1207–1217.

Wakschlag, L. S., Briggs-Gowan, M. J., Choi, S., Nichols, S., Kestler, J., Burns, J., Carter, A., & Henry, D. (2014). Advancing a multidimensional, developmental spectrum approach to preschool disruptive behavior. *Journal of the American Academy of Child and Adolescent Psychiatry, 53* (1), 82–96. doi:http://dx.doi.org/10.1016/j.jaac.2013.10.011

Wessel, J. R., Danielmeier, C., & Ullsperger, M. (2011). Error awareness revisited: Accumulation of multimodal evidence from central and autonomic nervous systems. *Journal of Cognitive Neuroscience, 23*, 3021–3036.

Woodman, G. F. (2010). A brief introduction to the use of event-related potentials (ERPs) in studies of perception and attention. *Attention, Perception & Psychophysics, 72*, 2031–2046. doi:10.3758/APP.72.8.2031

Zisner, A., & Beauchaine, T. P. (2016). Neural substrates of trait impulsivity, anhedonia, and irritability: Mechanisms of heterotypic comorbidity between externalizing disorders and unipolar depression. *Developmental Psychopathology, 28*, 1177–1208. doi:10.1017/S0954579416000754

Developmental Considerations

5

Early Childhood Irritability

USING A NEURODEVELOPMENTAL FRAMEWORK TO
INFORM CLINICAL UNDERSTANDING

M. Catalina Camacho, Lauren S. Wakschlag,
and Susan B. Perlman

The preschool age (3–6), also referred to as early childhood, is a unique period for the development of emotion regulation (Carroll & Steward, 1984; Cole, Michel, & Teti, 1994; Diamond, 2002; Tsujimoto, 2008). The ability to regulate emotion during this period is a burgeoning and rapidly maturing process, with the emotions of anger and frustration, both common substrates of irritability, occurring relatively frequently (Wakschlag et al., 2007, 2012, 2017). However, although irritability is common, there is still extensive variability in irritable temperament within children. This juxtaposition of normative misbehaviors (e.g., tantrums, grumpy mood) with stable irritable temperament presents unique challenges to the differentiation of normative variation from the onset of clinical problems (Wakschlag et al., 2012). However, as technologies for measuring neural function and structure improve, neuroimaging, in combination with behavioral and clinical assessment, has provided an additional tool for assessing pediatric irritability and its relationship with common substrates of impaired psychiatric functioning. Although not yet integrated into clinical assessment, we believe that, ultimately, joint consideration of brain–behavior atypticalities will enhance early identification (Leibenluft, 2017; Wakschlag et al., 2017). Here we present the current observational, parent-report, and neuroimaging research in this young population through a neurodevelopmental framework. In this chapter, we aim to (1) summarize the relevant rapid development occurring in the preschool years and the unique challenges posed in assessing irritability in this age group, (2) describe the advancements in measuring irritability and creating developmentally appropriate diagnostic assessments for preschool children, and (3) integrate these measurements within a neurodevelopmental framework to maximize differentiation of normative and non-normative irritability.

Challenges in the Assessment of Irritability During the Preschool Years

IMPORTANCE OF THE PRESCHOOL PERIOD

Preschool is a significant developmental time period as children transition to increased independence from caregivers. Beginning in toddlerhood, children are expected to demonstrate increasing personal agency and self-control as they progress into school age, which requires top-down modulation of actions, thoughts, and feelings (Brownell & Kopp, 2007; McClelland & Cameron, 2011). This increased independence coincides with rapid growth in linguistic abilities (Luu et al., 2009; McCarthy, 1930; Pungello, Iruka, Dotterer, Mills-Koonce, & Reznick, 2009), socioemotional expression (Duncan et al., 2007; Rhoades, Warren, Domitrovich, & Greenberg, 2011), and brain structural and functional development (Diamond, 2002; Giedd et al., 2009; Tsujimoto, 2008). Disruptions to the development of these systems and skills can have serious ramifications as children progress through adolescence and into adulthood, including conduct problems (Bennett et al., 1999), poorer socialization and anger control (Kochanska, Murray, & Harlan, 2000), and depression and anxiety symptoms (Phillips, Hammen, Brennan, Najman, & Bor, 2005). For these reasons, early childhood identification and treatment of behavioral and emotional concerns is of particular importance. Irritability as a dimensional symptom spans many psychiatric and behavioral concerns across development (Stringaris, 2011; Stringaris & Goodman, 2009; Wakschlag et al., 2015), can present at clinically significant levels in children as young as 2 years (Achenbach, Edelbrock, & Howelp, 1987; Wakschlag et al., 2012; Wakschlag, Tolan, & Leventhal, 2010), and is predictive of later functioning and psychiatric outcomes (Dougherty et al., 2013). Detection and treatment of clinically significant irritability is therefore a critical component of early intervention.

DEVELOPMENTAL CONSIDERATIONS

The rapid pace of maturation across the early childhood period introduces unique challenges to the definition and measurement of key constructs. Of particular relevance to contextualizing pediatric irritability is the rapid development of executive function during the preschool years, which is at the heart of emotion regulation and correlates with specific changes in neural function in this age group (Bernier, Carlson, & Whipple, 2010; Denham et al., 2017; Hofmann, Schmeichel, & Baddeley, 2012; Perlman, Huppert, & Luna, 2016).

Second only to the first 2 years of life, the preschool years include the most rapid neural development as the brain reaches approximately 95% of its final size by age 6 (Giedd et al., 2009). Timing for peak development varies by region and index of brain development (Giedd et al., 2009; Gogtay et al., 2004; Huttenlocher, de Courten, Garey, & Van der Loos, 1982; Shaw et al., 2008). In terms of synaptic density, the visual cortex peaks during the first year of life with a rapid decrease in density in early childhood and a slower decrease into adolescence and adulthood (Huttenlocher et al., 1982). In terms of cortical thickness and volume, however, peak development of both the parietal and frontal regions occurs in middle child-hood (9–12 years) and temporal cortex development peaks during adolescence (16–17 years), while occipital regions increase steadily into adulthood without a clear single peak (Giedd et al., 1999; Lenroot & Giedd, 2006). The greatest relative gains made in early childhood are therefore made in the frontal cortex, regions of the brain associated with executive function (Diamond, 2002; Tsujimoto, 2008). Peak developmental age in frontal cortical thickness varies within functionally and structurally defined subregions (Shaw et al., 2008). Most of the frontal cortex, including the dorsolateral prefrontal cortex (DLPFC) and the medial prefrontal cortex (MPFC), peaks in thickness from 9 to 11 years of age, while the anterior cingulate cortex (ACC) peaks further in puberty, between 11 and 14 years of age (Shaw et al., 2008).

Of particular note, there is evidence that orbitofrontal cortex (OFC) thickness peaks before age 5 (Shaw et al., 2008). The OFC is associated with top-down con-trol over social and emotional regulation and has innervations from visceral sen-sation signaling regions of the midbrain and brainstem (Pessoa, 2017) making it strategically placed to relate feelings to socioemotional context. Additionally, the prefrontal cortex peaks in synaptogenesis at around age 2–4 years, and synaptic pruning continues into mid-adolescence (Casey, Tottenham, Liston, & Durston, 2005). Taken together, this evidence supports the notion that the preschool years are an important period for development of neural regions associated with socioemotional regulation and executive function.

Concurrent with these changes in frontal cortex structure, the preschool years are marked by dramatic improvements across major domains of execu-tive function including working memory, inhibitory control, and cognitive flex-ibility (Diamond, 2002; Garon, Bryson, & Smith, 2005; Luciana & Nelson, 1998; Tsujimoto, 2008). The success that children have in developing these cognitive skills relates to their abilities to identify and regulate emotion (Carroll & Steward, 1984). Taken together, it seems that the preschool years are a sensitive period for foundational frontal lobe development, which not only sets the stage for selective pruning and refinement of the structure throughout preschool development, but also provides neurodevelopmental support for changes in executive function that can contribute to improved emotion regulation. Since irritability is associated with poor emotion regulation (i.e., temper tantrums and irritable mood), these cogni-tive measures and the associated neural structures and functional pathways are of particular interest in examining preschool irritability and in delineating developmentally expectable versus clinically concerning irritable behavior (Wakschlag et al., 2007).

DATA COLLECTION CHALLENGES

Acquiring neurodevelopmental data in preschool children requires a developmentally sensitive approach (Perlman, 2012; Wakschlag & Danis, 2012). First, preschool children are limited in their ability to express abstract concepts, such as intentions, thoughts, and feelings, making standard clinical interviews inappropriate for this young age. Young children are also limited in fine motor skills and vocabulary, limiting the tasks they can perform to simple experiments requiring decisions between few responses. By nature of the developmental stage, preschool children have limited attention spans and limited ability to take complex direction, requiring assessments to be administered in a highly engaging manner with rapid pacing. Finally, and a significant concern for neuroimaging research, preschool age children possess limited motor control and often are unable to stay still for extended periods for functional magnetic resonance imaging (fMRI) scans or neuropsychological testing (Johnson, 2001; Perlman, 2012).

Although modifications can be made to accommodate verbal challenges, such as simple and short questionnaires administered orally, language level and density of questioning achieved is not comparable between preschoolers and older children. Thus, many questionnaires cannot be adapted without compromising the measurement of the intended construct. Irritability is an emotion with both self and social components, and there is evidence that preschool children are still developing self and socially conscious emotional vocabulary (Bosacki & Moore, 2004). A more fruitful modification that can retain construct integrity for behavioral symptoms includes a behavior-based, rather than interview-based, clinical assessment. This might include a clinician observing a child interacting with a caregiver and coding behaviors of clinical interest (Campbell et al., 1986; Wakschlag, et al., 2008b) or a child interacting with an experimenter who elicits desired emotional behavior through child-appropriate probes (Gagne, Van Hulle, Aksan, Essex, & Goldsmith, 2011). As a result, direct observation is a critical aspect of early childhood irritability assessment (Wakschlag et al., 2005). To evaluate specific developmental constructs such as executive function, developmental scientists may employ colorful, animated, and child-appropriate computerized games based on classic assessment techniques in order to acquire needed data in a developmentally engaging manner. A classic go/no-go paradigm or Stroop task, for example, can be adjusted to include cartoon characters or animals rather than words (Briggs-Gowan et al., 2014; Li, Grabell, Wakschlag, Huppert, & Perlman, 2017; Perlman, 2012).

One final data collection challenge in assessing preschool irritability is the strong dependence on parent report. Due to a child's difficulties in accurately reporting past events or emotional information, parent report is weighed heavily in assessing irritability, which introduces both richness and limitations to the data. Parents have the ability to respond to many more questions and at a more abstract level than their young children and to provide historical context and greater ecological validity than laboratory assessments. Furthermore, parents can also provide clinicians with a richer insight into both the home and school environments as well as to certain events that may act as a precipitant to concerning behavior, such as the loss of a loved one or moving to a new home. Particularly important is that parents spend more time with children of this age than any other adult in their environment and thus can comment on difficulties in the home environment that may not be present in a clinician's office (i.e., challenges with bedtime). However, as with any self-report data, parent-reported data are filtered through the lens of the informant and may vary based on differences in parent knowledge of what is developmentally normative. Furthermore, given the nascent literature on the genetic basis of irritability (Coccaro, Bergeman, Kavoussi, & Seroczynski, 1997; Coccaro, Bergeman, & Mcclearn, 1993; Roberson-Nay et al., 2015; Savage et al., 2015) and intergenerational transmission (Sparks et al., 2014; Wiggins, Mitchell, Stringaris, & Leibenluft, 2014), the parent may be struggling with his or her own challenges with irritability or mental illness and thus may experience the child's irritability within a heightened emotional context. As a result, the integration of parent report with performance-based assessments is especially key in early childhood, when the differentiation of normative misbehavior from clinical patterns is especially challenging (Wakschlag et al., 2005).

DEFINING WHAT'S NORMAL

Clinical irritability criteria comprise phasic lapses in emotion regulation (e.g., temper tantrums) as well as persistent irritable or angry mood. While irritability may present as a symptom of multiple disorders, severe irritability has recently been included in the *Diagnostic and Statistical Manual of Mental Disorders* (DSM-5) as a unique disorder—*disruptive mood dysregulation disorder* (DMDD)—to be diagnosed when irritability presents as the primary cause for clinical concern (American Psychiatric Association, 2013). Currently, however, children under 6 are excluded from this diagnosis despite evidence of its validity at younger ages (Dougherty et al., 2017). A central challenge to differentiating normal from abnormal irritability in preschoolers is the fact that many of the behaviors that define irritability are quite common during this developmental stage. This illustrates the complicated nature of making psychiatric determinations in preschool children when symptoms and normative behaviors are so overlapping. The issue of developmentally appropriate clinical criteria has been the subject of much psychiatric research over the past few decades, with recent investigations seeking to delineate developmentally expected misbehaviors (those elicited from the context) and clinically concerning behavior (unexpected or unprovoked temper loss) (Wakschlag et al., 2012, 2017).

The Normal–Abnormal Boundaries of Irritability

DEFINING IRRITABILITY DIMENSIONALLY
AND CONTEXTUALLY

The differentiation of normative from clinically salient irritability at a behavioral level requires a developmental specification approach. The central feature of this approach is pinpointing those features that enhance normal/abnormal distinctions within a developmental period (Wakschlag et al., 2010). For example, since temper tantrums occur in the vast majority of preschool children, the mere presence of tantrums is not clinically salient at this age, and the DSM symptom "often loses temper" may overidentify young children. The DSM typically emphasizes the presence or absence of a symptom rather than its qualitative features; the latter have been determined as key to accurate clinical identification in young children (Wakschlag et al., 2007).

To address these issues, we have generated a developmentally sensitive toolkit specifically designed to differentiate early childhood normative misbehavior from emergent disruptive behavior (Biedzio & Wakschlag, 2018). Specifically, these are the Multidimensional Assessment Profile of Disruptive Behavior (MAP-DB) survey and the Disruptive Behavior Diagnostic Observation Schedule (DB-DOS) standardized clinical observation (Wakschlag et al., 2008a, 2008b, 2014). Both measures are derived from a shared developmental specification framework emphasizing features that more effectively enable a normal–abnormal irritability distinction within the developmental context (e.g., frequency, (dys)regulation, and developmental expectability in context) (Bufferd et al., 2016; Wakschlag et al., 2007a; Wakschlag et al., under review). *Frequency* assesses the regularity with which irritable behaviors occur since, while most children exhibit these behaviors, they are not the defining feature of day-to-day behavioral patterns (Wakschlag et al., 2014). For example, while 83.7% of preschoolers have had a tantrum over the past month, less than 10% of children at this age tantrum daily (Wakschlag et al., 2012). *Regulation* encompasses the intensity, flexibility, and organization of irritable behavior. *Expectability in context* assesses whether it is typical for a context to elicit an irritable response or not (Cole, Martin, & Dennis, 2004; Goldsmith & Davidson, 2004). The MAP-DB has the efficiency advantages of a survey, enabling population-level norms. In contrast, the DB-DOS is a more intensive, performance-based assessment designed for laboratory administration. Table 5.1 provides examples of information derived from the MAP-DB and DB-DOS for irritability. Ideally, information from these instruments could be combined for clinical assessment, but they are also designed to be administered independently for utility across varied settings and research designs.

TABLE 5.1 Exemplars of reported and observed features of preschool irritability

Temper Loss (MAP-DB)	Observed Anger Modulation (DB-DOS)
Have temper tantrums . . . when tired/hungry, during routines, that last > 5 min. out of the blue *Irritable mood* . . . , stay angry long time, have a short fuse, act irritable	*(Dys)regulation of irritability* (e.g., ease of elicitation, rapidity of escalation, capacity to make use of internal/external strategies to recover, pervasiveness across contexts)

From Wakschlag et al., 2008, 2012.

QUESTIONNAIRE ASSESSMENT: THE MAP-DB

The MAP-DB translates many of the qualitative constructs and importance of contextual variation gleaned from the DB-DOS into a survey tool. For each MAP-DB dimension, the survey includes both normative misbehaviors (e.g., has a temper tantrum) and dysregulated behaviors (e.g., tantrums until exhausted). The temper loss spectrum is depicted in Figure 5.1. Behaviors are queried across a range of contexts (e.g., with parents, with other adults) and eliciting triggers (e.g., "when tired, hungry or sick," "out of the blue"). The MAP-DB framework emphasizes a dimensional approach that characterizes behavior across an ordered spectrum from normative, commonly occurring behaviors to severe, rarely occurring behaviors using item response theory (IRT) methods. To enable generation of empirically derived parameters of abnormality, the MAP-DB uses a 6-point objective frequency scale (from 0 = never in past month to 5 = many times/day) (Wakschlag et al., 2014). The MAP-DB has been administered to more than 5,000 parents of diverse infants, toddlers, and preschoolers, demonstrating a robust severity spectrum

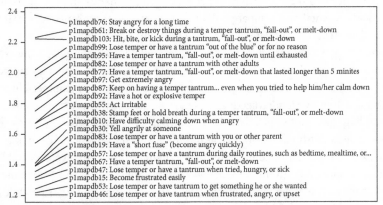

FIGURE 5.1 *Psychometric severity spectrum of early childhood irritability (MAP-DB Temper Loss in Early Childhood). Measured with the MAP-DB temper loss scale in early childhood. Data are derived from the MAPS replication sample (N = 1,857) and analyzed using item response theory (IRT). Theta (θ) scores (y-axis) are akin to z scores: mean = 0, SD = 1. A higher θ score indicates more reliable association the temper loss trait.*

from mild, normatively occurring irritable behaviors to severe, dysregulated irritability (Biedzio & Wakschlag, 2018; Wakschlag et al., 2017). Most strikingly, we have
demonstrated normal–abnormal differentiation of irritability in two independent
samples of preschoolers based on developmental features (Wakschlag et al., 2017).
These patterns demonstrated that (1) tantrums and mild irritability normatively
occur in most young children (83.7%) and under expectable circumstances (e.g.,
when frustrated, hungry, at times of transition) (Wakschlag et al., 2017). However,
dysregulated tantrums (e.g., until exhausted) and prolonged irritability (e.g., stays
angry for a long time) occur in less than 10% of young children, and (2) objective
frequency is a meaningful metric for differentiating normal versus abnormal expression. For example, daily or near daily occurrence of irritable behaviors is not
normative and occurs in less than 10% of preschoolers. Recently, we have used
a mixed-methods approach to demonstrate interesting qualitative differences in
these MAP-DB patterns (Shaunfield et al., in preparation). While daily irritability
is not normative for any sociodemographic group, at "normative" (milder) levels
there are distinct differences. Specifically, relative to white and Hispanic mothers,
African American mothers showed less tolerance for tantrum behavior and
explained that it was the parent's role to set limits which would prevent tantrums
from occurring in the first place (Shaunfield et al., in preparation). While needing
replication, these findings have implications for socioculturally tuned assessments.

PERFORMANCE-BASED ASSESSMENT: THE DB-DOS

The DB-DOS uses "presses" to increase the likelihood that irritability will actually be observed during clinical assessment (e.g., compliance demands, frustration, waiting). It provides unique information about contextual variation in the
child's capacity to regulate behavior across varying demands and social contexts
(e.g., with parental and nonparental adults). Interactions with parent maximize
the ecological validity of data obtained on how child irritability naturally unfolds
and is managed within the parent–child context, while interactions with the examiner provide a window on the child's capacity to make use of regulatory supports
from an adult (e.g., redirecting) (Wakschlag et al., 2005). Examiner/clinician
behavior is loosely standardized; specifically, a hierarchy of prompts is used for
responding to disruptive behavior to ascertain the minimal level of support a child
needs to reestablish equilibrium (Danis, Hill, &Wakschlag, 2009). Behaviors are
coded along a qualitative continuum (0–3) ranging from normative/expectable to
clinically concerning. In this way, across multiple contexts, we can systematically
observe what type of demands or transitions trigger young children's irritable behavior, the extent to which its expression is proportionate to context, and their
capacity to make use of both internal strategies (e.g., distraction, self-talk) and/
or external supports (e.g., parental reassurance or redirection). Observed irritability is coded separately for each context within the domain of problems in anger
modulation. These codes capture variations in the extent to which frustration/

anger/tantrums/upset is in response to expectable demands or transitions (e.g., cleaning up toys) versus pervasive regardless of the situation (e.g., even during fun activities). Qualitative features assessed include the ease with which irritability is elicited (e.g., "reflexive response" vs. gradual build-up), its rapidity of escalation, intensity, dysregulation, pervasiveness, and observed coping strategies. Contextual variation on the DB-DOS has proved to be informative across multiple independent samples (Bunte et al., 2013; Frost et al., 2017; Gray et al., 2012; Petitclerc et al., 2015; Tseng et al., 2015). For example, young children at-risk due to family history or stressful life experiences display heightened irritability during the DB-DOS Parent Context relative to low-risk peers. Contextual variation has also proved to be clinically informative (Frost et al., 2017; Tseng et al., 2015). In particular, preschoolers who showed lower decreases in irritability with the examiner versus their parent (the tendency to be more inhibited with unfamiliar vs. familiar adults is the developmentally expectable pattern) have poorer inhibitory control relative to peers (Petitclerc et al., 2015). We and others have demonstrated clinical validity of irritability ratings on the DB-DOS and its incremental utility above and beyond DSM symptoms (Bunte et al., 2013; Wakschlag et al., 2008).

CLINICAL UTILITY AND DIAGNOSIS

This dimensional spectrum of irritability severity has demonstrated clinical utility. Dimensional patterns indicate that clinically significant irritability is not an either/or phenomenon, with children well below traditional clinical cut points having significant clinical risk. For example, preschoolers with MAP-DB Temper Loss scores typically considered normative (i.e., 1 standard deviation [SD] above the population mean) have a 67% probability of clinically impairing symptoms, a risk that increased to 83% at 2 SD above the mean (Wakschlag et al., 2015). It has been suggested that categorical approaches resting on extreme scores are adequate for identifying children with severely dysregulated irritability but less so for those children falling at the normal–abnormal boundary. While this approach has some merit, our findings about developmental variability in irritability patterning in young children suggests that such patterns are less stable than assumed. Approximately one-third of preschoolers exhibit meaningful change in level of irritability within an approximately 1-year period (Wakschlag et al., 2015). Preschoolers who are low in irritability, those with clinical levels, and those at the normal–abnormal boundary are all equally likely to exhibit meaningful changes in irritability patterns. Furthermore, of the 6.5% of children exhibiting extremely high irritability (>2 SD above the population mean), less than one-third of these preschoolers remained at this level for more than one assessment. Accounting for this developmental variability improves clinical prediction (Wakschlag et al., 2015).

Thus, we have rigorously demonstrated the psychometric validity of these developmentally sensitive tools. Because the extent to which irritability interferes with young children's ability to learn, play, and engage with the world around them adaptively is crucial to clinical determination (Wakschlag et al., under review), we have also recently developed a companion impairment interview for this developmental irritability assessment toolkit (Wakschlag et al., under review). Additionally, because these patterns emerge very early in life, we have also adapted the MAP-DB for use with infants/toddlers. Preliminary findings indicate that similar developmental features are distinguishing in children as young as 12 months of age but that specific parameters defining the normal–abnormal boundary may shift (Biedzio & Wakschlag, in press). For example, 86% of infants/toddlers tantrum during daily routines versus 59% of preschoolers, but it is uncommon for young children at any age to hold their breath during a tantrum.

Neurodevelopment: Breakthroughs in Understanding the Neural Substrates of Preschool Irritability

As previously discussed, the rapid developmental growth and extensive normative variation of the preschool period present challenges to clinical and neurodevelopmental assessment. Although many of these challenges arise from short attention spans and motion-related issues, neurodevelopmental measurement techniques, such as fMRI, functional near-infrared spectroscopy (fNIRS), and event-related potentials (ERPs), often have the benefit of bypassing immature linguistic development to present a picture of the neural underpinnings of affective and cognitive function in irritable children. Most notably, fNIRS, a technique for measuring the hemodynamic blood oxygen-level dependent (BOLD) response using near-infrared light (Jobsis, 1977) has been a particularly useful tool in this pursuit (Aslin & Mehler, 2005). The fNIRS probe is placed on the child's head in the form of a cap or headband, which limits motion sensitivity. Although measuring a similar construct as fMRI (Cui, Bray, Bryant, Glover, & Reiss, 2011), fNIRS is notably less expensive in comparison, allowing researchers to collect larger samples and, in the case of a lab-purchased machine, more easily adapt to schedules for busy families. Further, fNIRS data can be collected in a simple research lab or the child's naturalistic location (e.g., home, school, clinic) and allows for interaction with an experimenter, computer screen, or even a family member. The following is a discussion of the emerging literature on the neural substrates of irritability. We mostly focus on the fNIRS imaging technique as it has provided the most reliable data in the preschool age range, with attention to emerging datasets using fMRI and ERP measurement.

NEURODEVELOPMENT OF IRRITABILITY WITHIN THE TEMPERAMENT DOMAIN

Understanding the neural substrates of irritable temperament in preschoolers has generally taken two interwoven approaches. First, research has probed the domain of emotional reactivity, generally focusing on frustration (i.e., the negative feelings associated with a blocked goal), as this is generally considered a prominent emotion in highly irritable children. In the first fNIRS study to examine frustration in preschool children, our research team introduced 3- to 6-year-old children with no personal or parental history of psychopathology to a computer game in which they raced a "very sneaky dog" to capture bones (The Frustrative Emotion Task for Children - FETCH; Perlman, Luna, Hein, & Huppert, 2014). Children slowly built up the necessary amount of bones to win a desired prize, but rapidly lost all their earnings when the dog became faster and stole all their bones back. During the experience of frustration, we recorded increased activation in the lateral prefrontal cortex (LPFC), which was positively correlated with parent-rated irritable temperament on the Child Behavior Questionnaire (CBQ), a widely used measure of childhood temperament (Rothbart, Ahadi, Hershey, & Fisher, 2001). We reasoned that children who are more irritable than their peers, but not impaired, may engage this region, which is often related to executive function and emotion regulation, in order to modulate their intense response to frustration while playing an enjoyable game. This finding has now been replicated and extended in a larger study ($n = 56$) where children were taught a specific emotion regulation strategy to use during a second frustration task (Grabell et al., under review). We found that use of the strategy correlated with increased LPFC activation and decreased negative facial expressions and that, while most children were effectively able to increase LPFC activation during frustration, change from pre- to post-test was largest in children with the least irritable temperament. A recent fMRI experiment that examined general emotional reactivity neural circuitry as a function of both age and temperament scanned children aged 4–12 during naturalistic viewing of children's movie scenes (Karim & Perlman, 2017). An age by temperament interaction was found in the LPFC and striatum, a region activated during the experience of reward and frustration, such that age-related increases in activation during negative scenes were observed but only in those children high in irritable temperament. This finding supports the hypothesis that typically developing but temperamentally irritable children may develop increased function of emotional reactivity and regulatory regions when faced with negative emotional challenges.

The second approach to probing the development of neural circuitry as a function of irritability in children has turned to the domain of executive function, as this grouping of basic skills is thought to comprise components of regulatory behaviors (Hofmann, Schmeichel, & Baddeley, 2012). Specifically, researchers have postulated that the emerging executive function skill of cognitive flexibility, defined as the ability to mentally switch between two or more demands (Scott, 1962), forms the basis of early emotion regulation strategies (Kopp, 1982; Zelazo & Cunningham, 2007). This skill may be particularly dysfunctional in children with high irritability who cannot easily shift their attention away from an undesirable outcome when goals are blocked or toward desirable possibilities when plans unexpectedly change. A recent fNIRS study used a novel cognitive flexibility task in which 46 3- to 5-year-old children were given the task of putting the animals of an escaped pet store back into their cages (Li et al., 2017). The "tricky" animals, however, liked to pretend to be other animals in order to trick the children, thus children were required to listen to the sound that the animal made in order to identify its true breed (e.g., a dog who says "meow" would really be a cat), creating a pre-school version (The Pet Store Stroop) of the classic Stroop paradigm (Stroop, 1935). We found that LPFC activation was highest during the Stroop condition in which animals did not make their correct sound and that children highest in irritability, but still within the normative, unimpaired range, also had the highest LPFC activation during this condition. Similar to the FETCH frustration findings described earlier, we suspected that those children who are more susceptible to frustration during challenge have developed effective use of this executive function region in order to manage challenge during a difficult task.

NEURODEVELOPMENT OF IRRITABILITY WITHIN THE CLINICAL DOMAIN

As extreme forms of irritability are a substrate of a range of psychopathologies, understanding its neurodevelopment in early childhood is important for uncovering the underpinnings of early childhood onset psychopathology. To illustrate, we again measured LPFC activation during the FETCH frustration task in a separate sample of 92 children aged 3–7 (Grabell et al., 2017). In this sample, however, children were recruited from both the community and local psychiatric clinics in order to sample as many highly irritable children experiencing related impairing symptoms as possible. Replicating our earlier findings (Perlman et al., 2014), we found that LPFC activation during frustration increased as a function of irritability, but only to the point of clinical impairment. Above the 91st percentile of irritability score based on the MAP-DB (Wakschlag et al., 2012), LPFC activation decreased as a function of irritability, creating an inverted U-shaped relationship. Interestingly, the apex MAP-DB score of this inverted U was a 42.5, which corresponds to the 96th percentile score on the MAP-DB in a community sample (Wakschlag et al., 2015). This implies a correspondence between neural indicators of irritability-related impairment and parent-reported irritability severity. An example of the relationship between irritability and executive function–related neural predictors of psychopathology was found by Kessel and colleagues (2016). Among children who were high in irritability at age 3, an enhanced ΔERN during a go/no-go task at age 6 (measured through ERP) predicted the development of internalizing symptoms at age 9, while a blunted ΔERN predicted the development of externalizing symptoms. In older samples, fMRI studies suggest that school-age children and adolescents presenting with clinically salient forms of irritability experience deficits in cognitive flexibility (Dickstein et al., 2007) with underlying deficits in PFC activation (Adleman et al., 2011). Though cognitive performance was not assessed, a study of 6- to 9-year-olds with severe temper outbursts found reduced cingulate cortex functional connectivity (measured by resting state fMRI) and that reduced anterior midcingulate cortex (a frontal region associated with emotion regulation) to precuneus (a posterior region associated with thinking about the self) connectivity was related to elevated mood dysregulation (Roy et al., 2017). Taken together, these findings indicate that neural differences between irritable temperament and clinical levels of irritability can be found in the domains of modulation of frustration and deployment of executive functions, potentially predicting a transition from the normal to abnormal boundary.

FUTURE NEURODEVELOPMENT RESEARCH WITHIN THE FAMILY SYSTEM

As technology improves, we propose the consideration of preschool irritability neurodevelopmental research within the family system. Parental support is a critical aspect of the development of executive function and emotion regulation during the preschool period (Hughes & Ensor, 2009). However, optimal parent support might be more challenging to achieve with highly irritable children. Furthermore, Belsky, Bakermans-Kranenburg, & IJzendoorn (2007) have proposed a differential susceptibility hypothesis in which children high in negative emotionality (e.g., irritability) are hypothesized to be more vulnerable to both positive and negative parental influences. Thus, it is critical that we examine the neurodevelopment of executive function and emotion regulation as a moderator for clinical outcome within the context of parent–child interaction. fNIRS has the ability to examine the correlation between the rise and fall of the hemodynamic response in order to characterize "interpersonal neural synchronization" (Jiang et al., 2015). Our team is currently in the process of employing this methodology to examine parent–child interpersonal neural synchronization using an adaptation of the DB-DOS as a mechanistic measure for scaffolding the development of emotion regulation and executive function, which are likely to buffer highly irritable children from the later onset of psychopathology symptoms.

Conclusion

Recent advances in preschool irritability research have been essential for demonstrating both that the normative misbehaviors that are part and parcel of irritability in young children (e.g., tantrums) can be distinguished from clinically concerning patterns (e.g., in frequency and quality) and that neuroimaging can provide clinically relevant insight into psychiatric concern at this young age. Translation to clinical application is a critical next step, requiring an approach that embraces the complexity of early development and also integrates these varying sources of information in a clinically feasible and meaningful manner. For example, using receiver operating curve (ROC) analyses, we have recently demonstrated that 2 of the 22 MAP-DB Temper Loss items may serve as effective irritability screeners (Wiggins et al., 2018). These two items, one a normative, commonly occurring misbehavior (i.e., becoming easily frustrated) and one an abnormal severe behavior (i.e., having destructive tantrums) identify irritability-related DSM disorders with good sensitivity (70–73%) and specificity (74–83%) as well as predict persistent irritability and elevated risk of disorders at early school age. We are also working toward algorithms for integrating the multifaceted information gathered via different irritability assessment methods as these provide unique sources of information and are only modestly correlated. Finally, we have theorized that joint consideration of brain–behavior markers of atypical irritability, as well as accounting for developmental change and parental contribution, will reduce the "developmental noise" and enhance the accuracy of early identification. Methods for incorporating this multilevel information in clinical decision-making have not yet been validated, and therein lies the next steps in preschool irritability research.

References

Achenbach, T. M., Edelbrock, C., & Howelp, C. T. (1987). Empirically based assessment of the behavioral/emotional problems of 2-and 3-year-old children. *Journal of Abnormal Child Psychology*, 15(4), 629–650. Retrieved from https://link.springer.com/content/pdf/10.1007%2FBF00917246.pdf

Adleman, N. E., Kayser, R., Dickstein, D., Blair, R. J. R., Pine, D., & Leibenluft, E. (2011). Neural correlates of reversal learning in severe mood dysregulation and pediatric bipolar disorder. *Journal of the American Academy of Child & Adolescent Psychiatry*, 50(11), 1173–1185.e2. Retrieved from http://doi.org/10.1016/j.jaac.2011.07.011

American Psychiatric Association. (2013). *Diagnostic and Statistical Manual of Mental Disorders* (5th ed.). Arlington, VA: American Psychiatric Association.

Aslin, R. N., & Mehler, J. (2005). Near-infrared spectroscopy for functional studies of brain activity in human infants: Promise, prospects, and challenges. *Journal of Biomedical Optics*, 10(1), 11009. Retrieved from http://doi.org/10.1117/1.1854672

Belsky, J., Bakermans-Kranenburg, M. J., & IJzendoorn, M. H. van. (2007). For better and for worse differential susceptibility to environmental influences. *Current Directions in Psychological Science*, 16(6), 300–304. Retrieved from http://doi.org/10.1111/j.1467-8721.2007.00525.x

Bennett, K. J., Lipman, E. L., Brown, S., Racine, Y., Boyle, M. H., & Offord, D. R. (1999). Predicting conduct problems: Can high-risk children be identified in kindergarten and grade 1? *Journal of Consulting and Clinical Psychology*, 67(4), 470–480.

Bernier, A., Carlson, S. M., & Whipple, N. (2010). From external regulation to self-regulation: Early parenting precursors of young children's executive functioning. *Child Development*, 81(1), 326–339. Retrieved from http://doi.org/10.1111/j.1467-8624.2009.01397.x

Biedzio, D., & Wakschlag, L. S. (2018). Developmental emergence of disruptive behaviors beginning in infancy: Delineating normal:abnormal boundaries to enhance early identification. In Charles Zeanah (Ed.), *Handbook of Infant Mental Health* (Fourth). New York: Guilford.

Bosacki, S. L., & Moore, C. (2004). Preschoolers' understanding of simple and complex emotions: Links with gender and language. *Sex Roles, 50*(9), 659–675. Retrieved from https://link.springer.com/content/pdf/10.1023%2FB%3ASERS.0000027568.26966.27.pdf

Briggs-Gowan, M. J., Nichols, S. R., Voss, J., Zobel, E., Carter, A. S., McCarthy, K. J., . . . Wakschlag, L. S. (2014). Punishment insensitivity and impaired reinforcement learning in preschoolers. *Journal of Child Psychology and Psychiatry, and Allied Disciplines, 55*(2), 154–61. Retrieved from http://doi.org/10.1111/jcpp.12132

Brownell, C. A., & Kopp, C. B. (2007). Transitions in toddler socioemotional development: Behavior, understanding, relationships. In C. A. Brownell & C. B. Kopp (Eds.), *Socioemotional development in the toddler years: Transitions and transformations* (pp. 1–40). New York: The Guilford Press.

Bufferd, S., Dyson, M., Hernandez, I., & Wakschlag, L. (2016). Explicating the "developmental" in preschool psychopathology. In D. Cichetti (Ed.), *Handbook of Developmental Psychopathology* (3rd Ed.), New York: Wiley.

Bunte, T. L., Laschen, S., Schoemaker, K., Hessen, D. J., van der Heijden, P. G. M., & Matthys, W. (2013). Clinical usefulness of observational assessment in the diagnosis of DBD and ADHD in preschoolers. *Journal of Clinical Child and Adolescent Psychology, 42*(6), 749–761. Retrieved from http://doi.org/10.1080/15374416.2013.773516

Campbell, S. B., Breaux, A. M., Ewing, L. J., Szumowski, E. K., Pierce, E. W., Baldwin, D., . . . Sell, E. (1986). Parent-identified problem preschoolers: Mother-child interaction during play at intake and 1-year follow-up. *Journal of Abnormal Child Psychology, 14*(3), 425–440.

Carroll, J. J., & Steward, M. S. (1984). The role of cognitive development in children's understandings of their own feelings. *Child Development, 55*(4), 1486–1492. Retrieved from http://www.jstor.org/stable/1130018

Casey, B. J., Tottenham, N., Liston, C., & Durston, S. (2005). Imaging the developing brain: What have we learned about cognitive development? *Trends in Cognitive Sciences, 9*(3), 104–110. Retrieved from http://doi.org/10.1016/j.tics.2005.01.011

Coccaro, E. F., Bergeman, C. S., Kavoussi, R. J., & Seroczynski, A. D. (1997). Heritability of aggression and irritability: A twin study of the Buss-Durkee Aggression Scales in adult male subjects. *Biological Psychiatry, 41*, 273–284. Retrieved from https://doi.org/10.1016/j.biopsych.2006.08.024

Coccaro, E. F., Bergeman, C. S., & Mcclearn, G. E. (1993). Heritability of irritable impulsiveness: A study of twins reared together and apart. *Psychiatry Research, 48*, 229–242. Retrieved from https://doi.org/10.1016/0165-1781(93)90074-Q

Cole, P., Michel, M., & Teti, L. (1994). The development of emotion regulation and dysregulation: A clinical perspective. In N. Fox (Ed.), *The development of emotion regulation: Biological and behavioral considerations* (pp. 73–102). Chicago: University of Chicago Press.

Cole, P. M., Martin, S. E., & Dennis, T. A. (2004). Emotion Regulation as a Scientific Construct: Methodological Challenges and Directions for Child Development Research. *Child Development, 75*(2), 317–333. http://doi.org/10.1111/j.1467-8624.2004.00673.x

Cui, X., Bray, S., Bryant, D. M., Glover, G. H., & Reiss, A. L. (2011). A quantitative comparison of NIRS and fMRI across multiple cognitive tasks. *Neuroimage*, *54*(4), 2808–2821. Retrieved from http://doi.org/10.1016/j.neuroimage.2010.10.069

Danis, B., Hill, C., & Wakschlag, L. (2009). In the eye of the beholder: Critical components of observation when assessing disruptive behaviors in young children. *Zero-to-Three*, *29*, 24–30.

Denham, S. A., Bassett, H. H., Way, E., Mincic, M., Zinsser, K., Graling, K., & Ayers Denham, S. (2017). Preschoolers' emotion knowledge: Self-regulatory foundations, and predictions of early school success Preschoolers' emotion knowledge: Self-regulatory foundations, and predictions of early school success. *Cognition and Emotion*, *26*(4), 667–679. Retrieved from http://doi.org/10.1080/02699931.2011.602049

Diamond, A. (2002). Normal development of prefrontal cortex from birth to young adulthood: Cognitive functions, anatomy, and biochemistry. In D. Stuss & R. Knight (Eds.), *Principles of frontal lobe function* (pp. 466–503). New York: Oxford University Press. Retrieved from http://devcogneuro.com/Publications/ChapterinStuss&Knight.pdf

Dickstein, D. P., Nelson, E. E., McClure, E. B., Grimley, M. E., Knopf, L., Brotman, M. A., . . . Leibenluft, E. (2007). Cognitive flexibility in phenotypes of pediatric bipolar disorder. *Journal of the American Academy of Child and Adolescent Psychiatry*, *46*(3), 341–355. Retrieved from http://doi.org/10.1097/chi.0b013e31802d0b3d

Dougherty, L. R., Smith, V. C., Bufferd, S. J., Carlson, G. A., Stringaris, A., Leibenluft, E., & Klein, D. N. (2017). DSM-5 disruptive mood dysregulation disorder: Correlates and predictors in young children. *Psychological Medicine*, *44*, 2339–2350. Retrieved from http://doi.org/10.1017/S0033291713003115

Dougherty, L. R., Smith, V. C., Bufferd, S. J., Stringaris, A., Psych, M. R. C., Leibenluft, E., . . . Klein, D. N. (2013). Preschool irritability: Longitudinal associations with psychiatric disorders at age 6 and parental psychopathology. *Journal of the American Academy of Child and Adolescent Psychiatry*, *52*, 1304–1313. Retrieved from http://doi.org/10.1016/j.jaac.2013.09.007

Duncan, G. J., Dowsett, C. J., Claessens, A., Magnuson, K., Huston, A. C., Klebanov, P., . . . Zill, N. (2007). School readiness and later achievement. *Developmental Psychology*, *43*(6), 1428–1446. Retrieved from http://dx.doi.org/10.1037/0012-1649.43.6.1428.supp

Frost, A., Jelinek, C., Bernard, K., Lind, T., Dozier, M., & Allison, C. (2017). Longitudinal associations between low morning cortisol in infancy and anger dysregulation in early childhood in a CPS-referred sample. *Developmental Science*. Retrieved from http://doi.org/10.1111/desc.12573

Gagne, J. R., Van Hulle, C. A., Aksan, N., Essex, M. J., & Goldsmith, H. H. (2011). Deriving childhood temperament measures from emotion- eliciting behavioral episodes: Scale construction and initial validation. *Psychological Assessment*, *23*(2), 337–353. Retrieved from http://doi.org/10.1037/a0021746

Garon, N., Bryson, S. E., & Smith, I. M. (2005). Executive function in preschoolers: A review using an integrative framework. *Psychological Bulletin*, *134*(1), 31–60. Retrieved from http://doi.org/10.1037/0033-2909.134.1.31

Giedd, J. N., Blumenthal, J., Jeffries, N. O., Castellanos, F. X., Liu, H., Zijdenbos, A., . . . Rapoport, J. L. (1999). Brain development during childhood and adolescence: A longitudinal MRI study. *Nature Neuroscience*, *2*(10), 861–863. Retrieved from http://doi.org/10.1038/13158

Giedd, J. N., Lalonde, F. M., Celano, M. J., White, S. L., Wallace, G. L., Lee, N. R., & Lenroot, R. K. (2009). Anatomical brain magnetic resonance imaging of typically developing children and adolescents. *Journal of American Academy Child and Adolescent Psychiatry*, 48(5), 465–470. Retrieved from http://doi.org/10.1097/CHI.0b013e31819f2715

Gogtay, N., Giedd, J. N., Lusk, L., Hayashi, K. M., Greenstein, D., Vaituzis, A. C., . . . Thompson, P. M. (2004). Dynamic mapping of human cortical development during childhood through early adulthood. *Proceedings of the National Academy of Sciences of the United States of America*, 101(21), 8174–8179. Retrieved from http://doi.org/10.1073/pnas.0402680101

Goldsmith, H. H., & Davidson, R. J. (2004). Disambiguating the Components of Emotion Regulation. *Child Development*, 75(2), 361–365. http://doi.org/10.1111/j.1467-8624.2004.00678.x

Grabell, A. S., Huppert, T. J., Li, Y., Hlutkowsky, C. O., Jones, H. M., Wakschlag, L. S., & Perlman, S. B. (under review). Mechanics of early deliberate emotion regulation: Elucidating young children's responses to therapeutic scaffolding.

Grabell, A. S., Li, Y., Barker, J. W., Wakschlag, L. S., Huppert, T. J., & Perlman, S. B. (2017). Evidence of non-linear associations between frustration-related prefrontal cortex activation and the normal:abnormal spectrum of irritability in young children. *Journal of Abnormal Child Psychology*. Retrieved from http://doi.org/10.1007/s10802-017-0286-5

Gray, S. A. O., Carter, A. S., Briggs-Gowan, M. J., Hill, C., Danis, B., Keenan, K., & Wakschlag, L. S. (2012). Preschool children's observed disruptive behavior: Variations across sex, interactional context, and disruptive psychopathology. *Journal of Clinical Child and Adolescent Psychology*. Retrieved from http://doi.org/10.1080/15374416.2012.675570

Hofmann, W., Schmeichel, B. J., & Baddeley, A. D. (2012). Executive functions and self-regulation. *Trends in Cognitive Sciences*, 16(3), 174–180. Retrieved from http://doi.org/10.1016/j.tics.2012.01.006

Hughes, C. H., & Ensor, R. A. (2009). How do families help or hinder the emergence of early executive function? *New Directions for Child and Adolescent Development*, 2009(123), 35–50. Retrieved from http://doi.org/10.1002/cd.234

Huttenlocher, P. R., de Courten, C., Garey, L. J., & Van der Loos, H. (1982). Synaptogenesis in human visual cortex: Evidence for synapse elimination during normal development. *Neuroscience Letters*, 33(3), 247–252. Retrieved from http://doi.org/10.1016/0304-3940(82)90379-2

Jiang, J., Chen, C., Dai, B., Shi, G., Ding, G., Liu, L., & Lu, C. (2015). Leader emergence through interpersonal neural synchronization. *Proceedings of the National Academy of Sciences*, 112(14), 4274–4279. Retrieved from http://doi.org/10.1073/pnas.1422930112

Jobsis, F. F. (1977). Noninvasive, infrared monitoring of cerebral and myocardial oxygen sufficiency and circulatory parameters. *Science*, 198(4323), 1264–1267. Retrieved from http://doi.org/10.1126/science.929199

Johnson, M. H. (2001). Functional brain development in humans. *Nature Reviews Neuroscience*, 2(7), 475–483. Retrieved from http://doi.org/10.1038/35081509

Karim, H. T., & Perlman, S. B. (2017). Neurodevelopmental maturation as a function of irritable temperament. *Human Brain Mapping*. Retrieved from http://doi.org/10.1002/hbm.23742

Kessel, E. M., Meyer, A., Hajcak, G., Dougherty, L. R., Torpey-Newman, D. C., Carlson, G. A., & Klein, D. N. (2016). Transdiagnostic factors and pathways to multifinality: The error-related negativity predicts whether preschool irritability is associated with internalizing versus externalizing symptoms at age 9. *Development and Psychopathology*, *28*(4 Pt 1), 913–926. Retrieved from http://doi.org/10.1017/S0954579416000626

Kochanska, G., Murray, K. T., & Harlan, E. T. (2000). Effortful control in early child-hood: Continuity and change, antecedents, and implications for social development. *Developmental Psychology*, *36*(2), 220–232. Retrieved from http://dx.doi.org/10.1037/0012-1649.36.2.220

Kopp, C. B. (1982). Antecedents of self-regulation: A developmental perspective. *Developmental Psychology*, *18*(2), 199–214. Retrieved from http://doi.org/10.1037/0012-1649.18.2.199

Leibenluft, E. (2017). Pediatric irritability: A systems neuroscience approach. *Trends in Cognitive Sciences*, *21*(4), 277–289. Retrieved from http://doi.org/10.1016/j.tics.2017.02.002

Lenroot, R. K., & Giedd, J. N. (2006). Brain development in children and adolescents: Insights from anatomical magnetic resonance imaging. *Neuroscience & Biobehavioral Reviews*, *30*(6), 718–729. Retrieved from http://doi.org/10.1016/j.neubiorev.2006.06.001

Li, Y., Grabell, A. S., Wakschlag, L. S., Huppert, T. J., & Perlman, S. B. (2017). The neural substrates of cognitive flexibility are related to individual differences in preschool ir-ritability: A fNIRS investigation. *Developmental Cognitive Neuroscience*, *25*, 138–144. Retrieved from http://doi.org/10.1016/j.dcn.2016.07.002

Luciana, M., & Nelson, C. A. (1998). The functional emergence of prefrontally guided working memory systems in four- to eight-year-old children. *Neuropsychologia*, *36*(3), 273–293. Retrieved from http://doi.org/10.1016/S0028-3932(97)00109-7

Luu, T. M., Vohr, B. R., Schneider, K. C., Katz, K. H., Tucker, R., Allan, W. C., & Ment, L. R. (2009). Trajectories of receptive language development from 3 to 12 years of age for very preterm children. *Journal of Pediatrics*, *124*(1), 333–341. Retrieved from http://doi.org/10.1542/peds.2008-2587

McCarthy, D. (1930). *The language development of the preschool child*. Westport, CT: University of Minnesota Press. Retrieved from http://pubman.mpdl.mpg.de/pubman/item/escidoc:2359021/component/escidoc:2390055/McCarthy_1930_Language_development.pdf

McClelland, M. M., & Cameron, C. E. (2011). Self-regulation and academic achievement in elementary school children. *New Directions for Child and Adolescent Development*, *2011*(133), 29–44. Retrieved from http://doi.org/10.1002/cd.302

Perlman, S. B. (2012). Neuroimaging in child clinical populations: Considerations for a suc-cessful research program. *American Academy of Child and Adolescent Psychiatry*, *51*(12), 1232–1235. Retrieved from http://doi.org/10.1016/j.jaac

Perlman, S. B., Huppert, T. J., & Luna, B. (2016). Functional near-infrared spectroscopy ev-idence for development of prefrontal engagement in working memory in early through middle childhood. *Cerebral Cortex (New York, N.Y. : 1991)*, *26*(6), 2790–2799. Retrieved from http://doi.org/10.1093/cercor/bhv139

Perlman, S. B., Luna, B., Hein, T. C., & Huppert, T. J. (2014). fNIRS evidence of prefrontal regulation of frustration in early childhood. *Neuroimage*, *85 Pt 1*, 326–34. Retrieved from http://doi.org/10.1016/j.neuroimage.2013.04.057

Pessoa, L. (2017). A network model of the emotional brain. *Trends in Cognitive Neuroscience*, *21*(5), 357–371. Retrieved from http://doi.org/10.1016/j.tics.2017.03.002

Petitclerc, A., Briggs-Gowan, M. J., Estabrook, R., Burns, J. L., Anderson, E. L., McCarthy, K. J., & Wakschlag, L. S. (2015). Contextual variation in young children's observed disruptive behavior on the DB-DOS: Implications for early identification. *Journal of Child Psychology and Psychiatry and Allied Disciplines*. Retrieved from http://doi.org/10.1111/jcpp.12430

Phillips, N. K., Hammen, C. L., Brennan, P. A., Najman, J. M., & Bor, W. (2005). Early adversity and the prospective prediction of depressive and anxiety disorders in adolescents. *Journal of Abnormal Child Psychology*, *33*(1), 13–24. Retrieved from http://doi.org/10.1007/s10802-005-0930-3

Pungello, E. P., Iruka, I. U., Dotterer, A. M., Mills-Koonce, R., & Reznick, J. S. (2009). The effects of socioeconomic status, race, and parenting on language development in early childhood. *Developmental Psychology*, *45*(2), 544–557. Retrieved from http://doi.org/10.1037/a0013917

Rhoades, B. L., Warren, H. K., Domitrovich, C. E., & Greenberg, M. T. (2011). Examining the link between preschool social-emotional competence and first grade academic achievement: The role of attention skills. *Early Childhood Research Quarterly*. Retrieved from http://doi.org/10.1016/j.ecresq.2010.07.003

Roberson-Nay, R., Leibenluft, E., Brotman, M. A., Myers, J., Larsson, H., Lichtenstein, P., & Kendler, K. S. (2015). Longitudinal stability of genetic and environmental influences on irritability: From childhood to young adulthood. *American Journal of Psychiatry*, *172*(7), 657–664. Retrieved from http://doi.org/10.1176/appi.ajp.2015.14040509

Rothbart, M. K., Ahadi, S. A., Hershey, K. L., & Fisher, P. (2001). Investigations of temperament at three to seven years: The Children's Behavior Questionnaire. *Child Development*, *72*(5), 1394–1408.

Roy, A. K., Bennett, R., Posner, J., Hulvershorn, L., Castellanos, F. X., & Klein, R. G. (2017). Altered intrinsic functional connectivity of the cingulate cortex in children with severe temper outbursts. *Development and Psychopathology*, 1–9. Retrieved from http://doi.org/10.1017/S0954579417001080

Savage, J., Verhulst, B., Copeland, W., Althoff, R. R., Lichtenstein, P., & Roberson-Nay, R. (2015). A genetically informed study of the longitudinal relation between irritability and anxious/depressed symptoms. *Journal of the American Academy of Child & Adolescent Psychiatry*, *54*, 377–384. Retrieved from http://doi.org/10.1016/j.jaac.2015.02.010

Scott, W. A. (1962). Cognitive complexity and cognitive flexibility. *Sociometry*, *25*(4), 405–414. Retrieved from http://doi.org/10.2307/2785779

Shaunfield, S., Petitclerc, A., Kaiser, K., Greene, G., Condon, D., Estabrook, R., & Wakschlag, L. S. (in preparation). "In their own voices": A mixed methods study of socio-cultural differences in maternal perceptions of young children's disruptive behavior.

Shaw, P., Kabani, N. J., Lerch, J. P., Eckstrand, K., Lenroot, R., Gogtay, N., . . . Wise, S. P. (2008). Neurodevelopmental trajectories of the human cerebral cortex. *Journal of Neuroscience*, *28*(14). Retrieved from http://doi.org/10.1523/JNEUROSCI.5309-07.2008

Sparks, G. M., Axelson, D. A., Yu, H., Ha, W., Ballester, J., Diler, R. S., . . . Birmaher, B. (2014). Disruptive mood dysregulation disorder and chronic irritability in youth at familial risk for bipolar disorder. *Journal of the American Academy of Child & Adolescent Psychiatry*, *53*, 408–416. Retrieved from http://doi.org/10.1016/j.jaac.2013.12.026

Stringaris, A. (2011). Irritability in children and adolescents: A challenge for DSM-5. *European Child and Adolescent Psychiatry, 20*, 61–66. Retrieved from http://doi.org/ 10.1007/s00787-010-0150-4

Stringaris, A., & Goodman, R. (2009). Longitudinal outcome of youth oppositionality: Irritable, headstrong, and hurtful behaviors have distinctive predictions. *Journal of the American Academy of Child and Adolescent Psychiatry, 48*(4), 404–412.

Stroop, J. R. (1935). Studies of interference in serial verbal reactions. *Journal of Experimental Psychology, 18*(6), 643–662. Retrieved from http://doi.org/10.1037/h0054651

Tseng, W. L., Guyer, A. E., Briggs-Gowan, M. J., Axelson, D., Birmaher, B., Egger, H. L., . . . Brotman, M. A. (2015). Behavior and emotion modulation deficits in preschoolers at risk for bipolar disorder. *Depression and Anxiety.* Retrieved from http://doi.org/ 10.1002/da.22342

Tsujimoto, S. (2008). The prefrontal cortex: Functional neural development during early childhood. *Neuroscientist, 14*(4), 345–358. Retrieved from http://doi.org/10.1177/ 1073858408316002

Wakschlag, L., Estabrook, R., Hlutkowsky, C., Anderson, E., Briggs-Gowan, M. J., Petitclerc, A., & Perlman, S. B. (under review). The Early Childhood-Related Impairment Interview (E-CRI): A novel method for assessing clinical significance of young children's irritability within developmental context.

Wakschlag, L. S., Briggs-Gowan, M. J., Carter, A. S., Hill, C., Danis, B., Keenan, K., . . . Leventhal, B. L. (2007). A developmental framework for distinguishing disruptive behavior from normative misbehavior in preschool children. *Journal of Child Psychology and Psychiatry, 48*(10), 976–987. Retrieved from http://doi.org/10.1111/ j.1469-7610.2007.01786.x

Wakschlag, L. S., Briggs-Gowan, M. J., Choi, S. W., Nichols, S. R., Kestler, J., Burns, J. L., . . . Henry, D. (2014). Advancing a multidimensional, developmental spectrum approach to preschool disruptive behavior. *Journal of the American Academy of Child & Adolescent Psychiatry, 53*, 82–96.e3. Retrieved from http://doi.org/10.1016/ j.jaac.2013.10.011

Wakschlag, L. S., Briggs-Gowan, M. J., Hill, C., Danis, B., Leventhal, B. L., Keenan, K., . . . Carter, A. S. (2008a). Observational assessment of preschool disruptive behavior, part II: Validity of the Disruptive Behavior Diagnostic Observation Schedule (DB-DOS). *Journal of the American Academy of Child & Adolescent Psychiatry, 47*(6), 632–641. Retrieved from http://doi.org/10.1097/CHI.0b013e31816c5c10

Wakschlag, L. S., Choi, S. W., Carter, A. S., Hullsiek, H., Burns, J., McCarthy, K., . . . Briggs-Gowan, M. J. (2012). Defining the developmental parameters of temper loss in early childhood: Implications for developmental psychopathology. *Journal of Child Psychology and Psychiatry, 53*(11), 1099–108. Retrieved from http://doi.org/10.1111/ j.1469-7610.2012.02595.x

Wakschlag, L. S., & Danis, B. (2012). Characterizing early childhood disruptive behavior. In J. Charles H. Zeanah (Ed.), *Handbook of infant mental health* (3rd Edition) (pp. 392– 408). New York: Guilford Press.

Wakschlag, L. S., Estabrook, R., Petitclerc, A., Henry, D., Burns, J. L., Perlman, S. B., . . . Briggs-Gowan, M. L. (2015). Clinical implications of a dimensional approach: The normal:abnormal spectrum of early irritability. *Journal of the American Academy of*

Child & Adolescent Psychiatry, *54*(8), 626–634. Retrieved from http://doi.org/10.1016/j.jaac.2015.05.016

Wakschlag, L. S., Hill, C., Carter, A. S., Danis, B., Egger, H. L., Keenan, K., . . . Briggs-Gowan, M. J. (2008b). Observational assessment of preschool disruptive behavior, part I: Reliability of the Disruptive Behavior Diagnostic Observation Schedule (DB-DOS). *Journal of the American Academy of Child & Adolescent Psychiatry*, *47*(6), 622–631. Retrieved from http://doi.org/10.1097/CHI.0b013e31816c5bdb

Wakschlag, L. S., Leventhal, B. L., Briggs-Gowan, M. J., Danis, B., Keenan, K., Hill, C., . . . Carter, A. S. (2005). Defining the "disruptive" in preschool behavior: What diagnostic observation can teach us. *Clinical Child and Family Psychology Review*, *8*(3). Retrieved from http://doi.org/10.1007/s10567-005-6664-5

Wakschlag, L. S., Perlman, S. B., Blair, R. J., Leibenluft, E., Briggs-Gowan, M. J., & Pine, D. S. (2017). The neurodevelopmental basis of early childhood disruptive behavior: Irritable and callous phenotypes as exemplars. *The American Journal of Psychiatry* (epub ahead of print). Retrieved from http://doi.org/10.1176/appi.ajp.2017.17010045

Wakschlag, L. S., Tolan, P. H., & Leventhal, B. L. (2010). "Ain't misbehavin': Towards a developmentally specified nosology for preschool disruptive behavior. *Journal of Child Psychology and Psychiatry*, *51*(1), 3–22. Retrieved from http://doi.org/10.1111/j.1469-7610.2009.02184.x

Wiggins, J., Briggs-Gowan, M., Estabrook, R., Brotman, M., Pine, D., Leibenluft, E., & Wakschlag, L. S. (2018). Identifying clinically significant irritability in early childhood. *Journal of the American Academy of Child and Adolescent Psychiatry. 57*(3), 191–199.e2

Wiggins, J. L., Mitchell, C., Stringaris, A., & Leibenluft, E. (2014). Developmental trajectories of irritability and bidirectional associations with maternal depression. *Journal of the American Academy of Child & Adolescent Psychiatry*, *53*, 1191–1205.e4. Retrieved from http://doi.org/10.1016/j.jaac.2014.08.005

Zelazo, P. D., & Cunningham, W. A. (2007). Executive function: Mechanisms underlying emotion regulation. In James Gross (Ed.) *Handbook of emotion regulation* (pp. 135–158). New York: Guilford Press.

6

Irritability Development from Middle Childhood Through Adolescence

TRAJECTORIES, CONCURRENT CONDITIONS, AND OUTCOMES

Cynthia Kiefer and Jillian Lee Wiggins

Introduction

Irritability is a symptom dimension characterized by angry mood and temper outbursts and conceptualized as a low threshold for anger (Brotman, Kircanski, Stringaris, Pine, & Leibenluft, 2016). Irritability cuts across multiple psychiatric disorders, including depressive, anxiety, and disruptive behavior disorders, as well as typical development (Stringaris, 2011; Cornacchio et al., 2016). Indeed, severe, chronic irritability is the cardinal symptom of disruptive mood dysregulation disorder (DMDD), which was added to the fifth edition of the *Diagnostic and Statistical Manual of Mental Disorders* (DSM-5; American Psychiatric Association [APA], 2013), as well as DMDD's precursor, severe mood dysregulation (SMD), a phenotype defined by persistent and severe irritability developed for research purposes (Brotman et al., 2006).

Irritability predicts internalizing and externalizing symptoms, psychiatric disorders, and functional impairment at every major developmental period (Dougherty et al., 2014, 2015; Wakschlag et al., 2015). Broadly speaking, SMD, DMDD, and dimensional measures of irritability symptoms in youth predict concurrent and prospective mood (anxiety, depressive) and disruptive behavior disorders (attention deficit/hyperactivity disorder [ADHD], oppositional defiant disorder, conduct disorder) through adulthood (Brotman et al., 2006; Deveney et al., 2015; Stringaris, Zavos, Leibenluft, Maughan, & Eley, 2012). Furthermore, pediatric irritability has long-term negative outcomes, including adult psycho-pathology (Fichter, Kohlboeck, Quadflieg, Wyschkon, & Esser, 2009; Stringaris, Cohen, Pine, & Leibenluft, 2009), impoverishment, lower educational attainment, worse health outcomes, self-reported police contact, and increased suicidality, above and beyond other disorders (Copeland, Shanahan, Egger, Angold, & Costello, 2014; Pickles et al., 2010). Thus, an exploration of the longitudinal associations of pediatric irritability may aid in the early prevention of serious outcomes and impairment in adulthood.

The purpose of the current review is to trace the longitudinal course of irritability in youth. We included studies that focused on trajectories of pediatric irritability from middle childhood through adolescence and irritability's relation to other childhood problems. We did not include studies focusing on adulthood except as an outcome of pediatric irritability because addressing irritability in earlier developmental stages may prevent later adult consequences (Vidal-Ribas, Brotman, Valdivieso, Leibenluft, & Stringaris, 2016). Furthermore, we did not include the vast literature on aggression, callous/unemotional traits, or other aspects of disruptive behavior in this review as irritability (i.e., low threshold for anger rather than the aggressive or disruptive behavior component), while highly correlated, is separate from these other constructs (Stringaris et al., 2012; Vidal-Ribas et al., 2016).

Prevalence and Stability of Irritability Symptoms from Middle Childhood Through Adolescence

Overall, studies have shown that irritability is fairly common in middle childhood through adolescence, with rates for clinical levels of irritability on par with other pediatric mood disorders (Brotman et al., 2006; Copeland, Brotman, & Costello, 2015). Prevalence rates for chronic, severe levels of irritability (i.e., defined using DMDD criteria) in childhood and adolescence range from 2% to 5% (Brotman et al., 2006; Mayes et al., 2015). Mayes et al. (2015) examined maternal-rated irritability symptoms in a population-based sample of 376 children aged 6–12 years (mean age = 9 years) and at an 8-year follow-up (mean age = 16 years) and found that maternal-rated irritability symptoms were "often" a problem for 9% of youths at baseline, 6% at follow-up, and 3% at both baseline and follow-up. Brotman et al. (2006) used data from the longitudinal, epidemiological Great Smoky Mountains Study, a community-based sample of children from 9 to 16 years of age ($N = 1,420$), to estimate irritability prevalence. Brotman et al. (2006) generated SMD classification from items on the Child and Adolescent Psychiatric Assessment (CAPA) and found the weighted lifetime prevalence of SMD in children aged 9–19 years to be 3.3% (Brotman et al., 2006); 1.8% of the children with SMD also evidence severe functional impairment due to their chronic irritability. This prevalence rate is similar to other rates of pediatric mood disorders, such as pediatric depression (approximately 2% prevalence rate) (Brotman et al., 2006). Additionally, irritability may be conceptualized as having tonic (persistent, angry mood) and phasic (temper outbursts) components (Copeland et al., 2015). Copeland, Brotman, and

Costello (2015) investigated the prevalence and developmental course of normative tonic and phasic irritability from childhood to adolescence using Great Smoky
Mountains Study data. Tonic or phasic irritability were considered present if either
the child or parent reported the presence of at least one symptom as measured
by the CAPA (Copeland et al., 2015). They found that, in childhood and adolescence, 51.4% report phasic irritability, 28.3% report tonic irritability, and 22.8% report both (Copeland et al., 2015). Of note, their data moreover suggest that tonic
and phasic aspects are highly related as both phasic and tonic irritability predict
one another over time. Of note, whereas in the Brotman et al. (2006) study, irritability was defined by endorsing many items on the CAPA to meet criteria for the
clinical presentation of SMD, and thus prevalence rates for severe irritability were
lower; in a study of normative irritability, tonic or phasic irritability was defined
by endorsing just one item on the CAPA, thus the prevalence rates for normative
irritability were considerably higher (Copeland et al., 2015). Collectively, this work
shows that normative levels of irritability are fairly common in childhood and
adolescence, while more severe, clinical levels of irritability demonstrate a prevalence rate consistent with that of other pediatric mood disorders.

Irritability maintains a somewhat stable course throughout adolescence,
with mild overall declines over time but the potential to increase in a subset of
individuals (Brotman et al., 2006; Leibenluft & Stoddard, 2013; Mayes et al., 2015).
Prevalence rates of both tonic and phasic irritability decrease over time, and the
degree of decrease does not vary by gender (Copeland et al., 2015). Mayes et al.
(2015) also found that irritability is more likely to decrease than increase from
early to later school age (i.e., ages 6–12 at baseline with 8-year follow-up). Indeed,
of children diagnosed with DMDD at baseline, 71% are in remission by follow-up.
However, 55% of the DMDD cases at follow-up have onset after baseline (Mayes
et al., 2015).

Some evidence suggests that specific developmental trajectories of irritability
may differ in later adolescence based on gender and the adolescent's initial levels
of irritability. Although Wiggins, Mitchell, Stringaris, and Leibenluft (2014) and
Copeland, Brotman, and Costello (2015) did not document gender differences in
irritability trajectory structure following toddlers through middle childhood or
early to middle childhood, respectively, some gender differences appear to emerge
in adolescence. In particular, Caprara, Paciello, Gerbino, and Cugini (2007)
investigated the developmental trajectories of irritability throughout adolescence
in a longitudinal study of 500 youths aged 12–20 years. They found that irritability
tends to decrease in adolescence in males but not females, whose irritability levels
tend to remain more stable while demonstrating higher irritability levels than
males over time (Caprara et al., 2007). Four types of developmental trajectories
were identified: youths whose irritability levels start at either a low or high level
tend to demonstrate more stability over time, whereas those whose irritability
symptoms start at a medium level either remained stable or declined (Caprara
et al., 2007). Youths in the high irritable trajectory are associated with physical

aggression and, to a lesser extent, verbal aggression and violence (Caprara et al., 2007). Adolescents who start with high levels of irritability and whose irritability increases over time become more ruminative 2 years later (Caprara et al., 2007), which is consistent with research demonstrating that irritability is associated with the emergence of internalizing symptoms in later adolescence (Copeland et al., 2015; Stringaris & Goodman, 2009). They also found that irritability is more related to verbal aggression in girls than boys from early to late adolescence, whereas irritability is more related to physical aggression and violence for boys than girls over the same time period (Caprara et al., 2007).

Importantly, even relatively low, nonclinical levels of irritability are associated with impairment and negative outcomes through adolescence. Copeland, Brotman, and Costello (2015) found that endorsing at least one tonic or phasic irritability symptom characterizes youth who experience impaired functioning (Copeland et al., 2015). Indeed, normative levels of phasic and tonic irritability are associated with increased risk of dysfunction, including parental burden, school suspensions, and service use, as well as concurrent and future emotional symptoms (Copeland et al., 2015). Furthermore, despite the declines over time in clinical levels of irritability, a large proportion of youths with prior diagnoses for DMDD/SMD who later fail to meet clinical criteria for DMDD/SMD (i.e., "remitted") still report clinically significant functional impairment (Deveney et al., 2015; Mayes et al., 2015). Thus, even normative or subthreshold levels of irritability are associated with social and emotional impairment at school and at home.

Irritability and the Emergence of Externalizing and Internalizing Symptoms from Middle Childhood into Adolescence

Although irritability in early childhood is primarily associated with externalizing problems such as aggression and anger outbursts, irritability in adolescence is largely associated with internalizing disorders. Indeed, irritability is at the intersection of internalizing and externalizing behaviors as irritability incorporates the emotional aspects of internalizing symptoms such as the angry, emotional response to blocked goals (i.e., frustration), but also externalizing components (i.e., anger leading to aggression). Increases in irritability from middle childhood to adolescence are preceded by worse externalizing behavior (Mulraney, Zendarski, Mensah, Hiscock, & Sciberras, 2016). Mulraney et al.'s (2016) study on children at mean age 10.2 years with ADHD investigated the relationship between early internalizing and externalizing problems and later irritability in adolescence at mean age 13.8 years. They found that externalizing symptoms in childhood significantly predict parent-reported irritability in early adolescence, even after controlling for age, ADHD symptom severity, concurrent externalizing problems, ADHD medication use, and neighborhood disadvantage (Mulraney et al., 2016).

Although irritability is present in childhood externalizing disorders (ODD, conduct disorder), irritability in adolescence is also associated with depression. Indeed, irritable mood is present in more than one-third of cases of adolescent depression (Stringaris et al., 2013). In addition, childhood irritability symptoms, above and beyond other externalizing symptom profiles such as the headstrong/hurtful component of ODD, predict distinct internalizing outcomes in adolescence (Stringaris & Goodman, 2009), as found in data combined from two British national surveys on children aged 5–16 years and their respective 3-year follow-ups. In particular, the irritability dimension predicts prospective emotional disorders including depression and anxiety, above and beyond the headstrong and hurtful dimensions of ODD, even after controlling for baseline psychopathology (Stringaris & Goodman, 2009). Importantly, the irritable dimension does not predict conduct disorder after holding age and gender constant (Stringaris & Goodman, 2009). Overall, irritability in adolescence is highly tied to depression and other internalizing problems.

The association between childhood irritability and the development of internalizing symptoms in adolescence may be explained by common genetic factors (Savage et al., 2015; Stringaris et al., 2012). Stringaris, Zavos, Leibenluft, Maughan, and Eley (2012) examined the genetic components of the irritable and headstrong/hurtful dimensions of ODD and their relation to depression and delinquency using a UK sample of twins and siblings aged 12–19 years at baseline and at an average of 8–33 months after initial contact. They found that irritability demonstrates significantly higher genetic correlations with depression ($r =.70$) than with delinquency ($r =.57$), suggesting a distinction between the dimension of irritability and the headstrong/hurtful behaviors (Stringaris et al., 2012). Furthermore, they found that the genetic relationship between depression and irritability at baseline fully accounts for the longitudinal relationship between irritability at baseline and depression at time two (Stringaris et al., 2012). In addition, Savage et al. (2015) studied the relations between irritability and depressed/anxious symptoms from the Swedish Twin Study of Child and Adolescent Development that began in childhood (8–9 years) and ended in young adulthood (19–20 years). They found that baseline irritability significantly predicts anxious/depressed symptoms at ages 13–14, and this effect is larger than the converse effect of anxiety/depression on irritability (Savage et al., 2015). They also found that the largest proportion of the variance in irritability and anxiety/depression, including their covariance over time, is primarily due to genetic factors (41–74%), with smaller effects associated with unique and common environmental factors (Savage et al., 2015). Taken together, these studies suggest that the link between pediatric irritability and internalizing disorders may be due to genetic factors common to both.

The relation between irritability and depression may differ by gender (Stringaris et al., 2013). Stringaris et al. (2013) utilized data from the Great Smoky Mountains Study to examine children and adolescents aged 9–16 years who met clinical criteria for depression. These children were divided into three groups: those with irritability but no depressed mood, depressed mood but no irritability, and those with both irritability and depressed mood (Stringaris et al., 2013). They found that girls are more likely to present with depression but not irritability, whereas boys are significantly more likely than girls to present with comorbid irritability and depression (Stringaris et al., 2013). Girls, but not boys, with both depression and irritability have significantly higher rates of comorbid conduct disorder versus girls with non-irritable depression (Stringaris et al., 2013). Taken together, these findings suggest that whereas irritability comorbid with depression is more common in boys, when girls have both irritability and depression, their symptom profile is more likely to also include conduct disorder.

Adolescence to Early Adulthood/Long-Term Outcomes

Overall, irritability symptoms in adolescence are highly predictive of later adult depression and anxiety (Fichter et al., 2009; Stringaris, Cohen, Pine, & Leibenluft, 2009). Indeed, using the Great Smoky Mountains longitudinal data, Brotman et al. (2006) found that pediatric irritability is a better predictor than pediatric depression of later adult depression. Stringaris et al. (2009) investigated the long-term associations between adolescent irritability and adult outcomes using a longitudinal community-based study involving parent interviews for adolescent participants (mean age = 13.8 years) and interviews with the participants 20 years later (mean age = 33.2 years). They found parent-reported irritability in adolescent youths predicts depressive disorders (major depression, dysthymia) and generalized anxiety disorder but not bipolar disorder or other anxiety disorders at a 20-year follow-up, controlling for baseline psychopathology (Stringaris et al., 2009). Importantly, even a 1 standard deviation increase in adolescent irritability doubles the risk of generalized anxiety disorder at the 20-year follow-up, after controlling for other psychopathology at baseline (Stringaris et al., 2009). Copeland, Shanahan, Egger, Angold, and Costello (2014) utilized a population-based study to assess youths aged 10–16 years up to six times for DMDD symptoms and three times in adulthood (ages 19, 21, and 24–26 years) for functional and psychiatric outcomes. A childhood history of DMDD is linked to increased risk of adult psychopathology, especially anxiety and depression, compared to healthy controls and those with a history of psychiatric disorders other than DMDD (Copeland et al., 2014). Althoff, Verhulst, Rettew, Hudziak, and Van Der Ende (2010) investigated the longitudinal outcomes of irritability as measured by the Child Behavior Checklist dysregulation profile (CBCL-DP). Using data from Dutch birth registries in youths aged 4–16 years assessed every 2 years for 14 years total (Althoff et al., 2010), they found that irritability predicts anxiety and disruptive behavior disorders, controlling for co-occurring psychopathology in adulthood (Althoff et al., 2010). However, while irritability is significantly associated with concurrent internalizing and externalizing in adolescence, Stringaris et al.

(2009) found that adolescent irritability predicts generalized anxiety disorder and depressive disorders, but not other externalizing disorders, at age 33. Leibenluft, Cohen, Gorrindo, Brook, and Pine (2006) used data from a longitudinal, epidemiological study that included approximately 700 children assessed three times over 9 years using the Diagnostic Interview Schedule for Children to assess for chronic irritability, defined as "generally present," and episodic irritability, defined as present "a lot more than usual" during specific time periods (Leibenluft et al., 2006). Children were assessed for psychiatric diagnosis at time 1 (mean age = 13.8 years), time 2 two years later (mean age = 16.2 years), and time 3 seven years later (mean age = 22.1 years) (Leibenluft et al., 2006). They found that episodic and chronic irritability are relatively distinct and stable constructs that vary in their associations with later psychopathology (Leibenluft et al., 2006). In particular, episodic irritability at time 1 is associated with mood and anxiety disorders at time 2, whereas chronic irritability at time 1 is associated with disruptive behavior disorders (ADHD) at time 2, even when adjusting for ADHD symptoms at time 1 (Leibenluft et al., 2006). Additionally, chronic irritability at time 1 is also associated with major depressive disorder at time 3 (Leibenluft et al., 2006). Of note, chronic irritability peaks in mid-adolescence and decreases into adulthood (Leibenluft et al., 2006). Collectively, these studies suggest that the link between irritability and externalizing problems is prominent in adolescence but attenuates over time, whereas the relationship between irritability and internalizing problems persists into adulthood (Leibenluft et al., 2006; Stringaris et al., 2009). Of note, however, an important limitation in these findings may be the lack of an adult equivalent to ODD (Stringaris et al., 2009).

Furthermore, adolescent irritability symptoms, above and beyond other psychopathology, predict increased suicidality (Pickles et al., 2010). Pickles et al. (2010) investigated predictors of lifetime suicidality using data from a representative, epidemiological community sample of adolescents first assessed in 1968 (aged 14–15 years) and again in 1999 (aged 44–45 years). In this landmark study, they collected data on adolescent psychopathology and ratings of psychiatric symptoms, adversity, and family functioning in adolescence, as well as adult assessments of lifetime suicidality and psychiatric history (Pickles et al., 2010). Irritability was assessed using a single item from the Eysenck Personality Questionnaire (Pickles et al., 2010). They found that adolescent irritability strongly predicts adult suicidality, above and beyond other affective disorders in adolescence, and irritability in adulthood is broadly related to adult psychopathology and increased internalizing problems (Pickles et al., 2010). Thus, irritable youth are at an increased risk for suicidality in adulthood.

In addition to adult psychopathology, adolescent irritability also predicts other serious problems in adulthood. Youths with a history of DMDD are more likely to experience impoverishment, negative health outcomes, and low educational attainment and to report police contact in adulthood compared with either controls or other psychiatric groups (Copeland et al., 2014). Youths with DMDD history are at higher risk for illicit or risky behaviors compared to youths without a history of DMDD (Copeland et al., 2014). Irritable males in particular are more likely to develop increased rates of drug abuse in adulthood (Althoff et al., 2010). Furthermore, Stringaris et al. (2009) found that adolescent irritability predicts lower income and educational attainment at the 20-year follow-up, and this association is not mediated by concurrent generalized anxiety disorder or major depression in adulthood. Overall, pediatric irritability predicts worse outcomes across a range of domains in adulthood.

Conclusion

To summarize, irritability is characterized by internalizing (angry mood) and externalizing (temper outbursts) symptoms and is fairly common in middle childhood through adolescence (Copeland et al., 2015). Although irritability generally demonstrates some decline over time (Brotman et al., 2006; Leibenluft & Stoddard, 2013; Mayes et al., 2015), both clinical and normative levels of irritability in middle childhood predict impairment and negative outcomes through adolescence (Copeland et al., 2015; Deveney et al., 2015; Mayes et al., 2015). While the association between irritability and externalizing problems is prominent from childhood to adolescence, it attenuates over time, whereas the link between irritability and internalizing problems persists into adulthood (Stringaris et al., 2009). From middle childhood to adolescence, irritability predicts concurrent and prospective internalizing disorders that persist into adulthood and shares genetic similarities to depression. Overall, irritability symptoms in adolescence significantly predict later adult psychopathology (Fichter et al., 2009; Stringaris, Cohen, Pine & Leibenluft, 2009). Irritability in youth is associated with impairment across a number of domains in adulthood, including impoverishment, negative health outcomes, low educational attainment, and police contact in adulthood (Copeland et al., 2014), and it predicts suicidality above and beyond other adult psychopathology (Pickles et al., 2010). Collectively, these findings suggest that irritability in middle childhood and adolescence has serious and lasting negative outcomes in adulthood. Taken together, these studies suggest that focus on early treatment and prevention of irritability symptoms in childhood is important to head off entrenched problems in adulthood.

Future Directions and Clinical Implications

Current research described in this chapter strongly indicates that irritability is associated with significant impairment and internalizing and externalizing disorders across development. Indeed, given that comorbid irritability symptoms worsen impairment (Copeland et al., 2015), clinicians should start assessing for concurrent irritability. Overall, the findings in this chapter under-score the need for effective interventions for irritability, of which there are very few (Brotman et al., 2016). Developing new, hypothesis-driven interventions will require identifying mechanisms (e.g., psychosocial, neural, genetic) across developmental periods that can be leveraged as moveable targets for preventive intervention and treatment. Other chapters in this book describe important work on identifying irritability mechanisms; such work must be continued and expanded to be leveraged for interventions. Additionally, whereas current work described here identifies detrimental adult outcomes associated with childhood and adolescent irritability, there are no disorders equivalent to DMDD or ODD in adulthood, which limits research on treatment for irritable adults. Overall, childhood and adolescent irritability represents an important area of research with clinical implications.

References

Althoff, R. R., Verhulst, F. C., Rettew, D. C., Hudziak, J. J., & Van Der Ende, J. (2010). Adult outcomes of childhood dysregulation: A 14-year follow-up study. *Journal of the American Academy of Child and Adolescent Psychiatry*, *49*(11), 1105–1116.e1. Retrieved from https://doi.org/10.1016/j.jaac.2010.08.006

American Psychiatric Association. (2013). *Diagnostic and statistical manual of mental disorders* (5th ed.). Arlington, VA: American Psychiatric Association. Retrieved from https://doi.org/10.1176/appi.books.9780890425596.744053

Brotman, M. A., Kircanski, K., Stringaris, A., Pine, D. S., & Leibenluft, E. (2016). Irritability in youth: A translational model. *American Journal of Psychiatry*, 18–20. Retrieved from https://doi.org/10.1176/appi.ajp.2016.16070839

Brotman, M. A., Schmajuk, M., Rich, B. A., Dickstein, D. P., Guyer, A. E., Costello, E. J., . . . Leibenluft, E. (2006). Prevalence, clinical correlates, and longitudinal course of severe mood dysregulation in children. *Biological Psychiatry*, *60*(9), 991–997. Retrieved from https://doi.org/10.1016/j.biopsych.2006.08.042

Caprara, G. V., Paciello, M., Gerbino, M., & Cugini, C. (2007). Individual differences conducive to aggression and violence: Trajectories and correlates of irritability and hostile rumination through adolescence. *Aggressive Behavior*, *33*, 359–374. Retrieved from https://doi.org/DOI: 10.1002/ab.20192

Copeland, W. E., Brotman, M. A., & Costello, E. J. (2015). Normative irritability in youth: Developmental findings from the great smoky mountains study. *Journal of the American Academy of Child and Adolescent Psychiatry*, *54*(8), 635–642. Retrieved from https://doi.org/10.1016/j.jaac.2015.05.008

Copeland, W. E., Shanahan, L., Egger, H., Angold, A., & Costello, E. J. (2014). Adult diagnostic and functional outcomes of DSM-5 disruptive mood dysregulation disorder. *American Journal of Psychiatry*, *171*(6), 668–674. https://doi.org/10.1016/j.drugalcdep.2008.02.002.A

Cornacchio, D., Crum, K. I., Coxe, S., Pincus, D. B., & Comer, J. S. (2016). Irritability and severity of anxious symptomatology among youth with anxiety disorders. *Journal of* the *American Academy of Child and Adolescent Psychiatry*, 55(1), 54–61. Retrieved from https://doi.org/10.1016/j.jaac.2015.10.007

Deveney, C. M., Hommer, R. E., Reeves, E., Stringaris, A., Hinton, K. E., Haring, C. T., . . . Leibenluft, E. (2015). A prospective study of severe irritability in youths: 2- and 4-year follow-up. *Depression and Anxiety, 32*(5), 364–372. Retrieved from https://doi.org/10.1002/da.22336

Dougherty, L. R., Smith, V. C., Bufferd, S. J., Kessel, E., Carlson, G. A., & Klein, D. N. (2015). Preschool irritability predicts child psychopathology, functional impairment, and service use at age nine. *Journal of Child Psychology and Psychiatry, 56*(9), 999–1007. doi:10.1111/jcpp.12403

Fichter, M. M., Kohlboeck, G., Quadflieg, N., Wyschkon, A., & Esser, G. (2009). From childhood to adult age: 18-year longitudinal results and prediction of the course of mental disorders in the community. *Social Psychiatry and Psychiatric Epidemiology, 44*(9), 792–803. Retrieved from https://doi.org/10.1007/s00127-009-0501-y

Leibenluft, E., Cohen, P., Gorrindo, T., Brook, J. S., & Pine, D. S. (2006). Chronic versus episodic irritability in youth: A community-based, longitudinal study of clinical and diagnostic associations. *Journal of Child and Adolescent Psychopharmacology, 16*(4), 456–466. Retrieved from https://doi.org/10.1089/cap.2006.16.456

Leibenluft, E., & Stoddard, J. (2013). The developmental psychopathology of irritability. *Development and Psychopathology, 25*(4 Pt 2), 1473–1487. doi:10.1017/S0954579413000722

Mayes, S. D., Mathiowetz, C., Kokotovich, C., Waxmonsky, J., Baweja, R., Calhoun, S. L., & Bixler, E. O. (2015). Stability of disruptive mood dysregulation disorder symptoms (irritable-angry mood and temper outbursts) throughout childhood and adolescence in a general population sample. *Journal of Abnormal Child Psychology, 43*(8), 1543–1549. Retrieved from https://doi.org/10.1007/s10802-015-0033-8

Mulraney, M., Zendarski, N., Mensah, F., Hiscock, H., & Sciberras, E. (2016). Do early internalizing and externalizing problems predict later irritability in adolescents with attention-deficit/hyperactivity disorder? *Australian & New Zealand Journal of Psychiatry, 51*(4). Retrieved from https://doi.org/10.1177/0004867416659365

Pickles, A., Aglan, A., Collishaw, S., Messer, J., Rutter, M., & Maughan, B. (2010). Predictors of suicidality across the life span: The Isle of Wight study. *Psychological Medicine, 40*(9), 1453–1466. Retrieved from https://doi.org/10.1017/S0033291709991905

Savage, J., Verhulst, B., Copeland, W., Althoff, R. R., Lichtenstein, P., & Roberson-Nay, R. (2015). A genetically informed study of the longitudinal relation between irritability and anxious/depressed symptoms. *Journal of the American Academy of Child and Adolescent Psychiatry, 54*(5), 377–384. Retrieved from https://doi.org/10.1016/j.jaac.2015.02.010

Stringaris, A. (2011). Irritability in children and adolescents: A challenge for DSM-5. *European Child and Adolescent Psychiatry, 20*(2), 61–66. Retrieved from https://doi.org/10.1007/s00787-010-0150-4

Stringaris, A., Maughan, B., Copeland, W. S., Costello, E. J., & Angold, A. (2013). Irritable mood as a symptom of depression in youth: prevalence, developmental, and clinical correlates in the Great Smoky Mountains Study. *J Am Acad Child Adolesc Psychiatry, 52*(8), 831–840. doi:10.1016/j.jaac.2013.05.017

Stringaris, A., Cohen, P., Pine, D. S., & Leibenluft, E. (2009). Adult outcomes of youth irritability: A 20-year prospective community-based study. *American Journal of Psychiatry, 166*(9), 1048–1054. Retrieved from https://doi.org/10.1176/appi.ajp.2009.08121849.

Stringaris, A., & Goodman, R. (2009). Longitudinal outcome of youth oppositionality: Irritable, headstrong, and hurtful behaviors have distinctive predictions. *Journal of the American Academy of Child & Adolescent Psychiatry*, *48*(4), 404–412. Retrieved from https://doi.org/10.1097/CHI.0b013e3181984f30

Stringaris, A., Zavos, H., Leibenluft, E., Maughan, B., & Eley, T. C. (2012). Adolescent irritability: Phenotypic associations and genetic links with depressed mood. *American Journal of Psychiatry*, (169), 47–54.

Vidal-Ribas, P., Brotman, M. A., Valdivieso, I., Leibenluft, E., & Stringaris, A. (2016). The status of irritability in psychiatry: A conceptual and quantitative review. *Journal of the American Academy of Child and Adolescent Psychiatry*, *55*(7), 556–570. Retrieved from https://doi.org/10.1016/j.jaac.2016.04.014

Wakschlag, L. S., Estabrook, R., Petitclerc, A., Henry, D., Burns, J. L., Perlman, S. B., . . . Briggs-Gowan, M. L. (2015). Clinical Implications of a Dimensional Approach: The Normal:Abnormal Spectrum of Early Irritability. *Journal of the American Academy of Child and Adolescent Psychiatry*, *54*(8), 626–634. doi:10.1016/j.jaac.2015.05.016

Wiggins, J. L., Mitchell, C., Stringaris, A., & Leibenluft, E. (2014). Developmental trajectories of irritability and bidirectional associations with maternal depression. *Journal of the American Academy of Child and Adolescent Psychiatry*, *53*(11), 1191–1205.e4. Retrieved from https://doi.org/10.1016/j.jaac.2014.08.005

7

On Being Mad, Sad, and Very Young

Michael Potegal

Interest in children's temper tantrums has been renewed in the context of childhood irritability and the new diagnosis of disruptive mood dysregulation disorder (DMDD) in the latest edition of the *Diagnostic and Statistical Manual of Mental Disorders* (DSM-5), as chronicled by the other chapters in this volume. This chapter, with a side of data, is intended to place tantrums in broader cultural, behavioral, neurobiological, and evolutionary contexts. It describes what is known about the emotional/behavioral organization of tantrums and what remains unknown about their ontogeny, highlighting some of the lesser known, curious phenomenology. One aim is to note lines of investigation to be explored and discoveries yet to be made about young children's emotions and behavior. Sources for these musings include observations conveyed by parents in a number of tantrum research projects and/or seen on home videos that were collected, edited, and used to train parents to identify and record behaviors of interest. Some of my own personal observations are also included. What follows is mostly a meditation on tantrum emotions and behavior in typically developing children, with a few comments about parent guidance in tantrum management made along the way. Issues of psychopathology are addressed in the last section.

What Is a Tantrum?

Absent a generally agreed upon definition, Potegal (2000) defined tantrums operationally as transient episodes of affectively negative emotional behavior, usually a variable mix of anger and distress, with the negative affect shown by the child's facial expression. As is generally true, anger can lead to aggressive behavior. Some children in forager and village groups scream, throw things, and hit with hands and objects, often targeting the mother (Gorer, 1943; Hill & Hurtado, 1996; Maretzki & Maretzki, 1963) as do some children in industrialized societies (Belden,

Thomson, & Luby, 2008). Crying as part of tantrums appears universal. Tantrums typically involve interaction with parents, but because it is the children who have the tantrums, their emotions and behavior are the main focus of this essay.

Tantrums Are Common Across Cultures: Are They Universal?

Tantrums are a common phenomenon of early childhood. Surveys of young North American and British children published between 1954 and 1984 found that 50–83% had tantrums (Einon & Potegal, 1994). Based on an analysis of tantrum frequency distributions, the mean prevalence in these children from 18 months through 3 years of age was around 70% (Potegal & Archer, 2004). Tantrums are prevalent among young children in sites in the Netherlands (53%; Koot & Verhulst, 1991), rural and urban areas of China (59–71%; Li, Shi, Wan, Hotta, & Ushijima, 2001, Luk, Leung, Bacon-Shone, & Lieh-Mak, 1991), Canada (83%; Giesbrecht, 2008), and Finland (87%; Österman & Björkqvist, 2010). In a more recent community survey of almost 1,500 American preschoolers, parents reported that 84% had tantrums (Wakschlag et al., 2012).

According to Ward's (1970) remarkably detailed account of public tantrums in Kau Sai, a fishing village east of Hong Kong, it was common in 1952–53 and later, to see red-faced, kicking, screaming children (especially 5- to 10-year-old boys) lying on the public sidewalk with no one paying attention.

Although such detailed behavioral descriptions are often lacking, there are multiple reports of children's tantrums from non-Western cultures around the world; for example, in forager groups including the Aché in Paraguay (Hill & Hurtado, 1996), Matsigenkas in Peru (Johnson, 2003), Chewong of the Malaysian peninsula (at least occasionally, Howell, 1989), !Kung San of the Kalahari desert in northwestern Botswana (Konner, 1972), Hadza of north-central Tanzania (Marlowe, 2005), Utku Inuit in northern Canada (Briggs, 1970), and the aboriginal peoples of Australia (Myers, 1988; Peterson, 1993). Among the tribal groups of New Guinea, children of the Kahili (Schieffelin, 1986), Kapauka (Pospisil, 1971), Kubo (Dwyer & Minnegal, 2008), Sambia (Herdt, 1986), and Telefolmin (Jorgensen, 1984) have all been noted to tantrum. More localized differences in tantrum prevalence have also been reported between Gujarati and English children living in Manchester (Hackett & Hackett, 1993), Black 6-year-olds in the United States versus those in Johannesburg (Barbarin, 1999), and among ethnic minorities in China (Li et al., 2001).

Correspondingly, queries of native language speakers/professional translators/ language scholars suggest that there are words or phrases equivalent to the child-connoting English "tantrum" in the major languages of the world, including Arabic, Bengali, French, German, Portuguese, and Spanish. These words denote the emotion of anger and its concomitant behaviors, as well as crying and other indices of distress such as dropping to the floor. They are similar to English usage of "tantrum" in that, when applied to an adult, these words connote that the individual is acting childishly. This common usage in diverse language groups implies long experience with tantrums as a characteristic of children in many places around the world. A few of these words and phrases conjure visual images. The Spanish "pataleta" conveys a picture of stamping or kicking legs; "rabieta" evokes the madness of rabies. The most picturesque might be the Dutch "kinderlicht driftbui" with its image of a small childhood rainstorm that comes and goes. There are colloquialisms in Mandarin Chinese, Hindi, and Russian to denote/describe anger and tantrum behaviors, but they may be applied to adults and children equally and require adjectival or other modification to specify the childish nature of the behaviors.

Given that a number of major languages do have an equivalent of "tantrum," might those that lack one be associated with cultural traditions that consider the doings of children as less significant or name-worthy than the affairs of adults? Or, are there societies in which children have minimal to few tantrums? Anthropologists and other observers have noted that infants in a number of non-Western cultures, like the former agro-pastoralist Gusii of Western Kenya, cry much less than babies in Western cultures. This is attributed to child-rearing practices that include close and continual proximity to mothers who immediately attend to any signs of distress. However, this level of attention is relinquished during and after weaning, at which point Gusii children do have tantrums (LeVine & LeVine, 1963). Alternatively, might tantrums be even more common than the prevalence figures suggest, viewed as a necessary part of emotional development? For example, respondents in only 7 of 24 societies listed tantrums as among the top 10 behavioral problems of preschool-age children (Rescorla et al., 2011). This is not to say that children are not having tantrums but that they may not be viewed as problematic.

EMOTIONAL/BEHAVIORAL ORGANIZATION OF TANTRUMS: THE ANGER/DISTRESS MODEL

Anger and distress have been identified as the two major emotional/behavioral components of children's tantrums. Factor analyses of parent-reported tantrum behaviors of 335 typically developing American 18- to 60-month-olds (Potegal & Davidson, 2003) as well as staff-observed 5- to 12-year-old child psychiatry inpatients (Potegal, Carlson, Margulies, Gutkovitch, & Wall, 2009) consistently differentiated and characterized separate anger- and distress-related factors. The anger-related factors include the vocalizations *shout* and *scream* and the behaviors *stamp, throw, hit,* and *kick. Run away* is an unusual anger behavior in that it involves avoidance rather than approach (Eisenberg et al., 1999), while *arch/stiffen* is an anger behavior that has apparent reflex-like properties, as noted later.

Distress-related factors include the vocalizations *whine* and *cry* and the behaviors *down* and *comfort-seek. Down* is mostly about dramatic drops to the floor but is scored to include any major/showy lowering of the head and/or slumping of the body. *Comfort-seek* includes verbal or physical appeals such as asking to sit on a parent's lap, approaching and touching parent, and raising arms to be picked up. The major emotion in distress is sadness, but the term "distress" is used to cover behaviors that might not routinely be included in sadness, such as dropping to the floor.

The anger–distress distinction has been replicated in tantrums of Canadian 3- to 5-year-olds as the best fitting solution of exploratory-confirmatory factor analyses using oblique factors (Giesbrecht, Miller, & Muller, 2010) as well as in clinic referred 2.5- to 5.5-year-olds with behavior problems (Eisbach et al., 2014). Qualitatively similar findings in Prader–Willi syndrome (Tunnicliffe, Woodcock, Bull, Oliver, & Penhallow, 2014) suggest model utility in pathological populations. These confirmations of two independent emotional/behavioral processes retire older notions that tantrums may be driven by some single motivational process, with distress and anger behaviors being triggered at different levels of that process (Potegal et al., 2003).

Within the anger-distress model, the two emotions have been further factorially and temporally differentiated. Anger factors can be easily ordered into progressive levels of intensity based on their respective behaviors and their differential association with parent ratings of global severity and autonomic activation (Potegal et al., 2003). Low, intermediate, and high anger factors were identified in the tantrums of both typically developing younger children (Potegal & Davidson, 2003) and psychiatrically disturbed older children (Potegal et al., 2009); the individual behaviors included in each factor were similar in the two samples despite gross differences in age and psychopathological status (e.g., low anger included *stamp*, high anger included *scream*). Belden et al.'s (2008) destructive aggressive and nondestructive aggressive tantrum factors in clinical and nonclinical samples of 3- to 6-year-olds overlap with the high and low anger factors, respectively. Within distress, *whine* and *down* have been identified as indicating lower intensity sadness, whereas *cry* and *comfort seek* are associated with higher intensity sadness.

Discriminant analyses of the acoustic characteristics of tantrum vocalizations support these categorical and intensity classifications (Green, Whitney, & Potegal, 2011). Within the anger category, shouts and screams were acoustically similar, with steep frequency increases at onset reaching high peak frequencies. This pair of vocalizations differed markedly from the whines and cries of distress, which showed gradual frequency increase at onset and lower peak frequencies. Within categories, screams were more energetic than shouts while cries were more energetic than whines, consistent with the previous identification of behaviors indicating higher and lower levels of emotion.

Behavior Trajectories

Anger- and distress-related behaviors also follow different temporal trajectories. In general, anger peaks early in the tantrum, then declines, while distress remains relatively constant throughout. Variations on this theme include findings that the high, intermediate, and low anger behaviors of the older child psychiatry inpatients were all maximum at tantrum onset and declined in roughly exponential fashion (see figure 1 in Potegal et al., 2009). Cluster analysis of the slopes of the decline confirmed the factor-analytic grouping of anger behaviors by intensity. Slopes of distress behaviors were not different from 0. Distress behaviors in the parent-reported tantrums of 1- to 5-year-olds (Potegal et al., 2003) were distributed across the tantrum relatively evenly, but the *comfort-seeking* component increased as the tantrum neared its end.

More recently, the duration of all behaviors in 193 beginning-to-end videos of tantrums at home of 88 2- and 3-year-olds were measured to the nearest second; each brief behavior, like a hit, was assigned a duration of 1 sec (Potegal, unpublished data). Calculation of behavior rates as sec/min of tantrum further supported the anger-distress distinction. We found all anger behaviors to be brief and intermittent, whereas all distress behaviors were prolonged and semi-continuous. The mean rate of each anger behavior was less than 4.5 sec/min; the mean rate of each distress behavior was greater than 4.5 sec/min.

In these new tantrum video data, a cluster analysis identified three trajectory groups. Anger in one group was high and maximum at onset and declined substantially thereafter, as it did in the older child psychiatry inpatients (Potegal et al., 2009). In the second group, anger was lower at onset and rose to a major peak in the first half of the tantrum, as it did in the parent-reported 3- to 5-year-olds (Potegal et al., 2003). Anger in the third group declined slightly across the tantrum. Importantly, distress had the same flat profile in all three groups. In all cases, distress typically outlasts anger, so tantrums end when crying and whining stop. Temporal relations of anger and distress may be preserved independent of tantrum duration. We have incidentally observed micro tantrums in which a single brief anger display was followed by a single brief distress display (e.g., a shout followed by a head drop, with the whole sequence lasting only a few seconds).

While states of anger and distress expressed within a child's tantrum function as independent factors, children who are irritable are also prone to sadness and to tantrums, so these traits are correlated across children (Bufferd, Doughtery, & Olino, 2017). This correlation speaks to generalized negative affectivity and deficits in emotion regulation that promote tantrums.

Back Arching as an Emotion-Gated Reflex

When restrained or picked up, angry and resistant children may stiffen, arch their backs, and tilt their heads back (technically, an axial hyperextension). Arching was the only child behavior to have a statistically significant association with parent intervention (Potegal et al., 2003); this is because arching can be triggered by contact. Back arching clearly depends on emotional state; children who are picked up when in a positive mood do not arch and may even cling or cuddle. In fact, contact-elicited arching loaded heavily on high anger in the tantrum factor analysis (Potegal et al., 2003). Parent report as well as my personal observations indicate that arching occurs quite rapidly. In typical parent–child ventral-ventral holding, back arching may seem to function as an escape response, moving the child backward away from the parent. However, videotapes of a standard experimental arm restraint situation show 15-month-olds arching backward even when briefly restrained from behind by their mother, although arching brought them closer to her (Potegal, Robison, Anderson, Jordan, & Shapiro, 2007). One mother reported having lost front teeth while holding her young son whose arching caused his head to strike her jaw. Arching in response to contact is not an escape response but a forceful reflex-like reaction with relatively fixed topography.

In its rapid triggering by contact, stereotyped topography, and dependence on emotional state, arching resembles the "state-dependent" reflexes of attack that have been demonstrated in several animal species. Normally, animals will withdraw from a touch on the lips or paw, but when aggression-related areas of hypothalamus are stimulated, lip contact will elicit a bite while paw contact will provoke a paw strike (for review, see Kruk, 1991). Aggressive motivation gates these reflexes into an operational mode so that attack responses can be executed quickly. Tantrum anger may similarly gate reflex arching.

Autonomic/Endocrine Activation

Autonomic activation plays a prominent, if contentious, role in emotion (e.g., Levenson, 2014 vs. Quigley & Barrett, 2014). In tantrums, signs of autonomic activation may be visible on the child's face. In the parent reported tantrums of the 18- to 60-month-olds, 26% involved sympathetic facial flushing with or without sweating (c.f., Drummond & Quah, 2001); parasympathetic salivation (drooling and spitting) and rhinorrhea (nose-running) were each reported in 6% or less of these tantrums (Potegal, 2000; lacrimation (tears) are certainly the most common parasympathetic response in tantrums but were not recorded separately from crying in this study). Tantrums with flushing were significantly longer, contained more elements, and were more intense than those without flushing. Flushing was most closely correlated with high anger behaviors (cf. table 1 in Levenson, 2014). Accordingly, flushing first appeared toward the beginning of the tantrum, as it would if associated with anger, rather than toward the end, as it would if it were just associated with vigorous and protracted physical activity. These effects were stronger for the younger children. Negative post-tantrum mood was predicted by greater autonomic arousal during the tantrum. Because facial indicators of autonomic activation do not require physiological equipment to measure and are easy for parents to assess, they have a potential use in parent-report studies as a marker of autonomic arousal.

Secretion of the "stress" hormone cortisol has been associated with sadness, but not anger, during infants' reactions to goal blockage (Lewis, Ramsay, & Sullivan, 2006). In our small study of 3-year-olds who were having at least 1–2 tantrums/ week lasting at least 2–4 minutes, salivary cortisol was measured under three conditions: baseline (at 9 AM, 2 PM, and bedtime), post-tantrum (at 20, 40, and 60 minutes after a tantrum), and non-tantrum yoked time control (at the same times of day on the next day when the child did not have a tantrum; Potegal, 2003). Parents recorded all tantrums on a 6-week calendar. Mean salivary cortisol at baseline was correlated with tantrum frequency ($r = .47$) but not with mean duration. Cortisol secretion was increased by having a tantrum, as indicated by a 27% rise over the yoked control sample at the 20-minute point followed by an apparent drop below control levels at 40 minutes and a return to control levels at 60 minutes. These effects were stronger in boys than girls and in the morning than the afternoon. In these 3-year-olds, as in Spinrad et al's (2009) study of preschoolers, there were no specific associations of cortisol with anger or distress behaviors.

Measuring Tantrum Intensity

For any particular child, some tantrums appear more intense than others. Having a validated measure of tantrum intensity could prove useful in determining a given child's sensitivities and triggers as well as in identifying psychopathological extremes in a population. How, then, to measure intensity? Longer duration would seem to indicate greater intensity (Wakschlag et al., 2012). For example, tantrums that included *stamp* or *down* (i.e., low level anger or distress) within their first 30 sec were shorter than those that did not (Potegal et al., 2003); a similar result was obtained with low anger *push* in the video data. But the intensity–duration correlation may be true only up to a point. Some analyses suggest that tantrums of typically developing children longer than 15, 20, or 25 min (depending on the dataset) are less intense (Potegal & Qiu, 2010); these may be primarily weepy tantrums (Einon & Potegal, 1994). Autonomic activation of the face is another obvious potential indicator of intensity. However, there are likely to be substantial individual differences in autonomic reactivity; some children may flush with the slightest anger, others, particularly older children, may not visibly flush no matter how angry they become.

Belden et al. (2008) identified three levels of intensity in 3- to 6-year-olds: (1) tantrums that rarely escalate to excessive crying or shouting and include no throwing, hitting, or kicking directed at property or people; (2) tantrums that include crying, shouting, and/or nondirected flailing but no aggression against property or people; and (3) tantrums that do include aggression against property or people. The most systematic work on intensity has been Wakschlag et al's (2012) development of a temper loss scale for 3- to 5-year-olds. Behavior characteristics specific to tantrums that are above the 95th percentile for the population sampled on this scale are listed here in descending order of severity:

Hit, bite, or kick
Tantrum from "out of the blue"
Break or destroy things
Tantrum until exhausted

Tantrum in the presence of a nonparental adult
Tantrum longer than 5 min
Stamp feet or hold breath

Indeed, hit and kick are high anger behaviors in the anger-distress model while stamp is a low anger behavior (it is a bit surprising that stamp made the 95th percentile cut). "Out of the blue" is reminiscent of psychopathological adult anger responses to little or no provocation in, for example, intermittent explosive disorder. "Tantrum until exhausted" is a relatively rare extreme that has been associated with anxiety in aggressively abused children (Furman, 1986). In contrast, a 5-minute tantrum is just the upper end of the average range in estimates of tantrum duration for younger children and may be in the middle of the average range for older children. The significance of tantrums in the presence of a nonparental adult is that most tantrums occur at home and involve the parents (Einon & Potegal, 1994; Potegal & Davidson, 2003).

When tantrums are part of aversive/coercive child–parent interactions, their severity is very likely to increase with repetition (Snyder, 2015). In any event, from a research perspective, tantrums at the upper end of their severity range provide a window onto emotions so intense as to be otherwise unavailable to routine scientific observation. (A short questionnaire to assess the severity of a child's tantrums by their impact on family life is available from the author.)

How Behavior Classifications Might Be Used to Quantify Tantrum Severity

Grouping behaviors by level implies that stamping, pushing, and throwing are generated at lower levels of anger while screaming, hitting, and kicking are generated at higher levels. Under certain simplifying assumptions, this hypothesis predicts that a content analysis of sets of tantrums from individual children could be used to quantify intensity. To wit, as anger rises from its pre-tantrum baseline, it must pass through lower levels before reaching whatever maximum level it achieves during the tantrum. Similarly, anger must descend through lower levels during its return to baseline. Anger behaviors during a tantrum must therefore be a mix of those generated while anger is rising or descending through lower levels and others generated while anger is near or at the highest level it reaches in that tantrum. Consequently, if a tantrum features high anger behaviors, it is also likely to include lower level behaviors. However, a tantrum can contain lower level behaviors without including any higher level ones. Letting L = low anger and H = high anger behaviors, tantrums would be expected to contain L, or L and H, but not H alone. The assumption that sufficient time is spent at lower and higher levels for behaviors to be generated at those levels is justified by the long descent of tantrum anger. Suitable adjustment for different base rates of the various behaviors would need to be made. Because of individual differences, such analyses would need to be carried out on sets of tantrums for each child.

A more fully developed model, the *anger intensity-behavioral linkage function model*, fits the distribution of low and high anger behaviors across the tantrum by reconstructing the rise and fall of anger as a latent variable, Momentary anger [MA(t)], which reflects the intensity of anger at each time point in the tantrum, and a set of unique linkage functions through which MA(t) controls the probability of each angry behavior. MA(t) has been modeled as a beta function; the linkage functions were modeled as logistic-polynomial composites (Potegal & Qiu, 2010; Qiu, Yang, & Potegal, 2009).

Faking It

Finally, intensity assessments must take into account when the child might be faking. Parents report children doing things that suggest they are not necessarily or always caught up in irresistible emotion. Before dropping to the floor, they may look around for a soft place to fall. They may reduce crying when parents leave the room and increase it when they return. Our home videos revealed a little girl who stopped wailing long enough to take a bite of her bread, then resumed where she left off. One particular 3-year-old boy appeared to be a master of tantrum-as-manipulation. In one video in which he was seated with his face buried in the crook of his elbow, the camera caught his surreptitious glance up at his mother. While kneeling on the floor during another tantrum with his back to his mother, he said "You can't see the tears on my face." Her off-camera voice could be heard acknowledging this (while trying not to laugh). Tantrums with such indicators of faking should get the lowest intensity score, obviously.

TANTRUM DAILY TIMING, MOTIVATIONS, AND FUNCTIONS

Circadian Rhythms

Goodenough's (1931) pioneering diary study, *Anger in Young Children*, found what we would now recognize as a circadian rhythm in tantrums, with a morning peak (about 11 AM) and a late afternoon/early evening peak (roughly 4–7 PM). A probability analysis of tantrum time-of-day data collected in 1994–95, more than 60 years later, replicated the morning and late afternoon/early evening peaks (Potegal & Kosorok, 1995, see Figure 7.1). A late afternoon peak in discomfort is not unique to toddler tantrums. Positive affect in healthy adults reaches a peak around 2 PM and declines steadily through the rest of the day (Hasler, Mehl, Bootzin, & Vazire, 2008; Miller et al., 2015). Processes underlying such mood shifts may contribute to similar, temporally localized distress in vulnerable populations across the lifespan, such as the late afternoon/early evening crying in colicky infants (White, Gunnar, Larson, Donzella, & Barr, 2000) and a 3–4 PM peak in "sundowning" agitation in individuals with dementia (Cipriani, Lucetti, Carlesi, Danti, & Nuti, 2015).

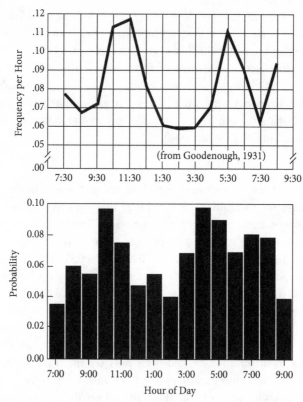

FIGURE 7.1 *Upper graph: Figure 2 from Goodenough (1931) shows tantrums per hour as a function of time of day calculated from diary accounts of 1,842 tantrums had by 45 children between infancy and 7 years of age. Lower graph: Poisson probability of a tantrum as a function of time of day, calculated from the Potegal and Davidson (2003) telephone survey of the most recent tantrum had by 991 children, 18 to 60 months old, with adjustment for the time of the telephone call.*

Upper graph reproduced with permission of the University of Minnesota Press. Florence L. Goodenough, *Anger in Young Children*, Institute of Child Welfare Monograph Series No. 9 (University of Minnesota Press, 1931). Copyright 1931 by the University of Minnesota. Renewed 1959.

Emotional Functions and Emotion Dynamics

From an individual perspective, anger functions to forestall or limit a threat while sadness mourns a loss that has already occurred (Lench, Tibbett, & Bench, 2016). Other views stress the social interactional functions of emotions. Even when prompted by internal experiences of hunger, fatigue, or discomfort, the vast majority of tantrums involve the young child's conflict with parents or siblings. From a social/emotional perspective, tantrum anger is about establishing or maintaining autonomy, demanding her way about this or that (or frustration about not getting his way), and/or resisting unwanted or intrusive demands. In this, it resembles adult anger, which has evolved as a more-or-less automatic reaction to fend off threat, forestall attack, and assert demands (Fessler, 2010; Sell, Cosmides, & Tooby, 2014). Anger mostly involves approach motivation, but angry adults actively avoid confrontation with socially dominant individuals and distance themselves from socially awkward encounters (Harmon-Jones, Gable, & Peterson, 2010; Kuppens, VanMechelen, & Meulders, 2004) much like the children who run away.

From a functional perspective, distress, which includes sadness, is about eliciting parental comfort-giving. Other things equal, we tend to comfort a child who is crying (Swain, Mayes, & Leckman, 2004). Because the distress components of a tantrum always outlast the anger, they function to generate child comfort-seeking and parental comfort-giving, repairing the social bonds broken by the child's preceding anger. Analysis of recorded marital exchanges suggest that anger and sadness in adult conflicts occur in the same combination and sequence and function in the same way, with the expression of sadness and distress reducing the partner's aggression and eliciting expressions of sympathy and support (Biglan, Lewin, & Hops, 1990; c.f. Katz, Jones, & Beach, 2000).

A noteworthy aspect of tantrum emotion dynamics revealed in the video recordings is the reciprocal relationship between anger and comfort-seeking. Although distress as a whole remained constant across the tantrum, the frequency of its comfort-seeking component accelerated in the last fraction of the tantrum as anger declined, suggesting that the decline in children's anger disinhibits their seeking for, and acceptance of, comforting.

Reconciliation (or Not) at Tantrum Termination

The most typical tantrum aftermath is for children to simply resume their usual activities. In 29–35% of parent reports, a young child's tantrum ended with a hug, cuddle, or other gesture of reconciliation, representing some intersection of child distress and parent comfort-giving (Einon & Potegal, 1994; Potegal & Davidson, 1997). In some cases, parents consoled children who passively accepted it. In others, reconciliation was solicited or initiated by the child who approached the parent (almost always the mother), leaned against her, raised arms up to her, or clutched her leg. Older children might apologize verbally. Various markers of stress and of physical separation between parent and child during the tantrum predicted reconciliation. Labeling such events "post-tantrum reconciliation," Potegal and Davidson (1997) treated them as if they had occurred after the tantrum was over. It might be more appropriate to consider them as a last stage of the tantrum in which distress is resolved.

"Therapeutic Holding" and Reconciliation

Therapeutic holding is a controversial procedure for enhancing child–parent attachment that was popularized by Welch (1989) and advocated by some attachment therapists for use with children with autism. The most recent report, with the largest sample, of what is now called Prolonged Parent-Child Embrace (PP-CE, Welch et al., 2006) defines four stages: (1) during confrontation, the adult (usually the mother) holds the child face to face, demands the child meet her gaze, and begins to express and elicit talk about feelings. (2) If the child was not already agitated when the adult began, her or his discomfort and irritability escalates into resisting and struggling in the conflict (formerly, "rejection") stage. During this stage, the adult forcefully holds the child no matter how strongly she or he fights. Parents are taught to tolerate the child's strongest emotional outbursts, to persist through the rejection, and to express their own intense feelings of fear, anger, or hurt, communicating that "nothing can come between us." Conflict/rejection stage restraint and struggling continue for 20–90 minutes, whereupon both mother and child reportedly experience (3) a sudden and profound transition to relaxation and strong feelings of bonding, marking the resolution stage of reciprocal embrace, caressing, kissing, and conversation. (4) Resolution is followed by synchrony, a state of calm arousal with attunement and reciprocity. "These latter stages were characterized by breathing in unison, deep mutual gaze, relaxation, reciprocal pleasure in each other's embrace, and open verbal and non-verbal communication" (Welch et al., 2006, p. 6). To Mercer's (2013) review of this literature should be added Stirling and McHugh's (1998) single case report and Sourander, Aurela, and Piha's (1994) report of nine child patients, all reportedly showing the four-stage sequence. Comments by a few Scottish adolescents who solicited therapeutic restraint by staff of the residential facilities to which they had been committed due to their aggressive behavior seem to confirm their experience of this sequence (Steckley, 2011).

Of course, physical restraint as in the PP-CE procedure is a classic trigger for tantrums (Watson & Watson, 1921). Indeed, the PP-CE Conflict stage is actually a tantrum. But, what is of greater theoretical interest is that the continuing restraint amplifies and prolongs the emotions of anger and distress such that reconciliation (the Resolution phase) then becomes more probable and more intense. This outcome is surprising. Perhaps forcing extreme and prolonged activation of neural networks that normally generate tantrum emotions and their associated behaviors creates some sort of opponent process situation in which the eventual exhaustion of intense anger against the background of continuing distress releases and amplifies impulses toward reconciliation, creating catharsis-like feelings.

To be sure, the methodology and reported successes of the published studies of therapeutic holding/PP-CE have been severely criticized, as have the ethics of such coercive procedures; fatalities have resulted from excessive restraint in related "therapeutic" situations (Mercer, 2013). While in no way advocating the use of therapeutic holding, the several reported replications of the sequence through the resolution phase imply that a complete theory of tantrum emotion dynamics must account for this striking phenomenon.

Are Tantrums Emotional Reactions, Behavioral Operants, or Both?

At first, tantrums may be primarily emotionally driven reactions over which the child has little control, an extension of infant crying. While retaining the emotional core, children learn through experience of outcomes to use tantrums as operants (albeit energetically and emotionally costly ones; McCurdy, Kunz, & Sheridan, 2006). Children may differ (or an individual child may differ from tantrum to tantrum) with regard to the mix of emotional push and reinforcer pull. Compare the tantrum in which the child stops abruptly when she or he is given what was demanded versus the one in which the child continues to tantrum after she or he is offered the originally desired item but then refuses it (Einon & Potegal, 1994).

In contrast to modeling tantrums as a mix of two emotions and the acts they engender, *applied behavior analysis* (ABA) treats tantrums as an operant, one among a number of undesirable/aversive behaviors that function either to obtain "tangibles" (preferred foods, objects, activities) and/or attention (negative attention being better than no attention; e.g., Harding et al., 2001) or to escape from unwanted demands (every second a child tantrums is a second he is not, e.g., getting ready for bed; Carr & Newsome, 1985; Ingvarsson, Hanley, & Welter, 2009). The functions just noted are listed in increasing order of their likelihood as tantrum motivators (Matson et al., 2011). Parenthetically, a tantrum in reaction to a demand to stop doing A and start doing B is better understood as an escape from demand rather than as a response to a "transition." ABA analyses are not always successful in establishing function, and it might be that tantrums motivated by tangibles, attention, or escape differ in particular behaviors, anger–distress ratio, overall severity, or other observable emotional/behavioral characteristics that would help identify their function.

Although ABA is a branch of behavioral psychology that mostly deals with individuals who are developmentally delayed or autistic, these categories are applicable to typically developing children. They suggest the approaches of *planned ignoring* for tantrums for tangibles or attention but *adult hand-over-child hand* physical guidance for escape-driven tantrums (Kern, Delaney, Hilt, Bailin, & Elliott, 2002). Planned ignoring requires not talking to or looking at the child, which parents may find difficult to do. Inadvertent parental attention, positive and/or negative, may explain the maintenance of tantrums despite their seeming cost. When planned ignoring is first introduced, an "extinction burst" of escalated tantrums is likely to follow (Vollmer et al., 1998) consistent with their identity as operants.

Tantrums and Oppositionality

Deliberate disobedience increases in the second year of life (Baillargeon, Keenan, & Cao, 2012; Lorber, Del Vecchio, & Slep, 2015). Tantrums may be immediately preceded by a period of oppositional behaviors, as I saw with my own daughter and as reported by other parents (Einon & Potegal, 1994), and as Eisbach et al. (2014) observed to precipitate 52% of the tantrums of 2- to 5.5-year-olds in the clinic. These children's oppositional behaviors included doing things they knew were against the rules as well as refusing to comply with specific parental commands.

The oppositionality–tantrum sequence may be interpreted as reflecting a child's escalating struggle for autonomy, irritable mood, or both. "Often loses temper" is one of the criteria for a diagnosis of oppositional defiant disorder (ODD), but how sensitive oppositional behaviors actually are as a predictor of tantrums (i.e., what percent of oppositional periods are followed by a tantrum) remains to be determined.

Parent Intervention

Tantrums can irritate parents and bystanders, too. Rhesus macaque mothers and their infants were attacked by other troop members more often when the infants were crying (Semple, Gerald, & Suggs, 2009). Although such attacks were rare, the mothers allowed infants to nurse significantly more often when around troop members who were likely to attack. Whining and crying can be aversive to human parents (Sokol, Webster, Thompson, & Stevens, 2005; Soltis, 2004), and the unpleasantness of tantrums for parents, especially mothers, has often been noted (e.g., Hill & Hurtado, 1996; Maretzki & Maretzki, 1963). In Western society, excessive infant crying can lead to infanticide, fantasied (Levitzky & Cooper, 2000) or actual (Porter & Gavin, 2010).

In a myth of the Yolngu of eastern Arnhem Land, a child having a tantrum was transformed into a sea-eagle (Morphy, 1989). When that doesn't happen, parents may intervene. While mothers in some cultures fend off blows without restraining the child or retaliating (e.g., Gorer, 1943; Peterson, 1993), even the tolerant Chewong, who routinely ignore tantrums, may shout at the child to stop (Howell, 1989). The less tolerant Matsigenkas reportedly subjected toddlers who tantrumed frequently to scalding baths (Johnson, 1981) while Gusii and Okinawan mothers may hit them (LeVine & LeVine, 1963; Maretzki & Maretzki, 1963). In some groups, an adult dressed as a ghost or local folklore monster appears to the terrified children who are told that the apparition will get them if they don't stop their tantrums (and other misbehavior; Maretzki & Maretzki, 1963; Nydegger & Nydegger, 1963).

In Potegal and Davidson's (2003) study, parents reported intervening in 79% of tantrums. Intervention probability was unrelated to the child's age or sex; it did increase with reported tantrum duration and intensity. Parent intervention was associated with higher rates of tantrum behavior, especially arch/stiffen, which is a response to being restrained, picked up, carried, or dressed (Potegal et al., 2003). These effects were confirmed in the video data by the finding that the tantrums in which anger rose and peaked during the first half all involved forcible parental intervention. The nature and consequences of parental action depend on culture, varying from those in which older children and adults may routinely tease younger children into tantrums (McSwain, 1981; Ward, 1970), to those in which parents ignore tantrums, to those in which children are punished for tantrums. In Western culture, harsh, punitive parenting is associated with child behavior problems, including tantrums, but these effects are moderated by the overall parent–child relationship and by subcultural context (Brenner & Fox, 1998; Deater-Deckard & Dodge, 1997).

TANTRUM ONTOGENY, AGE TRENDS, AND CESSATION

Episodes of generalized emotional distress have been claimed to differentiate into recognizable emotions, including anger, as early as 4–6 months of age (Potegal & Archer, 2004; Lewis, 2010; but see Camras, 2011); anger as a distinct emotion becomes more readily elicitable through 16 months (Braungart-Rieker, Hill-Soderlund, & Karrass, 2010). Some of these episodes may become recognizable as tantrums during the second year of life. They may persist for a few years, with the majority of children studied giving them up by age 4 or 5.

Frequency and Duration

Among the younger children who have tantrums, estimates of mean frequencies range between 1–9/week (Bufferd et al., 2017; Van Leeuwen, Bourgonjon, Huijsman, Van Meenen, & De Pauw, 2009, Sullivan & Lewis, 2012, Belden et al., 2008; Potegal & Davidson, 2003); modal rates across several older studies were 3–6/week (Potegal & Archer, 2004). Complementary to the 3–6/week mode, several authors have cited the percent of children having 1 or more tantrums/day as a marker of more extreme subpopulations. According to Grover (2008), at least 20% of 2-year-olds, 18% of 3-year-olds, and 10% of 4-year-olds have at least one temper tantrum every day. These figures may overestimate percentages of daily tantrumers in the older groups; Wakschlag et al. (2012) reported fewer than 9% among 3- to 5-year-olds. Potegal and Archer (2004, fig. 1) estimated less than 5% for 4-year-olds. Establishing the 95th percentile for tantrum frequency might provide a useful cutoff for clinical purposes. Per Bufferd et al. (2017, Table 2), 1.5 tantrums/day is at the 95th percentile for 3- to 5-year-olds as a group. Taken together, these reports suggest that the 95th percentile for tantrum frequency might be around 2/day for 3-year-olds falling to 1/day for 4-year-olds.

Grover's (2008) figures are consistent with the reduction in frequency with age reported in other cross-sectional data (Potegal & Davidson, 2003, see Figure 1 in Potegal & Archer, 2004). Reductions in tantrum frequency were accompanied by increases in mean duration, from 2 min in 18- to 24-month-olds to 5 min in 54- to 60-month-olds (Potegal & Davidson, 2003). The more accurate video data confirmed that the median tantrum duration for 2- to 3-year-olds was around 4 min. Such an increase in duration with age is consistent with mean durations of 12–16 min in studies that included children up to 6 or older (Belden et al., 2008; Österman & Björkqvist, 2010). However, an increase in mean duration with age in cross-sectional studies might result from children with shorter tantrums ceasing to tantrum earlier. A longitudinal study involving three reports at 6-month intervals by parents of 13- to 67-month-olds found both frequency and duration to decrease with age (Van Leeuwen et al., 2009; personal communication October 4, 2017). To complicate matters further, Goodenough (1931) found 1–4 min tantrum durations in children from infancy to 7 years, while Mireault and Trahan (2007) reported a mean 16 min duration in 3- to 5-year-olds. In these studies, standard deviations were large compared to means and/or a large percentage of tantrums were in the shorter end of the duration range, both effects being due to the long tails of the duration distributions (see Figure 1 in Potegal et al., 2003). Overall, tantrum frequency decreases with age while age effects on duration remain to be determined.

Tantrum Onset: Is There a "Transition Event?"

Episodes recognizable as tantrums emerge in the second year of life, for a few children as early as 12 months and for many more by 18 months. Three studies with direct home and/or lab observation or contemporaneous parent reports of children starting at 3–15 months found no or few tantrums before 15 months but numerous tantrums occurring from 18–30 months (Chen, Green, & Gustafson, 2009; Kopp, 1992; Minde & Tidmarsh, 1997). Chen et al.'s (2009) recordings of protest vocalizations against maternal prohibitions included no screams at 6 months but screaming in response to 34–35% of prohibitions at 12 and 18 months. If mothers count just screaming as a tantrum, then more children will be reported to tantrum at 12 months. This may account for mothers' reports of a mean age at tantrum onset as 53–58 weeks in Sullivan and Lewis's (2012) study. This interpretation is supported by a greater than doubling of the number of behaviors reported per tantrum from 12 to 20 months in this study. Tantrum frequency and the number of different contexts in which tantrums occurred also increased significantly from 12 to 20 months. Österman and Björkvist's (2010) retrospective parent survey of 105 past or current tantrumers (out of 132 children) up to 13 years old also found few tantrums before 12 months. However, 65% of onsets were reported to have occurred between 2 and 4 years, with the latest onset at 7 years. Such reports of later onset may be influenced by a memory bias related to the longer periods over which these parents were asked to recall early child behavior.

An apparent emergence or noticeable increase in tantrums for many children around 18 months may relate to improved motor control and ability to maintain attention to desired but unavailable objects and activities. Wenar (1982) noted a "negativity" beginning around this time and lasting for a few years that may have to do with new frustrations associated with emerging awareness of the self (Kopp, 1992). However, there are anecdotal reports of children who had tantrums for only a few weeks, only a few times, or, in several cases, only once. These time-limited events reportedly occurred around 18 months of age. Such accounts, together with Sullivan and Lewis's (2012) report of an increase in the number of tantrum elements from 12 to 20 months and observations of my own daughter suggest that various tantrum behaviors like hitting and dropping to the floor may come online and be practiced between 12 and 18 months (only after walking has become reliably independent at 13–15 months can parents discriminate voluntary dropping to the floor from accidental falling). Well-documented increases in physical aggression in the

TABLE 7.1 In-home observations of tantrum-related behavior onsets of a female child from 10 to 28 months

Age (Months)	First Observation of the Behavior
10	Began walking at 47 weeks
12–13	Stamping when restrained
15	Ran away when upset
15.5	When angry, hit parent within reach. Hitting continued over several weeks then stopped and kicking became more frequent
16.5	Dropped to floor - a few times in same day
19.5	First clearly recognizable tantrum, triggered by taking something away from her. No new behaviors, but more intense and much longer (5 min) event
21	1) Use of verbal "No" (learned from children at daycare), 2) Clearly deliberate disobedience, 3) Approached parent from a distance to hit
23	Spate of longer and more intense tantrums with extreme arching during a viral illness
25	1–2 tantrums/day, most brief, a few prolonged, triggered by trivial or undetectable events (given the wrong color pacifier?), with directed hitting, arching, dropping
28	Head butts, perhaps intended as play but painful, never occurred in tantrums

second year (Alink et al., 2006; Lorber et al., 2015) likely include the first appearance of intended/aimed aggressive hitting, kicking, etc. There then may be a developmental change indicated by a "transition event," perhaps the first fully formed, longest, and/or most intense tantrum up to that point, which heralds a period of more frequent, longer, and more intense tantrums in which the more recently developed behaviors are added to the whining, crying, and arching of earlier infancy. The order of appearance of new tantrum elements and how tantrums emerge is an interesting and unexplored aspect of tantrum ontogeny. A timeline of events for a personally observed female child is shown in Table 7.1, with what would count as a transition event at 19.5 months.

Notes Toward a Study of Transition Events/First Tantrums

Behavioral characteristics that differ before versus after a tantrum transition event might include (1) an increase in the number/kind of stimuli that trigger tantrums; (2) a step increase in the frequency, intensity, or duration of tantrums; (3) a new overlap/co-occurrence of formerly independent behaviors; or (4) introduction of new tantrum behaviors around which the others become organized. Longitudinal data could be collected by having parents complete a checklist of tantrum behaviors they had seen most recently, beginning when their child was 12 months old and continuing at 1- to 3-month intervals up to 24 or 36 months. They might also be asked to contact investigators when they see a first tantrum and/or a particularly long or intense tantrum. To generate more detailed records over shorter periods, we had success in having parents maintain a tantrum calendar in which they entered the onset time, duration, and relative intensity (on a 1–5 scale) of each tantrum the child had over 1–2 months. Randomized weekly check-in calls asking about the most recent tantrum during the recording period provided relia- bility data for comparison to the calendars once they were turned in. The statistical challenge is to detect step changes in the frequency, duration, intensity, number, or type of behaviors within each individual record. Nonparametric approaches like those of Van Dijk and Van Geert (2007), which focus on reliably identifying discontinuities in development, might be useful in this regard. Identification of a tantrum transition event would lend credence to the idea of a neurodevelopmental program that comes on line at a certain point in time.

Tantrums and Language Development

It has been claimed that toddlers' tantrums can be triggered by frustration with their language ability, which is inadequate to express their feelings and wishes. In most cases of normal development, however, parents understand what their children want or don't want well enough. By 3, which can be as terrible as 2, typ- ically developing children can understand what is said to them and can express themselves adequately. The lack of causal connection between communication problems and tantrums is true even for children with autism (Mayes, Lockridge, & Tierney, 2017; Sipes, Matson, Horovitz, & Shoemaker, 2011). Some older studies do suggest that children with delayed or abnormal language development are more prone to tantrum (Beitchman, 1985; Benasich, Curtis, & Tallal, 1993; Carlson, Potegal, Margulies, Gutkovich, & Basile, 2009; Caulfield, Fischel, Debaryshe, & Whitehurst, 1989; Vollmer, Northup, Ringdahl, Le Blanc, & Chauvin, 1996; but see Dominick, Davis, Lainhart, Tager-Flusberg, & Folstein, 2007). Whether these tantrums have to do with frustration around communication specifically or with more general emotional problems comorbid with problems in language develop- ment remains to be determined. This question notwithstanding, the "functional communication" approach of providing alternative modes of response to children with disabilities reportedly ameliorates tantrums and other undesirable behaviors (Durrand & Merges, 2001).

Tantrum Cessation or Another Transition?

The age at which children cease to tantrum is an interesting example of cultural influence on children's behavior. In prewar Japan, when young boys were taught to be subservient to older male relatives but were dominant over all female relatives, boys of 4 and 5 reportedly committed serious aggression against their mothers in their tantrums, kicking, punching, and biting her, which the mothers were culturally inhibited to defend against. This only stopped when the boys began school at age 6 or 7 and all aggression was mocked and/or punished (Gorer, 1943). Similar age limits on villagers' laissez-faire attitude to boys' misbehavior, including tantrums, prevailed on the Japanese island of Okinawa in the 1950s (Maretzki & Maretzki, 1963). In that era and later, Chinese boys in Kau Sai had public tantrums up to age 10 (Ward, 1971). In contemporary societies tantrums may persist for a few years with the majority of children giving them up by age 4 or 5. Thus, tantrum prevalence reported for children 6 and older ranges from 11% to 30% (Barbarin, 1999; Bhatia, Dhar, Singhal, & Nigam, 1990; Carlson, Danzig, Dougherty, Bufferd, & Klein, 2016; Hackett & Hackett, 1993; Österman & Björkvist, 2010); the drop to under 50% prevalence occurred at age 7 in MacFarlane, Allen, and Honzik's (1954) data.

We know even less about tantrum cessation than tantrum onset. Cessation in modern societies may be due in part to the noticeable increase in emotion regulation and its cross-situational consistency from 3–4 or 5 years of age (Kalpidou, Power, Cherry, & Gottfried, 2004; Ramani, Brownell, & Campbell, 2010). There was a significant decline in high anger behaviors and an increase in lower level anger behaviors in 3- and 4-year-olds in our tantrum survey (Figure 8.2 in Potegal, 2000). Alternatively, tantrums may never truly disappear but may morph into adult episodes of anger. Adults in the United States, Japan, and Russia report experiencing several episodes of anger per week, which typically last from a few minutes to about half an hour or, in more recent sociological surveys, up to an hour or more (Potegal, 2010; maybe longer in Romania: Kassinove & Broll-Barone, 2012). Although women (more than men) may cry when angry (Vingerhoets & Scheirs, 2000) adult episodes of anger are not typically thought of as associated with sadness. That is, the developmental changes include a major reduction in accompanying distress. But, the reduction may not be complete. Anger experiences facilitated facial expressions of sadness in 8- to 12-year-olds (Blumberg & Izard, 1991), while anger is often commingled with sadness in adults in Western societies (Scherer & Tannenbaum, 1986; Wickless & Kirsch, 1988) and in other cultures (Russell, 1991). Anecdotal inquiry suggests that some people's episodes of anger may end with discernable feelings of remorse, guilt, and/or other emotions not unrelated to sadness as well as sadness itself. Some events that provoke adult anger may also elicit sadness, but the sadness may be masked until the anger has subsided, much like the situation with anger and reconciliation in children's tantrums. Consider your own experiences of anger, dear reader, how often do they end with a tinge of sadness?

TANTRUMS IN THE BRAIN

A Conjecture About Lateralization of Tantrum Emotions

The apparent independence of tantrum anger and distress may take origin in separate specializations of the left cerebral hemisphere for anger and the right hemisphere for sadness and related emotions. There is evidence for greater left frontal activation associated with both state and/or trait anger in infants (Dawson, 1994; c.f. Baving, Laucht, & Schmidt, 2000) and adults (e.g., Harmon-Jones et al., 2010; Jaworska et al., 2013; Wang et al., 2016). Left hemisphere involvement is clearest for anger that is implicitly or explicitly allowed expression (i.e., that involves approach). Left hemisphere substrates for anger expressed in reactive aggression include the insula (Dambacher et al., 2014). Accordingly, left (but not right) frontal activity induced by transcranial direct current stimulation increases anger-related aggression (Hortensius, Schutter, & Harmon-Jones, 2011). When anger is associated with withdrawal, like running away in a tantrum, the right hemisphere becomes more active (Harmon-Jones et al., 2010).

Switching attention to that hemisphere, several lines of evidence suggest that relative right frontal activation is associated with a predominance of negative emotions that are most similar to the distress component of tantrums. Thus, stroke in left frontal cortex and/or basal ganglia may be acutely followed by depression (Robinson & Jorge, 2015; Shi, Yang, Zeng, & Wu, 2017), which has been interpreted to mean that the greater, unbalanced influence of the intact right hemisphere may predispose these individuals to emotional reactions including sadness. Such injury-related results have been disputed but are supported by studies of neurologically intact individuals, including children, in whom greater electroencephalographic (EEG) activation in right than left hemisphere is associated with sadness (Buss et al., 2003; Davidson & Slagter, 2000). In these studies, brain activation is indicated by EEG desynchronization, which is reciprocally related to EEG power. The right hemisphere has been specifically implicated in the motor act of crying (Parvizi et al., 2009; Wortzel et al., 2008).

Both hemisphere-emotion relationships were directly captured in a pilot study with 10 tantrum-prone and 11 non–tantrum-prone 4-year-olds whose resting EEG was recorded in one session and whose responses to anger-provoking (e.g., mild restraint) and sadness-provoking (e.g., disappointing prize) situations were behaviorally tested on a second occasion (Gagne, Van Hulle, Aksan, Essex, & Goldsmith, 2011). Right frontal activation was significantly associated with sad facial expressions across the groups. Left posterior temporal activation correlated with both parent-reported anger generally and with angry facial expressions in the testing situation; activation at this temporal site also differentiated the two groups (Figure 4.1 in Potegal & Stemmler, 2010). These results are consistent with evidence for simultaneous right ear advantage for anger detection and left ear advantage for sadness detection in dichotic listening studies in adults (Gadea, Espert, Salvador, & Marti-Bonmati, 2011).

Side and Sequence

Pulling together the various neurological bits and pieces, per Potegal and Stemmler (2010) and Potegal (2012), it may be that anger-related activity triggered in left temporal cortex is transmitted rostrally to orbitofrontal cortex (OFC) along the same pathways that seizures propagate from temporal to frontal lobe (Arain et al., 2016). Behaviors associated with OF "hypermotor" seizures resemble motor components of a tantrum (absent the corresponding emotional experience) with early autonomic activation (mostly flushing, as in tantrums) and vocalization (as in shouting and screaming) followed by bipedal movements (as in kicking, Alqadi,

Sankaraneni, Thome, & Kotagal, 2016; Wong et al., 2010). Subcortically directed signals originating in left OFC may disinhibit anger-related behaviors while callosal transmission to right frontal cortex activates distress-related feelings and behavior (Schutter & Harmon-Jones, 2013).

Potegal (2012) proposed that OFC normally exerts inhibitory control over impulses to anger and aggression generated in the temporal lobe. As noted earlier, temper loss is a defining feature of ODD, so Fahim, Fiori, Evans, and Pérusse's (2012) finding of a significant increase of gray matter density in left temporal cortex, together with a reduction in left OFC in 8-year-olds with ODD is quite consistent with the conjecture about emotion lateralization and within-hemisphere transmission in tantrums. OF cortex also processes effort/reinforcement contingencies, and it could be that the apparent emotional/energetic cost of tantrums does not fully register in immature OFC under conditions of high arousal. Perhaps the typical cessation of tantrums around 4 or 5 years results from an increasing inhibitory efficacy of OFC while their persistence in ODD and other conditions is associated with a developmental failure to increase such efficacy.

There are, of course, nonlateralized explanations for how the brain simultaneously maintains the opposing tendencies of anger, involving approach, and sadness, involving withdrawal (e.g., Petrican, Saverino, Rosenbaum, & Grady, 2015). One of these is the striking difference in the neural networks associated with anger, which are seemingly the most extensive and interconnected, versus those associated with sadness, which are the sparsest and least interconnected (Wager et al., 2015). Might tantrums involve the simultaneous activation of the dorsal anterior cingulate within the anger network and the rostral, precallosal cingulate within the sadness network?

Role(s) of Cingulate Cortex

The dorsal anterior cingulate cortex is also active in adult anger (e.g., Denson, Pedersen, Ronquillo, & Nandy, 2009), as well as in impulsivity and frustration. A specific role for the cingulate in tantrum circuitry is suggested by the reportedly intense tantrums of adults with seizures originating in this locus (Mazars, 1970) and recent findings of altered cingulate function and/or connections in disruptive children (Gavita, Capris, Bolno, & David, 2012) and, more specifically, those with severe tantrums (Roy et al., 2017). Loud vocalizations are a primary component of tantrums (Green et al., 2011), and cingulate control of vocalization, including crying, is well established (Holstege & Subramanian, 2016; Newman, 2007). As it does for other types of vocalizations, the cingulate likely generates tantrum vocalizations through a descending series of subcortical circuits, including those in hypothalamus (as suggested by dacrystic crying seizures associated with hypothalamic hamartomas) [Moise, Leary, Morgan, Papanastassiou, & Szabó, 2017]) and periaqueductal gray caudally to an inferred central pattern generator for crying in the basal pons (Wang et al., 2016). This description fits a tidy neurological scheme for control of emotion responses (Lauterbach, Cummings,

& Kuppuswamy,2013), but it must be noted that the organization of circuitry for crying based on localization of rare dacrystic seizures is speculative at present (Moise et al., 2017).

A Neurodevelopmental Program for Tantrums?

Do transition events, if and when they occur, represent the emergence of a neurodevelopmental program for tantrums that comes on line, ready to be activated, with the blossoming of a final synapse that completes a neural circuit for tantrum behaviors around 18 months? Arguments for why such a program might have evolved are presented next.

BIOLOGICAL ROOTS OF TANTRUMS: INTERGENERATIONAL CONFLICT, WEANING, AND THE TERRIBLE TWOS

Evolution of Tantrums

Evidence that tantrums are quite common, if not ubiquitous, across cultures and that tantrum behaviors may be generated by dedicated brain circuits suggests that they may have deep evolutionary roots. Infant and juvenile monkeys (Li, Ren, Li, Zhu, & Li, 2013; Weaver & de Waal, 2003) and apes (Slocombe, Townsend, & Zuberbühler., 2009; van Noordwijk & van Schaik, 2005) engage in behaviors recognizable as tantrums to human observers. Rhesus macaque and baboon infants emit specific scream calls after being rejected by their mothers (Wallez & Vauclair, 2012); chimpanzees distinguish tantrum screams from other types of screams (Slocombe et al., 2009). Howler monkey tantrums include screaming, body jerking, and biting the mother (Pavé, Kowalewski, Peker, & Zunino, 2010); baboon infants repeatedly drop to a prone position on the ground during their tantrums (Wallez & Vauclair, 2012). Tantrums in Yunnan snub-nosed monkeys (Li et al., 2013) and baboons (Altmann, 1983) first occur and/or become particularly intense when infants are 5 months old, preceding increased maternal rejection 1–3 months later when the mothers resume sexual activity. The mother's resumption of sexual activity, changes in her behavior during pregnancy, and the birth of new siblings trigger tantrums in the young of other primates species as well (Pavé, Kowalewski, Zunino, & Giraudo, 2015). Importantly, mothers in various monkey species, as well as chimpanzees often alter their ongoing behavior in response to their infant's tantrum (Nishida, 1990).

Tantrums have been observed in laboratory-reared juvenile chimps that had no opportunity to learn how to tantrum by watching others (Hebb, 1945). Similar stories are told about singleton human children whose very first observed tantrum had the classic elements of crying, falling to the floor, and kicking. Are the formats for tantrum behaviors genetically programed? Trivers (1974, 1985) proposed that tantrums may be a solution to a basic intergenerational conflict between offspring who benefit by maintaining parental nurturance for as long as possible and their mothers, whose inclusive fitness would be better served, after a point, by spending less time with this infant and more time producing the next one. Primate youngsters tantrum when they cannot keep up with their mother's travels, just as children in human forager groups do. But for both their progeny and ours, being denied the opportunity to suckle for milk is a major psychological and physiological stressor and a trigger for tantrums (Mandalaywala, Higham, Heistermann, Parker, & Maestripieri, 2014). In Trivers's view, weaning was a crux of the intergenerational conflict in response to which tantrums evolved as the infants' negotiating tool. However, tantrums appear to be optional, at least for some primate young. Thus, only 3 of 10 chacma baboon infants, closely observed in the wild for the first 2 years of life, including the period of weaning, engaged in tantrums (Barrett, Peter Henzi, & Lycett, 2006). Two of these did so only when their attempts at independent feeding were thwarted by a seasonal reduction in forageable food. Five other closely observed baboon infants living in a different, nutritionally richer natural environment were never observed to tantrum. Genetically programmed as their motor routines may be, tantrums are optional, not obligatory, for nonhuman primate infants. As Maestripieri (2002) argued, tantrums are an infant's means of negotiating when necessary; tantrum insistence and persistence is a marker of infant need.

The Human Condition

The extensive recent or contemporary evidence that weaning triggers children's tantrums comes from different places and cultures (e.g., African and South American forager groups; Fouts et al., 2005, Hill & Hurtado, 1996, Shostak, 1981), a pre-war Japanese village (Embree, 1939/2002), and so forth. For children in many nonindustrialized cultures weaning occurs during the mother's pregnancy with the next child. Thus, the weaning crisis is subsequently exacerbated by family attention shifting from the child to the new baby. This can also be the point at which mother and older sibs begin to refuse to carry the child around, so she or he must keep up with family moves and activities on his or her own. These combined stressors can trigger a period of frequent tantrums that occur with little or no additional provocation (e.g., Maretski & Maretski, 1963; Shostak, 1981).

Historically, 2 years has been the age of weaning in Western culture. Although there is considerable variation, the typical age at the end of weaning in nonindustrialized societies is about 2.5 years (Tsutaya & Yoneda, 2015). Biochemical analyses of ancient teeth yields dates of 2–4 years for the weaning period in forager groups during the middle Neolithic in Sweden (Howcraft, Eriksson, & Lidén, 2014) and in the same age range for even earlier periods in central California (Eerkens & Bartelink, 2013) and at the Matjes River Rock Shelter, South Africa (Clayton, Sealy, & Pfeiffer, 2006). A disposition to tantrum which develops at an age when weaning occurred over most of human history might well reflect an evolutionary strategy to retain parental attention if not nurturance.

Screaming, hitting, and biting during tantrums may be angry/aggressive behaviors inherited from our hominid ancestry. We humans are inventive in aggression as in other domains. At 28 months, my daughter added head butts to her aggression repertoire (they hurt!). Although she was still in the throes of tantrums at the time, she never head-butted during a tantrum. If there is a neurodevelopmental program for tantrums, does it just include a restricted range of behaviors that developed in evolution?

The distress component of tantrums likely has evolutionary roots as well. In general, young children's distress can elicit the parental succor and nurturance that is necessary for their survival. Among the specific distress behaviors, a noticeable lowering of head and/or body, which we labeled as *Down*, can be interpreted as a signal of submission. Ethologically, lowering the body is a sign of submission in many animal species including humans (e.g., in the subordinate postures assumed by adults; Burgoon & Dunbar, 2006; Tiedens & Fragale, 2003) and in the supine posture forced on the loser of play-fighting matches among human children in many cultures (Eibl-Eibesfeldt, 1989). Submission is also associated with the expression of infantile behaviors, which is the impression conveyed by a regression to the prone or supine crying and flailing of infancy.

End-of-tantrum reconciliation may not have evolved solely, or perhaps at all, in the context of parent–child conflicts that give rise to tantrums. Post-conflict reconciliation has been documented in species as diverse as ravens, domestic goats and wild sheep, spotted hyenas, and bottle-nosed dolphins, as well as in more than 24 species of nonhuman primates, in all major taxa within the primate order including prosimians, monkeys, apes, and humans. Different reconciliation styles among primate infants have been identified (Arnold & Aureli, 2007).

Thus, a neurodevelopmental program for tantrum behaviors and patterns may have evolved and be genetically programmed in contemporary humans. But, even if such a program exists, it need not be activated. A comparison between ethnically similar but culturally different Bofi farmers and foragers of the Congo Basin rain forest in the Central African Republic is instructive (Fouts et al., 2005). Among the farmers, mothers wean their children onto specially prepared rice gruels between 18 and 27 months of age by bandaging their nipples or painting them with red fingernail polish to imitate a wound and telling their children they can no longer nurse due to injury. The children respond to the abrupt weaning with "high levels of fussing and crying." In contrast, mothers among the foragers allow their children to self-wean, which they do between 36 and 53 months without a fuss. Differences in weaning practices are embedded in broader contrasts in cultural schemas and social relations. The more general observation, that at least 15% of children pass through early developmental challenges without tantrums, shows that, for humans as for other primates, tantrums are an option, not a necessity. Various biological, environmental, and family factors, and their interactions, make the expression of these emotions and their concomitant behaviors more or less likely. In psychopathology, the neurodevelopmental program is more easily triggered and excessively activated, generating tantrums that are insistent and persistent.

TANTRUMS AND PSYCHOPATHOLOGY, NEURODEVELOPMENTAL AND CENTRAL NERVOUS SYSTEM DISORDERS

When Tantrums Mean Trouble

Older surveys of 1- to 3-year-olds found prevalence rates of 5–7% for tantrums that were frequent, severe, or found troublesome by parents (Earls, 1980; Needlman, Stevenson, & Zuckerman, 1991; Richman, Stevenson, & Graham, 1975). According to Goldson and Reynolds (2011) 5–20% of children have tantrums that are severe, frequent, and/or disruptive. Severe tantrums at age 3 predict adult antisocial behavior (Stevenson & Goodman, 2001). Complementary to the normal dropoff in tantrum prevalence at ages 5–7, tantrums persisting to ages 8–10 predict antisocial behavior in later childhood (Stoolmiller, 2001) and adulthood (Caspi, Elder, & Bem, 1987).

How Frequent Is Too Frequent, How Long Is Too Long?

Belden et al. (2008) proposed that more than 5 tantrums a day outside the home and/or more than 10 tantrums a day at home on multiple days were indicators for psychiatric referral of 3- to 6-year-olds. These are above the 95th percentile rates tentatively estimated earlier. Roy et al. (2013) found a mean of 3 tantrums per week in 5- to 9-year-olds whose tantrums were disruptive.

Many children have the occasional long tantrum; but how long is too long on average? Varley and Smith (2003) noted that anxiety-triggered tantrums are often "extraordinarily long," while Carlson et al. (2009) recorded the mean duration of "rages" on a child psychiatry unit as 51 min. Cut points for duration at 5 min (Wakschlag et al., 2012), 15 min (Goldson & Reynolds, 2011), and 25 min (Belden et al., 2008) have been suggested. Given the mean tantrum durations reported for normal older children, a 25-minute cut point might be appropriate. In view of the developmental trends, both frequency and duration cut points need to be adjusted for age. At all ages, excessive aggression to property, to others, or to the self are likely indicators of externalizing disorder (Belden et al., 2008; Wakschlag et al., 2012).

Tantrums and Psychopathology

Tantrums are among the common reasons for a child's referral to a psychiatric facility (Sobel, Roberts, Rayfield, Barnard, & Rapoff, 2001); for example, 40% of 58 consecutive referrals of very young children with developmental delays to a mental health clinic were for tantrums (Fox, Keller, Grede, & Bartosz, 2007); 55% of 130 consecutive admissions to a child psychiatry unit were for "rages" (Carlson et al., 2009). Conversely, almost half the children being treated in an outpatient clinic had severe tantrums (Carlson et al., 2016).

As these observations suggest, tantrums are associated with psychopathology (e.g., they are routinely included on checklists of externalizing disorders like ODD). However, they are also associated with internalizing disorder. That is, children who tantrum excessively are at increased risk for anxiety and depression (Mireault & Trahan, 2007; Roy et al., 2013; Wakschlag et al., 2015). Conversely, depressed or anxious children are prone to excessive tantrums. "A child with [social anxiety disorder] SAD may have a temper tantrum to avoid school; a child with [obsessive compulsive disorder] OCD may have a tantrum to avoid wearing clothes with buttons; a child with phobia to dogs may have a tantrum to avoid a park" (Varley & Smith, 2003, p. 1110).

The parents of 18 internalizing, 17 externalizing, and 16 typically developing 4-year-olds, selected on the basis of Achenbach Child Behavior Checklist (CBCL) scores, recorded every tantrum their child had on tantrum calendars over 27–81 days (Potegal, 2005). The two psychopathological groups had significantly longer and more frequent tantrums than did the typical group ($p <.02$). There were no differences in tantrum characteristics between the two extreme groups. Calendar-derived tantrum frequency and duration were significantly correlated with Total CBCL score and Emotional Reactivity Scale scores. So, both externalizing and internalizing disorders may be associated with increased tantrum frequency, duration, and severity. The finding that a lower ratio of tantrum anger to distress may specifically reflect childhood anxiety (Potegal et al., 2009) suggests that the anger-distress model may help elucidate issues of psychopathology.

Bipolar Disorder

By the late 1990s and early 2000s, children with juvenile bipolar disorder had developed a reputation for very intense and prolonged "rages" (Carlson & Glovinsky, 2009). This led to the mistaken belief that severe tantrums were diagnostic of bipolar disorder and to inappropriate treatment of children having such tantrums with antipsychotic medication (Leibenluft, 2011). This is, among other things, a base rate issue, with bipolar prevalence estimated at 3% or less (Van Meter, Moreira, & Youngstrom, 2011) while tantrums are much more common. Although severe tantrums are among the symptoms reported for youth later diagnosed with bipolar disorder (Hernandez, Marangoni, Grant, Estrada, & Faedda, 2017), most children with severe tantrums do not have bipolar disorder (Carlson et al., 2009; Grimmer, Hohmann, & Poustka, 2014; Roy et al., 2013).

Tantrums as Symptoms of Disrupted Mood

DMDD was introduced in the DSM-5 in 2013 to characterize more adequately the condition of children who were previously being misdiagnosed with pediatric bipolar disorder. DMDD is defined as chronic irritability interspersed with at least three intense tantrums a week in children at least 6 years old. This age minimum is consistent with the normal dropoff in tantrum prevalence. DMDD prevalence in the middle childhood population is 8–9% (Dougherty et al., 2014; Mayes, Waxmonsky, Calhoun, & Bixler, 2016) while 45% of 4- to 5-year-olds admitted to an early childhood psychiatric day treatment program exhibited DMDD symptoms (Martin et al., 2017). This prevalence in clinic is consistent with the percentages of admissions-with-tantrums noted earlier. Patients with DMDD had a median of 4 tantrums per week according to a chart review (Tufan et al., 2016). DMDD is associated with multiple comorbidities including ODD, anxiety, and depression (Freeman, Youngstrom, Youngstrom, & Findling, 2016, Mayes et al., 2016) and predicts subsequent psychopathology (Dougherty, Barrios, Carlson, & Klein, 2017).

Other Conditions Associated with Tantrums

Tantrums have also been reported in association with a range of neurological and medical conditions too numerous for citation. Noted briefly here are a few conditions for which research results relate to some of the issues raised earlier.

Children on the autism spectrum (ASD) are well known for tantrums. Three- to 16-year-old children with ASD scored higher than those with attention deficit/hyperactivity disorder (ADHD) on both anger ("Easily becomes angry," "Destroys ones property") and distress (Crying, tearful, and weepy") aspects of tantrum behavior (Goldin, Matson, Tureck, Cervantes, & Jang, 2013). More severe ASD symptomatology is associated with more intense tantrums, especially with more distress behaviors (Konst, Matson, & Turygin, 2013a; 2013b). Anecdotal accounts from people who have worked with these children suggest that the comfort-seeking/reconciliation component of distress may be reduced or absent. While not surprising, such accounts remain to be validated by empirical observation.

The angry outbursts in Tourette syndrome reviewed in "Fits, Tantrums, and Rages in TS and Related Disorders" (Budman, Rosen, & Shad, 2015) do bear some similarity to tantrums as described; for example, a childhood onset of "episodes occur most frequently at home and are most commonly directed toward a parent, usually the child's mother although less frequently toward siblings, pets, and property" (p. 275). However, these events are not reported to contain a distress component but may feature elements of anxiety or panic. If so, and then despite the paper's title, these episodes may resemble anger attacks associated with adult depression and other psychopathologies (Painuly, Gover, Gupta, & Mattoo, 2011) more than childhood tantrums.

The developmental cessation of tantrums is delayed in individuals with Down syndrome, fragile X, Williams, and Prader-Willi syndromes (Rice et al., 2015). Tantrums are common in Prader-Willi syndrome, in which a failure of satiety mechanisms leads to hyperphagia and excessive demands for food, which is the motivation for some of their tantrums (Tunniclffe et al., 2010). Neurochemically, individuals with Prader-Willi syndrome who tantrum frequently have shown reduced cerebral γ-aminobutyric acid (GABA), which was associated with their outbursts (Rice, 2016). Parallel conclusions about the inhibitory role of GABA in aggression have been drawn from studies in rodents (e.g., Potegal, 1986; Potegal, Yoburn, & Glusman, 1983).

Tantrums may also be exacerbated in childhood medical conditions that result in discomfort or pain (e.g., reflux, headache, dental caries, and so forth). Thus, when a child's tantrums are not ameliorated through appropriate behavioral intervention, a medical workup might be advisable.

No Tantrums

Importantly, perhaps 10–30% of children in Western cultures never have tantrums or at least events that are intense and prolonged enough to be recognized by adults as tantrums. These non-tantrumers are typically described as temperamentally pleasant and easy going. Is the *absence* of childhood tantrums a marker of current, and perhaps future, emotional stability? Comparisons of temperament between children in the same families who do and do not tantrum would be of interest in this regard. Tantrums are sometimes a symptom of disorder; they are always a phenomenon of early childhood affect, exploration of which will increase our knowledge of processes and events in children's emotional lives. Hopefully, this chapter may intrigue a reader or two into generating testable hypotheses in formal study designs to elucidate such processes and events.

Acknowledgments

For information about "tantrums" in their native language, I thank Nazan Aksan, Mohamad Anwar, Drishadwati Bargi, Nadya Clayton, Chuqing Dong, Erdenetsetseg Dorjgotov, Jie He, Sungok Hong, Zoltán Kövecses, Erik McDonald, Larisa Polynskaya, Uplabdhi Scott, Yana Taets, and Luba Wiese among others; they bear no responsibility for the conclusions drawn from the information they kindly provided.

References

Alink, L. R., Mesman, J., Van Zeijl, J., Stolk, M. N., Juffer, F., Koot, H. M., ... Van IJzendoorn, M. H. (2006). The early childhood aggression curve: Development of physical aggression in 10- to 50-month-old children. *Child Development, 77*(4), 954–966.

Alqadi, K., Sankaraneni, R., Thome, U., & Kotagal, P. (2016). Semiology of hypermotor (hyperkinetic) seizures. *Epilepsy & Behavior, 54*, 137–141.

Altmann, J. (1983). Costs of reproduction in baboons (Papio cynocephalus). Behavioral Energetics: The Cost of Survival in Vertebrates. In W. P. Aspey & S. I. Lustick (Eds.), *Behavioral energetics: The costs of survival* (pp. 67–88). Ohio State University Press, Columbus, Ohio.

Arain, A. M., Azar, N. J., Lagrange, A. H., McLean, M., Singh, P., Sonmezturk, H., . . . Abou-Khalil, B. (2016). Temporal lobe origin is common in patients who have undergone epilepsy surgery for hypermotor seizures. *Epilepsy & Behavior, 64*, 57–61.

Arnold, K., & Aureli, F. (2007). Postconflict reconciliation. In C. J. Campbell, A. Fuentes, K. C. MacKinnon, M. Panger, & S. K. Bearder (Eds.), *Primates in Perspective* (pp. 592–608). Oxford University Press, Oxford.

Baillargeon, R. H., Keenan, K., & Cao, G. (2012). The development of opposition-defiance during toddlerhood: A population-based cohort study. *Journal of Developmental & Behavioral Pediatrics, 33*(8), 608–617.

Barbarin, O. A. (1999). Social risks and psychological adjustment: A comparison of African American and South African children. *Child Development, 70*(6), 1348–1359.

Barrett, L., Peter Henzi, S., & Lycett, J. E. (2006). Whose life is it anyway? Maternal investment, developmental trajectories, and life history strategies in baboons. In L. Swedell & S. R. Leigh (Eds.), *Reproduction and fitness in baboons: Behavioral, ecological, and life history perspectives* (pp. 199–224). New York: Springer.

Baving, L., Laucht, M., & Schmidt, M. H. (2000). Oppositional children differ from healthy children in frontal brain activation. *Journal of Abnormal Child Psychology, 28*(3), 267–275.

Beitchman, J. H. (1985). Therapeutic considerations with the language impaired preschool child. *The Canadian Journal of Psychiatry, 30*(8), 609–613.

Belden, A. C., Thomson, N. R., & Luby, J. L. (2008). Temper tantrums in healthy versus depressed and disruptive preschoolers: Defining tantrum behaviors associated with clinical problems. *Journal of Pediatrics, 152*(1), 117–122.

Benasich, A. A., Curtis, S., & Tallal, P. (1993). Language, learning and behavioral disturbance in children. *Journal of the American Academy of Child and Adolescent Psychiatry, 32*, 6–23.

Bhatia, M., Dhar, N., Singhal, P., & Nigam, V. (1990). Temper tantrums: Prevalence and etiology in a non-referral outpatient setting. *Clinical Pediatrics, 29*, 311–315.

Biglan, A., Lewin, L., & Hops, H. (1990). A contextual approach to the problem of aversive practices in families. In G. R. Patterson (Ed.), *Depression and Aggression in Family Interaction* (pp. 103–129). Hillsdale, NJ: Lawrence Erlbaum.

Blumberg, S. H., & Izard, C. E. (1991). Patterns of emotion experiences as predictors of facial expressions of emotion. *Merrill-Palmer Quarterly, 1982*, 183–197.

Braungart-Rieker, J. M., Hill-Soderlund, A. L., & Karrass, J. (2010). Fear and anger reactivity trajectories from 4 to 16 months: The roles of temperament, regulation, and maternal sensitivity. *Developmental Psychology, 46*(4), 791–804.

Brenner, V., & Fox, R. A. (1998). Parental discipline and behavior problems in young children. *Journal of Genetic Psychology, 159*, 251–256.

Briggs, J. L. (1970). *Never in anger: Portrait of an Eskimo family*. Cambridge, MA: Harvard University Press.

Budman, C. L., Rosen, M., & Shad, S. (2015). Fits, tantrums, and rages in TS and related disorders. *Current Developmental Disorders Reports, 2*(4), 273–284.

Bufferd, S. J., Dougherty, L. R., & Olino, T. M. (2017). Mapping the frequency and severity of depressive behaviors in preschool-aged children. *Child Psychiatry & Human Development, 48*(6), 934–943.

Burgoon, J. K., & Dunbar, N. E. (2006). Nonverbal expressions of dominance and power in human relationships. In V. Manusov & M. L. Patterson (Eds.), *The Sage handbook of nonverbal communication* (pp. 279–298). Thousand Oaks, CA: Sage.

Buss, K. A., Schumacher, J. R. M., Dolski, I., Kalin, N. H., Goldsmith, H. H., & Davidson, R. J. (2003). Right frontal brain activity, cortisol, and withdrawal behavior in 6-month-old infants. *Behavioral Neuroscience, 117*(1), 11.

Camras, L. A. (2011). Differentiation, dynamical integration and functional emotional development. *Emotion Review, 3*(2), 138–146.

Carlson, G. A., Danzig, A. P., Dougherty, L. R., Bufferd, S. J., & Klein, D. N. (2016). Loss of temper and irritability: The relationship to tantrums in a community and clinical sample. *Journal of Child and Adolescent Psychopharmacology, 26*(2), 114–122.

Carlson, G. A., & Glovinsky, I. (2009). The concept of bipolar disorder in children: A history of the bipolar controversy. *Child and Adolescent Psychiatric Clinics of North America, 18*(2), 257–271.

Carlson, G. A., Potegal, M., Margulies, D., Gutkovich, Z., & Basile, J. (2009). Rages: What are they and who has them?. *Journal of Child and Adolescent Psychopharmacology, 19*(3), 281–288.

Carr, E. G., & Newsom, C. (1985). Demand-related tantrums: Conceptualization and treatment. *Behavior Modification, 9*(4), 403–426.

Caspi, A., Elder, G. H., Jr, & Bem, D. J. (1987). Moving against the world: Life course patterns of explosive children. *Developmental Psychology, 23*, 308–313.

Caulfield, M. B., Fischel, J. E., Debaryshe, B. D., & Whitehurst, G. J. (1989). Behavioural correlates of developmental expressive language disorder. *Journal of Abnormal Child Psychology, 17*(2), 187–201.

Chen, X., Green, J. A., & Gustafson, G. E. (2009). Development of vocal protests from 3 to 18 months. *Infancy, 14*(1), 44–59.

Cipriani, G., Lucetti, C., Carlesi, C., Danti, S., & Nuti, A. (2015). Sundown syndrome and dementia. *European Geriatric Medicine, 6*(4), 375–380.

Clayton, F., Sealy, J., & Pfeiffer, S. (2006). Weaning age among foragers at Matjes River Rock Shelter, South Africa, from stable nitrogen and carbon isotope analyses. *American Journal of Physical Anthropology, 129*(2), 311–317.

Dambacher, F., Sack, A. T., Lobbestael, J., Arntz, A., Brugman, S., & Schuhmann, T. (2014). Out of control: Evidence for anterior insula involvement in motor impulsivity and reactive aggression. *Social Cognitive and Affective Neuroscience, 10*(4), 508–516.

Davidson, R. J., & Slagter, H. A. (2000). Probing emotion in the developing brain: Functional neuroimaging in the assessment of the neural substrates of emotion in normal and disordered children and adolescents. *Mental Retardation and Developmental Disabilities Research Reviews, 6*(3), 166–170.

Dawson, G. (1994). Frontal electroencephalographic correlates of individual differences in emotion expression in infants: A brain systems perspective on emotion. *Monographs of the Society for Research in Child Development, 59*(2–3), 135–151.

Deater-Deckard, K., & Dodge, K. A. (1997). Externalizing behavior problems and discipline revisited: Nonlinear effects and variation by culture, context, and gender. *Psychological Inquiry, 8*(3), 161–175.

Denson, T. F., Pedersen, W. C., Ronquillo, J., & Nandy, A. S. (2009). The angry brain: Neural correlates of anger, angry rumination, and aggressive personality. *Journal of Cognitive Neuroscience, 21*(4), 734–744.

Dominick, K. C., Davis, N. O., Lainhart, J., Tager-Flusberg, H., & Folstein, S. (2007). Atypical behaviors in children with autism and children with a history of language impairment. *Research in Developmental Disabilities, 28*(2), 145–162.

Dougherty, L. R., Barrios, C. S., Carlson, G. A., & Klein, D. N. (2017). Predictors of later psychopathology in young children with disruptive mood dysregulation disorder. *Journal of Child and Adolescent Psychopharmacology, 27*(5), 396–402.

Dougherty, L. R., Smith, V. C., Bufferd, S. J., Carlson, G. A., Stringaris, A., Leibenluft, E., & Klein, D. N. (2014). DSM-5 disruptive mood dysregulation disorder: Correlates and predictors in young children. *Psychological Medicine, 44*(11), 2339–2350.

Drummond, P. D., & Quah, S. H. (2001). The effect of expressing anger on cardiovascular reactivity and facial blood flow in Chinese and Caucasians. *Psychophysiology, 38*(2), 190–196.

Durrand, V. M., & Merges, E. (2001). Functional communication training: A contemporary behavioral analytic intervention for problem behaviors. *Focus on Autism & Other Developmental Disabilities, 16*, 110–119.

Dwyer, P. D., & Minnegal L. M. (2008, November). Fun for them, fun for us and fun for all: The "far side" of field work in the tropical lowlands. *Anthropological Forum, 18*(3), 303–308.

Earls, F. (1980). Prevalence of behavior problems in 3-year-old children. *Archives of General Psychiatry, 37*, 1153–1157.

Eerkens, J. W., & Bartelink, E. J. (2013). Sex-biased weaning and early childhood diet among middle Holocene hunter–gatherers in central California. *American Journal of Physical Anthropology, 152*, 471–483.

Eibl-Eibesfeldt, I. (1989). *Human ethology*. New York: Aldine de Gruyter.

Einon, D. F., & Potegal, M. (1994). Temper tantrums in young children. In Potegal, M. and Knutson, J. (Eds.), *The dynamics of aggression: Biological and social processes in dyads and groups* (pp. 157–194). Hillsdale NJ: Lawrence Erlbaum.

Eisbach, S. S., Cluxton-Keller, F., Harrison, J., Krall, J. R., Hayat, M., & Gross, D. (2014). Characteristics of temper tantrums in preschoolers with disruptive behavior in a clinical setting. *Journal of Psychosocial Nursing and Mental Health Services, 52*(5): 32–40.

Eisenberg, N., Fabes, R. A., Murphy, B. C., Shaepard, S., Guthrie, I. K., Maszk, P., . . . Jones, S. (1999). Prediction of elementary school children's socially appropriate and problem behavior from anger reactions at 4–6 years. *Journal of Applied Developmental Psychology, 20*, 119–142.

Embree, J. F. (1939/2002). *Suye Mura: A Japanese village*. Chicago: University of Chicago Press. Reprinted Routledge Oxon.

Fahim, C., Fiori, M., Evans, A. C., & Pérusse, D. (2012). The relationship between social defiance, vindictiveness, anger, and brain morphology in eight-year-old boys and girls. *Social Development, 21*(3), 592–609.

Fessler, D. M. (2010). Madmen: An evolutionary perspective on anger and men's violent responses to transgression. In M. Potegal, G. Stemmler, & C. Spielberger (Eds.), *International handbook of anger: Constituent and concomitant biological, psychological and social processes* (pp. 361–381). New York: Springer.

Fouts, H., Hewlett, B., Lamb, M., BirdDavid, N., Crespi, B., Gottlieb, A., . . . Wells, J. (2005). Parent-offspring weaning conflicts among the Bofi farmers and foragers of Central Africa. *Current Anthropology*, *46*(1), 29–50.

Fox, R. A., Keller, K. M., Grede, P. L., & Bartosz, A. M. (2007). A mental health clinic for toddlers with developmental delays and behavior problems. *Research in Developmental Disabilities*, *28*, 119–129.

Freeman, A. J., Youngstrom, E. A., Youngstrom, J. K., & Findling, R. L. (2016). Disruptive mood dysregulation disorder in a community mental health clinic: Prevalence, co-morbidity and correlates. *Journal of Child and Adolescent Psychopharmacology*, *26*(2), 123–130.

Furman, E. (1986). Aggressively abused children. *Journal of Child Psychotherapy*, *12*(1), 47–59.

Gadea, M., Espert, R., Salvador, A., & Martí-Bonmatí, L. (2011). The sad, the angry, and the asymmetrical brain: Dichotic listening studies of negative affect and depression. *Brain and Cognition*, *76*(2), 294–299.

Gagne, J. R., Van Hulle, C. A., Aksan, N., Essex, M. J., & Goldsmith, H. H. (2011). Deriving childhood temperament measures from emotion-eliciting behavioral episodes: Scale construction and initial validation. *Psychological Assessment*, *23*(2), 337.

Gavita, O. A., Capris, D., Bolno, J., & David, D. (2012). Anterior cingulate cortex findings in child disruptive behavior disorders.: A meta-analysis. *Aggression and Violent Behavior*, *17*(6), 507–513.

Giesbrecht, G. F. (2008). *Emotion regulation and temper tantrums in preschoolers: Social, emotional, and cognitive contributions* (Doctoral dissertation University of Victoria). Retrieved from https://dspace.library.uvic.ca/bitstream/handle/1828/1271/Gerry%20Giesbrecht%20Dissertation%20(Final%20version).pdf?sequence=1&isAllowed=y

Giesbrecht, G. F., Miller, M. R., & Muller, U. (2010). The anger-distress model of temper tantrums: Associations with emotional reactivity and emotional competence. *Infant and Child Development*, *19*, 478–497. doi.org/10.1002/icd.677

Goldin, R. L., Matson, J. L., Tureck, K., Cervantes, P. E., & Jang, J. (2013). A comparison of tantrum behavior profiles in children with ASD, ADHD and comorbid ASD and ADHD. *Research in Developmental Disabilities*, *34*(9), 2669–2675.

Goldson, E., & Reynolds, A. (2011). Child development and behavior. In J. M. Sondheimer, M. J. Levi, R. R. Deterding, & W. W. Hay (Eds.), *Current diagnosis & treatment: Pediatrics* (64–103). New York: McGraw-Hill.

Goodenough, F. (1931). *Anger in young children*. Minneapolis: University of Minnesota Press.

Gorer, M. G. (1943). Section of anthropology: Themes in Japanese culture. *Transactions of the New York Academy of Sciences*, *5*(5 Series II), 106–124.

Green, J. A., Whitney, P. G., & Potegal, M. (2011). Screaming, yelling, whining and crying: Categorical and intensity differences in vocal expressions of anger and sadness in children's tantrums. *Emotion*, *11*, 1124–1133. doi.org/10.1037/a0024173

Grimmer, Y., Hohmann, S., & Poustka, L. (2014). Is bipolar always bipolar? Understanding the controversy on bipolar disorder in children. *F1000prime Reports*, *6*.

Grover, G. (2008). Temper tantrums. In C. D. Berkowitz (Ed.), *Pediatrics: A primary care approach* (pp. 199–201). Philadelphia: Saunders.

Hackett, L., & Hackett, R. (1993). Parental ideas of normal and deviant child behaviour. A comparison of two ethnic groups. *British Journal of Psychiatry*, *162*(3), 353–357.

Harding, J. W., Wacker, D. P., Berg, W. K., Barretto, A., Winborn, L., & Gardner, A. (2001). Analysis of response class hierarchies with attention-maintained problem behaviors. *Journal of Applied Behavior Analysis, 34*(1), 61–64.

Harmon-Jones, E., Gable, P. A., & Peterson, C. K. (2010). The role of asymmetric frontal cortical activity in emotion-related phenomena: A review and update. *Biological Psychology, 84*(3), 451–462.

Hasler, B. P., Mehl, M. R., Bootzin, R. R., & Vazire, S. (2008). Preliminary evidence of diurnal rhythms in everyday behaviors associated with positive affect. *Journal of Research in Personality, 42*(6), 1537–1546.

Hebb, D. O. (1945). The forms and conditions of chimpanzee anger. *Bulletin of the Canadian Psychological Association, 5*(2), 32–35.

Herdt, G. (1986). Aspects of socialization for aggression in Sambia ritual and warfare. *Anthropological Quarterly, 59*, 160–204.

Hernandez, M., Marangoni, C., Grant, M., Estrada, J., & Faedda, L. G. (2017). Parental reports of prodromal psychopathology in pediatric bipolar disorder. *Current Neuropharmacology, 15*(3), 380–385.

Hill, K. R., & Hurtado, A. M. (1996). *Ache´ life history: The ecology and demography of a foraging people*. New York: Transaction Publishers.

Holstege, G., & Subramanian, H. H. (2016). Two different motor systems are needed to generate human speech. *Journal of Comparative Neurology, 524*(8), 1558–1577.

Hortensius R., Schutter D. J. L. G., & Harmon-Jones E. (2011). When anger leads to aggression: Induction of relative left frontal cortical activity with transcranial direct current stimulation increases the anger-aggression relationship. *Social Cognition and Affective Neuroscience, 7*, 342–347.

Howell, S. (1989). Chewong concepts of human nature. In S. Howell & R. Willis (Eds.), *Societies at peace: Anthropological perspectives* (pp. 45–59). Taylor & Frances/Routledge.

Howcroft, R., Eriksson, G., & Lidén, K. (2014). Infant feeding practices at the Pitted Ware Culture site of Ajvide, Gotland. *Journal of Anthropology and Archaeology, 34*, 42–53.

Ingvarsson, E. T., Hanley, G. P., & Welter, K. M. (2009). Treatment of escape-maintained behavior with positive reinforcement: The role of reinforcement contingency and density. *Education and Treatment of Children, 32*(3), 371–401.

Jaworska, N., Berrigan, L., Ahmed, A. G., Gray, J., Korovessis, A., Fisher, D. J., . . . Knott, V. J. (2013). The resting electrophysiological profile in adults with ADHD and comorbid dysfunctional anger: A pilot study. *Clinical EEG and Neuroscience, 44*(2), 95–104.

Johnson, A. (2003). *Families of the forest: The Matsigenka Indians of the Peruvian Amazon*. Berkeley: University of California Press.

Johnson, O. R. (1981). The socio-economic context of child abuse and neglect in native South America. In J. E. Korbin (Ed.), *Child abuse and neglect* (pp. 56–70). Berkeley: University of California Press.

Jorgensen, D. (1984). The clear and the hidden: Person, self, and suicide among the Telefolmin of Papua New Guinea. *OMEGA-Journal of Death and Dying, 14*(2), 113–126.

Kalpidou, M. D., Power, T. G., Cherry, K. E., & Gottfried, N. W. (2004). Regulation of emotion and behavior among 3-and 5-year-olds. *Journal of General Psychology, 131*(2), 159–178.

Kassinove, H., & Broll-Barone, B. (2012). Self-reported anger episodes in Romanian children, adolescents, and adults. *Romanian Journal of School Psychology, 5*(9), 13–30.

Katz, J., Jones, D. J., & Beach, S. R. (2000). Distress and aggression during dating conflict: A test of the coercion hypothesis. *Personal Relationships*, 7(4), 391–402.

Kern, L., Delaney, B. A., Hilt, A., Bailin, D. E., & Elliot, C. (2002). An analysis of physical guidance as reinforcement for noncompliance. *Behavior Modification*, 26(4), 516–536.

Konner, M. J. (1972). Aspects of the developmental ethology of a foraging people. *Ethological Studies of Child Behaviour*, 285–304.

Konst, M. J., Matson, J. L., & Turygin, N. (2013a). Exploration of the correlation between autism spectrum disorder symptomology and tantrum behaviors. *Research in Autism Spectrum Disorders*, 7(9), 1068–1074.

Konst, M. J., Matson, J. L., & Turygin, N. (2013b). Comparing the rates of tantrum behavior in children with ASD and ADHD as well as children with comorbid ASD and ADHD diagnoses. *Research in Autism Spectrum Disorders*, 7(11), 1339–1345.

Koot, H. M., & Verhulst, F. C. (1991). Prevalence of problem behavior in Dutch children aged 2-3. *Acta Psychiatrica Scandinavica*, 83(s367), 1–37.

Kopp, C. B. (1992). Emotional distress and control in young children. In N. Eisenberg & R. A. Fabes (Eds.), *Emotion and its regulation in early development* (pp. 41–56). New Directions for Child Development, no. 55. San Francisco: Jossey-Bass.

Kruk, M. R. (1991). Ethology and pharmacology of hypothalamic aggression in the rat. *Neuroscience & Biobehavioral Reviews*, 15(4), 527–538.

Kuppens, P., Van Mechelen, I., & Meulders, M. (2004). Every cloud has a silver lining: Interpersonal and individual differences determinants of anger-related behaviors. *Personality and Social Psychology Bulletin*, 30(12), 1550–1564.

Lauterbach, E. C., Cummings, J. L., & Kuppuswamy, P. S. (2013). Toward a more precise, clinically informed pathophysiology of pathological laughing and crying. *Neuroscience & Biobehavioral Reviews*, 37(8), 1893–1916.

Leibenluft, E. (2011). Severe mood dysregulation, irritability, and the diagnostic boundaries of bipolar disorder in youths. *American Journal of Psychiatry*, 168(2), 129–142.

Lench, H. C., Tibbett, T. P., & Bench, S. W. (2016). Exploring the toolkit of emotion: What do sadness and anger do for us? *Social and Personality Psychology Compass*, 10(1), 11–25.

Levenson, R. W. (2014). The autonomic nervous system and emotion. *Emotion Review*, 6(2), 100–112.

LeVine, R. A., & LeVine, B. B. (1963). Nyansongo: A Gusii community in Kenya. In B. B. Whiting (Ed.), *Six cultures: Studies of child rearing* (pp. 15–202). New York: Wiley.

Levitzky, S., & Cooper, R. (2000). Infant colic syndrome: Maternal fantasies of aggression and infanticide. *Clinical Pediatrics*, 39(7), 395–400.

Lewis, M. (2010). The development of anger. In M. Potegal, G. Stemmler, & C. Spielberger (Eds.), *International handbook of anger: Constituent and concomitant biological, psychological and social processes* (pp. 177–192). NY Springer.

Lewis, M., Ramsay, D. S., & Sullivan, M. W. (2006). The relation of ANS and HPA activation to infant anger and sadness response to goal blockage. *Developmental Psychobiology*, 48(5), 397–405.

Li, T., Ren, B., Li, D., Zhu, P., & Li, M. (2013). Mothering style and infant behavioral development in Yunnan Snub-Nosed monkeys (Rhinopithecus bieti) in China. *International Journal of Primatology*, 34(4), 681–695.

Li, Y., Shi, A., Wan, Y., Hotta, M., & Ushijima, H. (2001). Child behavior problems: Prevalence and correlates in rural minority areas of China. *Pediatrics International*, 43(6), 651–661.

Lorber, M. F., Del Vecchio, T., & Slep, A. M. S. (2015). The emergence and evolution of infant externalizing behavior. *Development and Psychopathology, 27*(3), 663–680.

Luk, S. L., Leung, P. W. L., Bacon-Shone, J., & Lieh-Mak, F. (1991). The structure and prevalence of behavioral problems in Hong Kong preschool children. *Journal of Abnormal Child Psychology, 19*(2), 219–232.

MacFarlane, J. W., Allen, L., & Honzik, M. P. (1954). *A developmental study of the behavior problems of normal children between twenty-one months and fourteen years.* Berkeley: University of California Press.

Maestripieri D. (2002). Parent-offspring conflict in primates. *International Journal of Primatology, 23*, 923–951.

Mandalaywala, T. M., Higham, J. P., Heistermann, M., Parker, K. J., & Maestripieri, D. (2014). Physiological and behavioural responses to weaning conflict in free-ranging primate infants. *Animal Behaviour, 97*, 241–247.

Maretzki, T. W., & Maretzki, H. (1963). Taira: An Okinawan village. In B. Whiting (Ed.), *Six cultures: Studies of child rearing* (pp. 363–540). New York: Wiley.

Marlowe, F. W. (2005). Who tends Hadza children?. In B. S. Hewlett & M. E. Lamb (Eds.), *Hunter – gatherer childhoods: evolutionary, developmental and cultural perspectives* (pp. 177–190). New Brunswick, NJ: Aldine Transaction.

Martin, S. E., Hunt, J. I., Mernick, L. R., DeMarco, M., Hunter, H. L., Coutinho, M. T., & Boekamp, J. R. (2017). Temper loss and persistent irritability in preschoolers: Implications for diagnosing disruptive mood dysregulation disorder in early childhood. *Child Psychiatry & Human Development, 48*(3), 498–508.

Matson, J. L., Sipes, M., Horovitz, M., Worley, J. A., Shoemaker, M. E., & Kozlowski, A. M. (2011). Behaviors and corresponding functions addressed via functional assessment. *Research in Developmental Disabilities, 32*(2), 625–629.

Mayes, S. D., Lockridge, R., & Tierney, C. D. (2017). Tantrums are not associated with speech or language deficits in preschool children with autism. *Journal of Developmental and Physical Disabilities, 29*(4), 587–596.

Mayes, S. D., Waxmonsky, J. D., Calhoun, S. L., & Bixler, E. O. (2016). Disruptive mood dysregulation disorder symptoms and association with oppositional defiant and other disorders in a general population child sample. *Journal of Child and Adolescent Psychopharmacology, 26*(2), 101–106.

Mazars, G. (1970). Criteria for identifying cingulate epilepsies. *Epilepsia, 11*, 41–47.

McCurdy, M., Kunz, G. M., & Sheridan, S. M. (2006). Temper tantrums. In G. G. Bear & K. M. Minke (Eds.), *Children's needs III: Development, prevention, and intervention* (pp. 149–157). Washington, DC US: National Association of School Psychologists.

McSwain, R. (1981). Care and conflict in infant development: An East-Timorese and Papua New Guinean comparison. *Infant Behavior and Development, 4*, 225–246.

Mercer, J. (2013). Holding therapy: A harmful mental health intervention. *Focus on Alternative and Complementary Therapies, 18*(2), 70–76.

Miller, M. A., Rothenberger, S. D., Hasler, B. P., Donofry, S. D., Wong, P. M., Manuck, S. B., . . . Roecklein, K. A. (2015). Chronotype predicts positive affect rhythms measured by ecological momentary assessment. *Chronobiology International, 32*(3), 376–384.

Minde, K., & Tidmarsh, L. (1997). The changing practices of an infant psychiatry program: The McGill Experience. *Infant Mental Health Journal, 18*, 135–144.

Mireault, G., & Trahan, J. (2007). Tantrums and anxiety in early childhood: A pilot study. *Early Childhood Research & Practice, 9*(2), n2.

Moise, A. M., Leary, L., Morgan, L. C., Papanastassiou, A. M., & Szabó, C. Á. (2017). Ictal laughter and crying: Should they be classified as automatisms? *Epilepsy & Behavior Case Reports, 7*, 31–33.

Morphy, H. (1989). On representing ancestral beings. In H. Morphy (Ed.), *Animals into Art* (pp. 144–160). University of Oxford, London.

Myers, F. R. (1988). The logic and meaning of anger among Pintupi Aborigines. *Man, 23*(3), 589–610.

Needlman, R., Stevenson, J., & Zuckerman, B. (1991). Psychosocial correlates of severe temper tantrums. *Journal of Developmental and Behavioral Pediatrics, 2*, 77–83.

Newman, J. D. (2007). Neural circuits underlying crying and cry responding in mammals. *Behavioural Brain Research, 182*(2), 155–165.

Nishida, T. (1990). Deceptive behavior in young chimpanzees: An essay. In Nishida, T. (Ed.), *The chimpanzees of the Mahale Mountains* (pp. 285–290). Tokyo: Tokyo University Press.

Nydegger, W. F., & Nydegger, C. (1963). Tarong: An Ilocos barrio in the Philippines. In B. Whiting (Ed.), *Six cultures: Studies of child rearing* (pp. 693–868). New York: Wiley.

Österman, K., & Björkqvist, K. (2010). A cross-sectional study of onset, cessation, frequency, and duration of children's temper tantrums in a nonclinical sample. *Psychological Reports, 106*(2), 448–454.

Painuly, N. P., Grover, S., Gupta, N., & Mattoo, S. K. (2011). Prevalence of anger attacks in depressive and anxiety disorders: Implications for their construct? *Psychiatry and Clinical Neurosciences, 65*(2), 165–174.

Parvizi, J., Coburn, K. L., Shillcutt, S. D., Coffey, C. E., Lauterbach, E. C., & Mendez, M. F. (2009). Neuroanatomy of pathological laughing and crying: A report of the American Neuropsychiatric Association Committee on Research. *The Journal of Neuropsychiatry and Clinical Neurosciences, 21*(1), 75–87.

Pavé, R., Kowalewski, M. M., Peker, S. M., & Zunino, G. E. (2010). Preliminary study of mother–offspring conflict in black and gold howler monkeys (Alouatta caraya). *Primates, 51*(3), 221–226.

Pavé, R., Kowalewski, M. M., Zunino, G. E., & Giraudo, A. R. (2015). How do demographic and social factors influence parent-offspring conflict? The case of wild black and gold howler monkeys (Alouatta caraya). *American Journal of Primatology, 77*(8), 911–923.

Peterson, N. (1993). Demand sharing: Reciprocity and the pressure for generosity among foragers. *American Anthropologist, 95*(4), 860–874

Petrican, R., Saverino, C., Rosenbaum, R. S., & Grady, C. (2015). Inter-individual differences in the experience of negative emotion predict variations in functional brain architecture. *NeuroImage, 123*, 80–88.

Porter, T., & Gavin, H. (2010). Infanticide and neonaticide: A review of 40 years of research literature on incidence and causes. *Trauma, Violence, & Abuse, 11*(3), 99–112.

Pospisil, L. (1971). *Kapauku Papuans and their law*. Publications No 54, Human Relations Area Files. New Haven, CT: Yale University Press.

Potegal, M. (1986). Differential effects of ethyl (R,S)-nipecotate on the behaviors of highly and minimally aggressive female hamsters. *Psychopharmacology, 89*, 444–448.

Potegal, M. (2000). Toddler tantrums: Flushing and other visible autonomic activity in an anger-crying complex. In R. Barr et al. (Eds.), *Crying as a sign, a symptom, and a* signal: Clinical, emotional, and developmental aspects of infant and toddler crying (pp. 121–136). Surrey, UK: MacKeith Press.

Potegal, M. (2003). *Preliminary observations on salivary cortisol baseline and transients associated with tantrums in 3-year-olds* (p. 195). Tampa, FL: Society for Research in Child Development.

Potegal, M. (2005, April). *Tantrums in externalizing, internalizing and typically developing 4-year-olds.* Poster presented at the biennial meeting of the Society for Research in Child Development: Atlanta, GA.

Potegal, M. (2010). The temporal dynamics of anger: Phenomena, processes and perplexities. In M. Potegal, G. Stemmler, & C. Spielberger (Eds.), *International handbook of anger* (pp. 385–402). New York: Springer.

Potegal, M. (2012). Temporal and frontal lobe initiation and regulation of the top-down escalation of anger and aggression. *Behavioural Brain Research. 231,* 386–395

Potegal, M., & Archer, J. (2004). Sex differences in childhood anger and aggression. *Child and Adolescent Psychiatric Clinics of North America: Sex and Gender. 13,* 513–528.

Potegal, M., Carlson, G., Margulies, D., Gutkovitch, Z., & Wall, M. (2009). Rages or temper tantrums? The behavioral organization, temporal characteristics, and clinical significance of angry-agitated outbursts in child psychiatry inpatients. *Child Psychiatry and Human Development 40,* 621–636

Potegal, M., & Davidson, R. J. (1997). Young children's post tantrum affiliation with their parents. *Aggressive Behavior (Special Issue on Appeasement and Reconciliation) 23,* 329–342.

Potegal, M., & Davidson, R. J. (2003). Temper tantrums in young children: 1) Behavioral composition. *Journal of Developmental and Behavioral Pediatrics, 24,* 140–147.

Potegal, M., & Kosorok, M. (1995). *Temper tantrums in young children.* Indianapolis, IN: Society for Research in Child Development.

Potegal, M. Kosorok, M. R., & Davidson R. J. (2003). Temper tantrums in young children: II) Tantrum duration and temporal organization. *Journal of Developmental and Behavioral Pediatrics, 24,* 148–154.

Potegal, M., & Qiu, P. (2010). Anger in children's tantrums: A new, quantitative, behaviorally based model. In M. Potegal, G. Stemmler, & C. Spielberger (Eds.), *International handbook of anger* (pp. 193–217). New York: Springer. doi.org/10.1007/978-0-387-89676-2_12

Potegal, M., Robison, S., Anderson, F., Jordan, C., & Shapiro, E. (2007). Sequence and priming in 15-month-olds' reactions to brief arm restraint: Evidence for a hierarchy of anger responses. *Aggressive Behavior, 33,* 1–11.

Potegal, M., & Stemmler, G. (2010). Constructing a neurology of anger. In M. Potegal, G. Stemmler, & C. Spielberger (Eds.), *International handbook of anger* (pp. 39–60). New York: Springer. doi.org/10.1007/978-0-387-89676-2_12

Potegal, M., Yoburn, C., & Glusman, M. (1983). Disinhibition of muricide and irritability by instraseptal muscimol. *Pharmacology, Biochemistry and Behavior, 19,* 663–669.

Quigley, K. S., & Barrett, L. F. (2014). Is there consistency and specificity of autonomic changes during emotional episodes? Guidance from the conceptual act theory and psychophysiology. *Biological Psychology, 98,* 82–94.

Qiu, P., Yang, R., & Potegal, M. (2009). Statistical modeling of the time course of tantrum anger. *Annals of Applied Statistics, 3,* 1013–1034.

Ramani, G. B., Brownell, C. A., & Campbell, S. B. (2010). Positive and negative peer interaction in 3-and 4-year-olds in relation to regulation and dysregulation. *Journal of Genetic Psychology, 171*(3), 218–250.

Rescorla, L. A., Achenbach, T. M., Ivanova, M. Y., Harder, V. S., Otten, L., Bilenberg, N., . . . Dobrean, A. (2011). International comparisons of behavioral and emotional problems in preschool children: Parents' reports from 24 societies. *Journal of Clinical Child & Adolescent Psychology, 40*(3), 456–467.

Rice, L. (2016). Understanding the characteristics and causal mechanisms of temper outbursts in Prader-Willi syndrome. (Doctoral dissertation.) University of Sydney. Retrieved from https://ses.library.usyd.edu.au/handle/2123/15932.

Rice, L. J., Gray, K. M., Howlin, P., Taffe, J., Tonge, B. J., & Einfeld, S. L. (2015). The developmental trajectory of disruptive behavior in Down syndrome, fragile X syndrome, Prader–Willi syndrome and Williams syndrome. *American Journal of Medical Genetics Part C: Seminars in Medical Genetics, 169*, 182–187.

Richman, N., Stevenson, J. E., & Graham, P. J. (1975). Prevalence of behaviour problems in 3-year-old children: An epidemiological study in a London borough, *Journal of Child Psychology and Psychiatry, 16*, 277–287.

Robinson, R. G., & Jorge, R. E. (2015). Post-stroke depression: A review. *American Journal of Psychiatry, 173*(3), 221–231.

Roy, A. K., Bennett, R., Posner, J., Hulvershorn, L., Castellanos, F. X., & Klein, R. G. (2017). Altered intrinsic functional connectivity of the cingulate cortex in children with severe temper outbursts. *Development and Psychopathology, 30*(2), 571–579.

Roy, A. K., Klein, R. G., Angelosante, A., Bar-Haim, Y., Leibenluft, E., Hulvershorn, L., . . . Spindel, C. (2013). Clinical features of young children referred for impairing temper outbursts. *Journal of Child and Adolescent Psychopharmacology, 23*(9), 588–596.

Russell, J. A. (1991). Culture and the categorization of emotions. *Psychological Bulletin, 110*(3), 426–450.

Scherer, K. R., & Tannenbaum, P. H. (1986). Emotional experiences in everyday life: A survey approach. *Motivation and Emotion, 10*(4), 295–314.

Schieffelin, B. B. (1986). Teasing and shaming in Kahili children's interactions. In B. B. Schieffelin & E. Ochs (Eds.), *Language Socialization Across Cultures* (pp. 165–181). Cambridge University Press.

Schutter, D. J., & Harmon-Jones, E. (2013). The corpus callosum: A commissural road to anger and aggression. *Neuroscience & Biobehavioral Reviews, 37*(10), 2481–2488.

Sell, A., Cosmides, L., & Tooby, J. (2014). The human anger face evolved to enhance cues of strength. *Evolution and Human Behavior, 35*(5), 425–429.

Semple, S., Gerald, M. S., & Suggs, D. N. (2009). Bystanders affect the outcome of mother–infant interactions in rhesus macaques. *Proceedings of the Royal Society of London B: Biological Sciences, 276*, 2257–2262.

Shi, Y., Yang, D., Zeng, Y., & Wu, W. (2017). Risk factors for post-stroke depression: A meta-analysis. *Frontiers in Aging Neuroscience, 9*, 218–225.

Shostak, M. (1981). *The life and words of a !Kung woman.* Cambridge, MA: Harvard University Press.

Sipes, M., Matson, J. L., Horovitz, M., & Shoemaker, M. (2011). The relationship between autism spectrum disorders and symptoms of conduct problems: The moderating effect of communication. *Developmental Neurorehabilitation, 14*(1), 54–59.

Slocombe, K. E., Townsend, S. W., & Zuberbühler, K. (2009). Wild chimpanzees (Pan troglodytes schweinfurthii) distinguish between different scream types: Evidence from a playback study. *Animal Cognition, 12*(3), 441–449.

Snyder, J. (2015). Coercive family processes in the development of externalizing behavior: Incorporating neurobiology into intervention research. In T. P. Beauchaine & S. P. Hinshaw (Eds.), *The Oxford Handbook of Externalizing Spectrum Disorders* (pp. 286–302). Oxford University Press.

Sobel, A. B., Roberts, M. C., Rayfield, A. D., Barnard, M. U., & Rapoff, M. A. (2001). Evaluating outpatient pediatric psychology services in a primary care setting. *Journal of Pediatric Psychology, 26*(7), 395–405.

Sokol, R. I., Webster, K. L., Thompson, N. S., & Stevens, D. A. (2005). Whining as mother-directed speech. *Infant and Child Development, 14*(5), 478–490.

Soltis J. (2004). The signal functions of early infant crying. *Behavioral and Brain Sciences, 27,* 443–458

Sourander, A., Aurela, A., & Piha, J. (1994). Therapeutic holding in child and adolescent psychiatric inpatient treatment. *Nordic Journal of Psychiatry, 50*(5), 375–379.

Spinrad, T. L., Eisenberg, N., Granger, D. A., Eggum, N. D., Sallquist, J., Haugen, R. G., . . . Hofer, C. (2009). Individual differences in preschoolers' salivary cortisol and alpha-amylase reactivity: Relations to temperament and maladjustment. *Hormones and Behavior, 56*(1), 133–139.

Steckley, L. (2011). Touch, physical restraint and therapeutic containment in residential child care. *British Journal of Social Work, 42*(3), 537–555.

Stevenson, J., & Goodman, R. (2001). Association between behaviour at age 3 years and adult criminality. *The British Journal of Psychiatry, 179*(3), 197–202.

Stirling, C., & McHugh, A. (1998). Developing a non-aversive intervention strategy in the management of aggression and violence for people with learning disabilities using natural therapeutic holding. *Journal of Advanced Nursing, 27*(3), 503–509.

Stoolmiller, M. (2001). Synergistic interaction of child manageability problems and parent-discipline tactics in predicting future growth in externalizing behavior for boys. *Developmental Psychology, 37,* 814–825.

Sullivan, M. W., & Lewis, M. (2012). Relations of early goal-blockage response and gender to subsequent tantrum behavior. *Infancy, 17*(2), 159–178.

Swain, J. E., Mayes, L. C., & Leckman, J. F. (2004). The development of parent-infant attachment through dynamic and interactive signaling loops of care and cry. *Behavioral and Brain Sciences, 27*(4), 472–473.

Tiedens, L. Z., & Fragale, A. R. (2003). Power moves: Complementarity in dominant and submissive nonverbal behavior. *Journal of Personality and Social Psychology, 84*(3), 558.

Trivers, R. L. (1974). Parent–offspring conflict. *American Zoology, 14,* 249–264.

Trivers, R. L. (1985). *Social evolution.* Benjamin/Cummings, Menlo Park, CA.

Tsutaya, T., & Yoneda, M. (2015). Reconstruction of breastfeeding and weaning practices using stable isotope and trace element analyses: A review. *American Journal of Physical Anthropology, 156*(S59), 2–21.

Tufan, E., Topal, Z., Demir, N., Taskiran, S., Savci, U., Cansiz, M. A., & Semerci, B. (2016). Sociodemographic and clinical features of disruptive mood dysregulation disorder: A chart review. *Journal of Child & Adolescent Psychopharmacology, 26,* 94–100.

Tunnicliffe, P., Woodcock, K., Bull, L., Oliver, C., & Penhallow, J. (2014). Temper outbursts in Prader-Willi syndrome: Causes, behavioural and emotional sequence and responses by carers. *Journal of Intellectual Disability Research*, *58*(2), 134–150.

Van Dijk, M., & Van Geert, P. (2007). Wobbles, humps and sudden jumps: A case study of continuity, discontinuity and variability in early language development. *Infant and Child Development*, *16*(1), 7–33.

Van Leeuwen, K., Bourgonjon, L., Huijsman, L., Van Meenen, M., & De Pauw, S. (2009). Temper tantrums in young children: Relations with child temperament, child problem behavior and parenting. Poster presented at the SRCD Biennial Meeting, April 2009, Location: Denver.

Van Meter, A., Moreira, A., & Youngstrom E. (2011). Meta-analysis of epidemiologic studies of pediatric bipolar disorder. *Journal of Clinical Psychiatry*, *72*, 1250–1256.

van Noordwijk, M. A., & van Schaik, C. P. (2005). Development of ecological competence in Sumatran orangutans. *American Journal of Physical Anthropology*, *127*(1), 79–94.

Varley, C. K., & Smith, C. J. (2003). Anxiety disorders in the child and teen. *Pediatric Clinics of North America*, *50*(5), 1107–1138.

Vingerhoets, A., & Scheirs, J. (2000). Sex differences in crying: Empirical findings and possible explanations. In Agneta H. Fischer (Ed.), *Gender and emotion* (pp. 143–165). Cambridge: Cambridge University Press.

Vollmer, T. R., Northup, J., Ringdahl, J. E., Le Blanc, L. A., & Chauvin, T. M. (1996). Functional analysis of severe tantrums displayed by children with language delays: An outclinic assessment. *Behavior Modification*, *20*, 97–115.

Vollmer, T. R., Progar, P. R., Lalli, J. S., Camp, C. M., Sierp, B. J., Wright, C. S., . . . Eisenschink, K. J. (1998). Fixed-time schedules attenuate extinction- induced phenomena in the treatment of severe aberrant behavior. *Journal of Applied Behavior Analysis*, *31*(4), 529–542.

Wager, T. D., Kang, J., Johnson, T. D., Nichols, T. E., Satpute, A. B., & Barrett, L. F. (2015). A Bayesian model of category-specific emotional brain responses. *PLoS Computational Biology*, *11*(4), e1004066.

Wakschlag, L. S., Choi, S. W., Carter, A. S., Hullsiek, H., Burns, J., McCarthy, K., . . . Briggs-Gowan, M. J. (2012). Defining the developmental parameters of temper loss in early childhood: Implications for developmental psychopathology. *Journal of Child Psychology and Psychiatry*, *53*(11), 1099–1108.

Wakschlag, L. S., Estabrook, R., Petitclerc, A., Henry, D., Burns, J. L., Perlman, S. B., . . . Briggs-Gowan, M. L. (2015). Clinical implications of a dimensional approach: The normal:abnormal spectrum of early irritability. *Journal of the American Academy of Child & Adolescent Psychiatry*, *54*(8), 626–634.

Wallez, C., & Vauclair, J. (2012). First evidence of population-level oro-facial asymmetries during the production of distress calls by macaque (Macaca mulatta) and baboon (Papio anubis) infants. *Behavioural Brain Research*, *234*(1), 69–75.

Wang, G., Teng, F., Chen, Y., Liu, Y., Li, Y., Cai, L., . . . Jin, L. (2016). Clinical features and related factors of poststroke pathological laughing and crying: A case–control study. *Journal of Stroke and Cerebrovascular Diseases*, *25*(3), 556–564.

Ward, B. E. (1970). Temper tantrums in Kau Sai: Some speculations upon their effects. In Mayer, P. (Ed.), *Socialisation: The approach from social anthropology* (pp. 109–126). London: Tavistock.

Watson, J. B., & Watson, R. R. (1921). Studies in infant psychology. *The Scientific Monthly*, *13*(6), 493–515.

Weaver, A., & de Waal, F. (2003). The mother-offspring relationship as a template in social development: Reconciliation in captive brown capuchins (Cebus apella). *Journal of Comparative Psychology*, *117*(1), 101.

Welch, M. G. (1989). *Holding time: How to eliminate conflict, temper tantrums, and sibling rivalry and raise happy, loving, successful children*. New York: Simon and Schuster.

Welch, M. G., Northrup, R. S., Welch-Horan, T. B., Ludwig, R. J., Austin, C. L., & Jacobson, J. S. (2006). Outcomes of prolonged parent–child embrace therapy among 102 children with behavioral disorders. *Complementary Therapies in Clinical Practice*, *12*(1), 3–12.

Wenar, C. (1982). On negativism. *Human Development*, *25*, 1–23.

White, B. P., Gunnar, M. R., Larson, M. C., Donzella, B., & Barr, R. G. (2000). Behavioral and physiological responsivity, sleep, and patterns of daily cortisol production in infants with and without colic. *Child Development*, *71*(4), 862–877.

Wickless, C., & Kirsch, I. (1988). Cognitive correlates of anger, anxiety, and sadness. *Cognitive Therapy and Research*, *12*(4), 367–377.

Wong, C. H., Mohamed, A., Larcos, G., McCredie, R., Somerville, E., & Bleasel, A. (2010). Brain activation patterns of versive, hypermotor, and bilateral asymmetric tonic seizures. *Epilepsia*, *51*(10), 2131–2139.

Wortzel, H. S., Oster, T. J., Anderson, C. A., & Arciniegas, D. (2008). Pathological laughing and crying: Epidemiology, pathophysiology and treatment. *CNS Drugs*, *22*, 531–545.

Etiological Mechanisms

8

Genetics of Pediatric Irritability

Meridith L. Eastman, Ashlee A. Moore, and Roxann Roberson-Nay

This chapter provides an overview of behavioral and molecular genetics of pediatric irritability. Irritability is a *transdiagnostic* dimensional construct that lends itself well to exploration with multiple methods across numerous levels of analysis in human and model organisms. Given its transdiagnostic nature, irritability has been explored in the context of numerous psychiatric phenotypes, but whether the genetic mechanisms of irritability in the context of these diverse psychopathologies differs, is not known. To untangle this question, molecular genetic studies of irritability manifest with and without comorbid internalizing or externalizing conditions may be compared to determine if genetic variants differ; however, this effort would undoubtedly require extremely large sample sizes. For this reason, another possible approach to elucidate genetic mechanisms is via genetically-informed multivariate models where the fit of models (i.e., independent pathway, common pathway) can be compared to test distinct hypotheses about the types of shared genetic and environmental pathways by which covariation between the phenotypes occur (Neale & Cardon, 1992). Ultimately, psychiatric genetics will provide estimates of genetic (and environmental) influences on irritable mood while molecular genetics studies will impart an understanding of its underlying biology.

For this chapter, we conducted searches on the PubMed and PsycInfo databases for the terms "Genes" or "Genetics" or "Heritability" AND "Irritability" or "Irritable Mood" to identify animal studies, behavioral genetic (BG) studies, and molecular genetic studies on irritability. This yielded 167 results in PsycInfo and 461 PubMed results. Two of the authors of this chapter (A. A. M. and M. L. E) examined abstracts for relevance and excluded case studies and studies on very specific adult and pediatric populations (e.g., drug-dependent, with Alzheimer's or Huntington's, Prader-Willi syndrome), studies on irritable infant temperament

TABLE 8.1. Summary of results from animal studies of irritability

Ref No.	Sample Characteristics	Irritability Measure	Results
17	Mice (male and female)	Aggressiveness (fights, behavior while handling) rated using observation	Both male and female ICR mice (not C57BL6J) showed increases in monoamine neurotransmitter levels from 4 weeks of age to 28–32 weeks of age. Only male ICR mice (not C57BL6J) showed increased aggression from 4 to 28–32 weeks of age.
32	41 rhesus monkeys 56% female	Primate Neonatal Neurobehavioral Assessment	Gene × environment interaction found that the short 5 HT transporter allele was associated with neonatal irritability in fetal alcohol–exposed monkeys, but not in non–fetal alcohol-exposed monkeys.
34	13 rats 100% male	Modified version of the Brady and Nauta Scale (measures behaviors such as resistance to capture and handling, muscle tension, and biting)	Septal lesions resulted in increased irritability in both strains; however, one strain, known to have lower whole brain synthesis rates of 5-HT (RLA/Verh) exhibited higher postop irritability than the other (RHA/Verh).
37	Mice (male and female)	Aggressiveness rated using wounding index and resident-intruder test	Two of the four mouse strains studied (BA and C47BL/6J lines) showed only slight increases in aggression after unpredictable chronic mild stress (UCMS), with the BA strain being particularly resistant to the effects of UCMS.

(i.e., fussiness), and studies related to genetic differences in drug efficacy. The final list of relevant articles included 4 animal studies, 13 BG studies, and 20 molecular genetics studies for a total of 37 unique studies on irritability (one study, Greenwood et al., 2013, included both behavioral and molecular genetics elements). These studies are summarized in Tables 8.1–8.3 and discussed in the sections that follow. A glossary of relevant terms italicized throughout the chapter is presented in Table 8.4.

Animal Studies

Animal models can be useful to study the genetic etiology of human traits. Using animals with genomic similarity to humans, scientists are able to manipulate study conditions (e.g., induce stress, provide enrichments, limit socialization) in a controlled environment (Simmons, 2008). Such manipulations and controls may be either unethical or too difficult to achieve in comparable human studies.

TABLE 8.2. Summary of results from twin and family studies of irritability

Ref No.	Sample Characteristics	Irritability Measure	Results
5	63 youth and 79 of their parents 25% female Mean youth age ≈ 12	Severe Mood Dysregulation (SMD) diagnosis via the Schedule for Affective Disorders and Schizophrenia for School-Age Children	Parents of children with bipolar disorder (BP) were more likely to have BP than parents of children with SMD.
11	60 youth from 37 families 52% female Mean youth age ≈ 11	Kiddie Schedule for Affective Disorders and Schizophrenia (KSADS)	Severity of irritable mood and problems with mood regulation were associated with bilineal risk of BP (two parents with BP).
12	600 twins 0% female Mean age ≈ 44	Irritability Scale from the Buss-Durkee Hostility Inventory	37% of variance due to dominant genetic effects, 63% due to nonshared environmental effects. Genetic correlation between irritability scale and direct hostility (.46), indirect hostility (.80), and verbal hostility (.71). Environmental correlation between irritability scale and direct hostility (.41), indirect hostility (.09), and verbal hostility (.46).
13	> 1,000 twins 60% female Mean age ≈ 59	Items from 1) Karolinska Scales of Personality, 2) Emotionality, Activity, and Sociability Temperament Survey, and 3) Type A Behavior Questionnaire	41% of variance due to dominant genetic effects, 54% due to nonshared environmental effects.
21	1,008 twins Approx. 50% female Participants were assessed at 8 months, 4 years, and 7 years old	Behavioral observation ratings by trained psychologists	For degree of irritability at age 4, MZ twins more correlated (.40) than DZ twins (.06). For irritable/negative mood at age 4, MZ twins more correlated (.45) than DZ twins (.17).
25	670 individuals from 101 families with bipolar proband 62% female Mean age = 45	Temperament Evaluation of Memphis, Pisa, Paris and San Diego-Autoquestionnaire (TEMPS-A)	52% of the variance due to genetic effects.

(continued)

TABLE 8.2. Continued

Ref No.	Sample Characteristics	Irritability Measure	Results
33	>5000 twins Approx. 51% female Participants were assessed at age 7 years, 10 years, and 12 years old	Irritable latent class of oppositional defiant disorder (ODD) via the oppositional subscale of the Connor's Parent Rating Scales Revised Short Form	At age 7, 25.2% and 33.3% of variance in irritable class membership due to genetic effects for females and males, respectively. At age 7, 39.5% and 27.9% of variance due to genetic effects for females and males, respectively. At age 7, 45% and 31% of variance due to genetic effects for females and males, respectively.
36	2510 twins 51% female Mean age ≈ 12	Irritable dimension of ODD via Diagnostic Interview for Children and Adolescents	54% of variance due to genetic effects, 46% due to nonshared environmental effects.
43	337 child-parent dyads 58% female youth Mean youth age ≈ 12	Child and Adolescent Psychiatric Assessment	Irritability predicts future MDD onset independent of family risk (family risk for MDD does not act on irritability directly).
45	2,620 twins 50% female Assessed at 8–9 years, 13–14 years, 16–17 years, and 19–20 years	Child Behavior Checklist	Quantitative, but not qualitative, genetic sex effects were found. For males, the percentage of variance explained by genetic effects at times 1, 2, 3, & 4 were 36%, 68%, 76%, & 89%, respectively. For females, the percentage of variance explained by genetic effects at waves 1–4 were 66%, 64%, 56%, & 46% respectively Genetic stability found in both sexes, with some new genetic innovations in males.
47	2,620 twins 50% female Assessed at 8–9 years, 13–14 years, 16–17 years, and 19–20 years	Child Behavior Checklist	Percentage of variance explained by genetic effects at times 1, 2, 3, & 4 were 42%, 51%, 48%, and 46%, respectively. The percentage of variance explained by nonshared environmental effects at times 1–4 was 49%, 47%, 50%, & 53%, respectively. Shared environmental effects explained the remaining variance. Evidence for stable genetic effects, as well as genetic innovations at each time point. Evidence for stable unique environmental effects and unique environmental innovations at each time point. Evidence for stable common environmental effects only (no innovations). Genetic correlation between irritability and depression/anxiety ranged from 57% - 67%, depending on wave.

40	242 individuals Approx. 38% female 12–30 years old	Kiddie Schedule for Affective Disorders and Schizophrenia Diagnostic Interview for Genetic Studies Family Interview for Genetic Studies	Irritability symptoms were not significantly different between those with and without high familial risk of bipolar disorder.
50	2,651 individuals Approx. 42% male Mean age at first irritability assessment ≈ 15	Irritable dimension of ODD via Achenbach System of Empirically Based Assessment	31% of variance due to genetic effects, 69% due to nonshared environmental effects. Genetic correlation between irritability and depression was .7. Genetic correlation between irritability and delinquency was .57, although this was due entirely to the overlap between ODD dimensions (irritable and hurtful/headstrong).

TABLE 8.3. Summary of results from molecular genetic studies of irritability

Ref No.	Sample Characteristics	Irritability Measure	Results
1	750 children Approx. 13% female 5–17 years old	Irritable dimension of ODD via the long form of the Conners parent rating scale	No association between irritability and 9 polymorphisms in the candidate gene/regions DRD4, OTR, and 5-HTTLPR. No genome-wide significant findings in GWAS.
4	390 adults 61% female Mean age = 52.5	Temperament Evaluation of Memphis, Pisa, Paris, and San Diego-Autoquestionnaire	No significant candidate gene associations with irritable temperament.
9	111 adults 61.3% female Mean age = 39.2	Questionnaire for Measuring Factors of Aggression	In candidate gene study, COMT rs932377 C/C genotype associated with lower irritability.
22	139 females Mean age = 31.39	Temperament Evaluation of Memphis, Pisa, Paris and San Diego-Autoquestionnaire	A significant association was found between the s allele of 5HTTLPR and the TEMPS scores of the depressive, anxious, irritable, and particularly the cyclothymic temperaments; no association was found with the hyperthymic temperament.
10	209 adults Approx. 36% female Age range 22–90	Karolinska Scales of Personality	No significant candidate gene associations after multiple testing corrections.
14	Sample 1: o 123 young adults o 60% female Sample 2: o 204 adults o 56% female o 30–63 years old	Sample 1: o Buss-Durkee Hostility Inventory Sample 2: o Multidimensional Personality Questionnaire	Sample 1: o 11 genotype (vs. 12 vs. 22) of promotor region SNP of ADRA2A candidate gene associated with irritability subscale. Sample 2: o Results from sample 1 replicated.
15	370 adults 44% female Mean age = 42	Swedish Universities Scales of Personality	Two long variants of the transcription factor polymorphism (intron 2) in the AP-2β gene associated with lower irritability in women, but not in men.
18	206 adults 60.7% female Mean age = 50.4	Diagnostic Interview for Genetic Studies	No significant linkage associations.

20	571 adults 56% female Age range 18–79	Questionnaire for the Measuring Factors of Aggression	Irritability associated with G allele carrier status for rs225374 in candidate gene ABCG1.
24	1,263 adults 64% female	Temperament Evaluation of Memphis, Pisa, Paris and San Diego-Autoquestionnaire	GWAS analysis revealed genome-wide significant associations for irritable temperament on chromosome 1 within INTS7 and DTL genes.
26	1,001 adults Approx. 60% female	Diagnostic Interview for Genetic Studies	GWAS analyses revealed no genome-wide significant differences between irritable mania and elated mania.
25	670 individuals from 110 families with bipolar proband	Temperament Evaluation of Memphis, Pisa, Paris, and San Diego-Autoquestionnaire	Linkage analysis did not reveal any regions of the genome significantly associated with irritability.
29	178 adults 60% female Mean age ≈ 40	Affective Disorders Evaluation	Irritability associated with rs17306779, rs3829125, and rs1090440 in candidate gene AKR1C4.
30	290 young adults 41% female Mean age ≈ 22	Temperament Evaluation of Memphis, Pisa, Paris and San Diego	4 repeats, vs. 2 repeats, of the VNTR polymorphism in the DRD4 candidate gene associated with irritable temperament in males, but not females.
41	94 adults 57% female Mean age = 39.2	Spielberger State-Trait Anger Expression Inventory-2	Rs4675690 in candidate gene CREB1 associated with anger expression score.
44	>5,500 children 4–9 years	Strengths and Difficulties Questionnaire	Polygenic risk score derived from schizophrenia Psychiatric Genetic Consortium GWAS associated with irritability at age 7, but this did not remain significant after controlling for sex and social class.
46	70 adults 71% female Mean age = 59	Temperament Evaluation of Memphis, Pisa, Paris and San Diego-Autoquestionnaire	No significant associations between irritable temperament and 38 SNPs in candidate genes CLOCK, ARNTL, TIM, and PER3.
51	517 adults 52% female Mean age = 45	Karolinska Scales of Personality	An allele of rs17577 in candidate gene MMP-9 associated with higher irritability in males, but not females.

(continued)

TABLE 8.3. Continued

Ref No.	Sample Characteristics	Irritability Measure	Results
53	44 adults 32% female Mean age = 27.4	Temperament Evaluation of Memphis, Pisa, Paris and San Diego-Autoquestionnaire	No significant association between temperament measures and SNPs within candidate genes BDNF, GSK3β, and Wnt.
55	172 adults 100% female 42 years old	Karolinska Scales of Personality	"Non-conformity" factor, including indirect aggression and irritability, associated with a polymorphic TA repeat in the estrogen receptor α gene.

TABLE 8.4. Glossary of important terminology

Term	Definition
Allele	One of two or more forms of a single gene.
Candidate gene / Candidate gene study	A gene that is suspected of being causally related to a trait or disease. Candidate gene studies test whether a statistical correlation exists between the phenotype of interest and variants of the candidate gene.
Gene × environment interaction	A difference in the magnitude or direction of effect of an environmental factor for people with different genotypes.
Genome-wide association study (GWAS)	An examination of a large number of SNPs across the genome to see if any are associated with a specific trait.
Heritability	The proportion of a trait's phenotypic variance that is due to genetic variance in the population.
Linkage analysis	Type of gene-mapping study based on co-segregation of a trait with a known genetic marker.
Pathway analysis	Type of study in which a set of genes corresponding to a biological pathway is tested for association with a phenotype.
Phasic irritability	The tendency to have developmentally inappropriate outbursts of intense anger.
Polygenic risk score (PRS)	A sum of trait-associated alleles across multiple genetic loci.
Single nucleotide polymorphisms (SNPs)	A variation of a single base pair at a specific genomic location.
Tonic irritability	Persistently angry, grumpy, or grouchy mood.
Transdiagnostic	Characteristic of multiple types of psychopathology.

Additionally, animals with shorter reproductive cycles and life spans offer the opportunity to conduct developmental studies in much briefer periods of time than would be possible with humans (Institute of Medicine, 2006). With these advantages, animal models can be an important first step in understanding heritability and genetic etiology of psychological traits.

Our literature search identified four animal studies that have examined the genetics of irritability (or related emotional constructs). Three of these involved rodent models and the fourth was conducted in rhesus monkeys. The rodent models (Everett, 1977; Lieblich & Driscoll, 1983; Mineur, Prasol, Belzung, & Crusio, 2003) examined differences in aggressive behavior or emotionality among genetically different inbred strains. Observed "aggressive behavior" and "emotionality" were essentially used as proxies for irritability in these studies. The earliest rodent study (Everett, 1977) found differences in aggressive behavior (operationalized as number of fights and aggressive behavior, such as biting and vocalizing while being handled) with age between two inbred strains of mice. The more aggressive strain also showed increased brain levels in monoamines, which suggests a role of dopaminergic, adrenergic, and serotonergic systems in comparable behavior in humans. A later study (Lieblich & Driscoll, 1983) induced septal lesions in two strains of rats and assessed emotionality through a scale that measured behaviors such as resistance to capture and handling, muscle tension, and biting. Authors noted that the strain that exhibited more post-lesion irritability had also exhibited higher base brain synthesis rates of serotonin in other studies. The final rodent study (Mineur et al., 2003) tested differential responses to unpredictable chronic mild stress (UCMS) in genetically different inbred mouse strains. Because the strains exhibiting different levels of UCMS-induced aggression were also known to differ in base rates of serotonin synthesis, the authors suggested that increased aggression observed in some depressed patients may be related to serotonin levels.

An extensive body of prior research on the role of serotonin dysfunction in a wide variety of psychopathology led one group of researchers (Kraemer, Moore, Newman, Barr, & Schneider, 2008) to test the role of serotonin transporter gene genotype and fetal alcohol exposure on irritability in newborn rhesus monkeys. They found that the short *allele* of the serotonin transporter gene was associated with increased irritability among fetal alcohol-exposed monkeys, whereas irritability did not differ as a function of genotype for non–fetal alcohol-exposed monkeys, demonstrating a *gene × environment interaction* that may also hold for human neonates who were prenatally exposed to alcohol.

By demonstrating strain differences (either alone or in combination with environmental manipulations) in behavioral proxies for irritability, rodent models suggest that the trait is, at least partially, genetically mediated, paving the way for studies of the heritability of irritability in humans. Furthermore, the rodent and primate models are all suggestive of a role for serotonin (alone or in concert with dopamine and noradrenaline; Everett, 1977) in the etiology of irritability, findings which have influenced selection of *candidate genes* in molecular genetics studies of irritability.

Behavioral Genetic Studies

The primary purpose of BG studies is to examine the relative influence of genes and environment on a behavioral trait or psychiatric phenotype. BG research can range from simple to complex models. A study using simple BG methodology might involve assessing whether children of parents with irritability are more at risk of developing irritability themselves. This type of family study is a common first step in BG research and is generally used to determine whether a trait has a basis that is familial in nature (i.e., influenced by genetics or shared family environment). At the other extreme, a study using more complex BG methodology might use longitudinal twin data to determine how genetic influences unfold over the life span, how the accumulation of environmental experiences influence behavior, and/or the amount of genetic influences that are common to two or more traits. The latter types of studies are able to answer more nuanced questions about a trait of interest and are generally performed only after the heritability of said trait has been determined.

Heritability is defined as the proportion of phenotypic variation within a population that is due to genetic variance (Neale & Cardon, 1992). The primary type of study used to determine heritability is the classical twin study. The twin study takes advantage of the fact that monozygotic (MZ) twins are genetically identical and therefore share 100% of their polymorphic alleles (i.e., those alleles that vary among individuals in a population). Alternatively, dizygotic (DZ) twins are about as similar as most other siblings, sharing about 50% of their polymorphic alleles. Furthermore, both MZ and DZ twins are unique from other family members in that they share nearly identical pre- and post- natal family environments (Kendler, Neale, Kessler, Heath, & Eaves, 1993). These known relationships allow for the difference in MZ versus DZ similarity to be interpreted as reflecting genetic influences. In the classical twin study, MZ and DZ correlations are used to decompose the overall trait variance into three separate sources of variance: additive genetic influences (A), common/familial environment (C), and unique environment (E). Genetic influences (A) reflect the additive effect of multiple genomic alleles. Common/family environment (C) reflects environmental factors that cause family members to be more alike, whereas unique environment (E) reflects aspects that are unique to one member of a twin pair and includes measurement error.

A modest number of BG studies have examined the heritability of irritability, although only a few have done so specifically in child populations. In a study using observational ratings of irritability in 504 4-year-old twin pairs, trained psychologists observed twins during mental and motor testing and during free play and rated them on several dimensions, including "degree of irritability." The heritability of observed irritability was approximately 68%, and a irritability/negative mood factor derived from several behavioral ratings was estimated slightly lower at 56% (Goldsmith & Gottesman, 1981). A more recent study used a longitudinal dataset of more than 2,500 Swedish twins to examine heritability throughout development as measured by an irritability scale created from the Child Behavior Checklist (CBCL). In this study, the heritability remained relatively stable over four waves of data collection and was estimated at 41%, 51%, 48%, and 46% (representing age groups of 8–9, 13–14, 16–17, and 19–20, respectively) (Savage et al., 2015). This same Swedish twin sample also has been used to examine the longitudinal course of genetic effects on pediatric irritability from childhood through adulthood (Roberson-Nay et al., 2015). Results of this study revealed significant quantitative genetic sex effects, indicating that there were different degrees of genetic influence for males and females. Specifically, males and females differed in their longitudinal genetic trajectories such that the heritability for males increased substantially over the four waves of data collection and was estimated at 36%, 68%, 76%, and 89%, respectively. On the other hand, the heritability decreased moderately for females, with heritabilities estimated at 66%, 64%, 56%, and 46%, respectively (Roberson-Nay et al., 2015). An illustration of this modeling approach (i.e., Cholesky decomposition) is illustrated in Figure 8.1, where only the additive genetic component is depicted for simplicity.

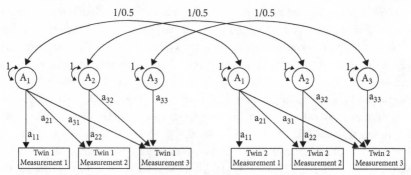

FIGURE 8.1 *Cholesky decomposition. For simplicity, only the additive genetic component is illustrated. In this figure, there are three measurements that can reflect either three different phenotypes or three longitudinal measures of the same phenotype across time. The Cholesky decomposition assumes that the latent variable A1 accounts for variation in Measurement 1 and may also explain variation in Measurement 2 and Measurement 3. The contribution of A1 to A2 and A3 is represented by the cross paths (e.g., a21, a31), which reflect shared genetic covariation.*

Although BG irritability research among juveniles is limited, research among other age groups may facilitate a better understanding of the genetic contributions to irritability in general. Among adult populations, the heritability of irritability has been estimated at between 37% and 58% (Coccaro, Bergeman, Kavoussi, & Seroczynski, 1997; Coccaro, Bergeman, & McClearn, 1993; Greenwood et al., 2013). Several adult twin studies also have reported a nonadditive (dominant) genetic effect, such that individual genetic alleles appear to have a multiplicative, rather than additive, effect. Although a potentially interesting finding, these dominant genetic effects might be better explained by these studies' reliance on hostility-related irritability measures (Cocarro et al., 1993, 1997), such as the irritability subscale from the Buss-Durkee Hostility Inventory (Buss & Durkee, 1957) and the anger subscale from the Emotionality, Activity, and Sociability Temperament Survey (Buss & Plomin, 1984).

It is not surprising that BG studies of irritability have most often been conducted in the context of psychiatric disorders, considering that *tonic irritability* and *phasic irritability* are prominent features of oppositional defiant disorder (ODD), disruptive mood dysregulation disorder (DMDD), and pediatric mood disorders (i.e., bipolar and unipolar depression), among others (American Psychiatric Association [APA], 2013). The heritability of the irritable dimension of ODD in juveniles suggests moderate heritability, ranging from 25% to 54% (Kuny et al., 2013; Mikolajewski, Taylor, & Iacono 2017; Perich Frankland, Roberts, Levy, Lenroot, & Mitchell, 2016; Stringaris, Zavos, Leibenluft, Maughan, & Eley, 2012). Furthermore, this irritable dimension of ODD appears to share genetic underpinnings with depression, with one study reporting a genetic correlation of 0.7 between the two traits (Stringaris et al., 2012).

Other studies have examined the relationship between mood disorders and irritability outside the context of ODD. In one family study, 337 high-risk families were studied where a parent had experienced at least two major depressive (MDD) episodes. This study found that both irritability and high levels of family risk (more relatives with MDD and/or more severe familial MDD) influenced future MDD onset (Rice et al., 2017). This finding was replicated and extended in another study using more than 2,500 Swedish twins (Savage et al., 2015). This study used a longitudinal design and reported a high genetic correlation between irritability and depression/anxiety (.57 to .67, depending on wave of data collection). Furthermore, the cross-lagged longitudinal model reported in this study revealed that irritability was associated with future risk for depression more than vice versa.

Unlike MDD, the results of studies investigating the relationship between irritability and bipolar disorder (BD) have been mixed. In a study of 60 children with at least one parent with BD, severity of irritable mood was associated with bilineal risk of BD (i.e., having two parents with BD; Chang, Steiner, & Ketter, 2000). However, another study reported that BD and severe mood dysregulation (i.e., a cluster of symptoms composed primarily of irritability [APA, 2013]) were distinct in terms of familial aggregation/clustering (Brotman et al., 2007; also see Fristad et al., 2016). Furthermore, another study showed no difference in irritability symptoms in controls versus individuals at high familial risk for developing BD (Perich et al., 2016).

Overall, BG studies indicate that pediatric irritability is likely influenced primarily by additive genetic and nonshared unique environmental factors, with little to no influence of dominant genetic or shared family environmental factors. However, the implications of these findings are not entirely assured due to the heterogeneous phenotypic definition of irritability used by researchers and the fact that the phenotype is often studied in the context of other psychiatric disorders.

Molecular Genetic Studies

Whereas twin and family studies identify how much variance in a trait is due to genetic factors, molecular genetic studies aim to identify which genes contribute significantly to variance in irritability.

To date, molecular genetic investigations of irritability have been largely limited to two approaches: *candidate gene studies* and *genome-wide association studies* (GWAS). Candidate gene studies a priori identify a gene that might have a role in the etiology of irritability and test whether a statistical correlation exists between the phenotype of interest and variants (often one or more *single nucleotide polymorphisms*, or SNPs) of a gene that may cause changes in its protein or expression (Tabor, Risch, & Myers, 2002). Candidate gene studies have been criticized because of a lack of replication and because the hypothesis-driven approach is limited by researchers' ability to use currently available science to identify biologically plausible candidate genes (Tabor et al., 2002). Nearly all (17 out of 18) candidate gene studies related to irritability were in adult, rather than pediatric, samples. One exception (Aebi et al., 2016) investigated the association between several different genes and the irritable subtype of ODD in children and adolescents with attention deficit/hyperactivity disorder (ADHD). However, the finding of a significant association between irritability and a gene in adults has implications for the genetics of pediatric irritability (assuming that there is a relationship between pediatric and adult phenotypic definitions of irritability) because of the DNA sequence's stability across the life course. Reflecting the transdiagnostic nature of irritability, candidate gene studies have examined irritability within the context of different types of psychopathology including BD (Johansson, Nikamo, Schalling, & Landén, 2011; Rybakowski et al., 2014), schizophrenia (Carmine et al., 2003), ODD and ADHD (Aebi et al., 2016), depression (Perlis et al., 2007), and suicidality (Calati et al., 2011; Gietl et al., 2007). No molecular genetic studies have been done on the trait of irritability in isolation.

Many different candidate genes have been investigated in an effort to identify genetic contributors to irritability. These include genes implicated in the dopaminergic and serotonergic systems such as *5-HTTLPR* (Aebi et al., 2016; Borkowska et al., 2015 Gonda et al., 2006; Kang, Namkoon, & Kim, 2008), *COMT* (Calati et al., 2011), *DRD4* (Aebi et al., 2016; Kang et al., 2008), and *AP-2ß* (Damberg et al., 2003); circadian rhythms (*CLOCK, ARNTL, TIM, PER3*; Rybakowski et al., 2014); learning and memory, such as *BDNF* (Tsutsumi et al., 2011) and MMP-9 (Suchankova, Pettersson, Nordenström, Holm, & Ekman, 2012); hormonal regulation such as *AKR1C4* (Johansson et al., 2011) and the estrogen receptor α gene (Westberg et al., 2003); cell signaling such as *GSK3β* (Tsutsumi et al., 2011), *CREB1* (Perlis et al., 2007), and *NOTCH4* (Carmine et al., 2003); the noradrenergic system (*ADRA2A;* Comings et al., 2000); and cholesterol homeostasis (*ABCG1*; Gietl et al., 2007). Candidate gene selection thus far implicates a wide range of biological systems and functions, a reflection of the lack of clarity regarding the biological etiology of irritable mood (see Chapters 8 and 9).

Nine of the 18 candidate studies we reviewed found significant associations between a candidate gene and a measure of irritability. Enthusiasm for these findings is tempered by the lack of replication of results among them and variability in defining the phenotype across studies. Six studies (Comings et al., 2000; Damberg et al., 2003; Gonda et al., 2006; Kang et al., 2008; Suchankova et al., 2012; Westberg et al., 2003) reported significant results among healthy samples. Among clinical samples, Gietl et al. (2007) found an association between *ABCG1* genotype and the irritability subscale of the Questionnaire for Measuring Factors of Aggression in a mixed sample of suicide attempters, completers, and healthy controls; Johansson et al. (2011) reported an association between *AKR1C4* genotype and manic/hypomanic irritability in male patients with BD; Perlis et al. (2007) reported an association between *CREB1* genotype and anger expression score of the Spielberger State-Trait Anger Expression Inventory-2 in a sample of MDD patients. Candidate gene findings thus span biological functions ranging from hormonal regulation (Perlis et al., 2007) to learning and memory (Suchankova et al., 2012).

Given the lack of replication and diverse phenotypic definitions across studies, results of the candidate gene literature on irritability are inconclusive, as has generally been the case for candidate gene studies on other complex traits. Due to the aforementioned limitations of candidate gene studies, such investigations are now often restricted to replication studies or to testing of candidate genes that have been identified through more rigorous gene-finding methods (such as GWAS, described below).

Another hypothesis-driven molecular genetics approach is *pathway analysis,* in which a set of genes corresponding to a biological pathway is tested for association with a phenotype (Ramanan, Shen, Moore, & Saykin, 2012). Genes within the tested pathway may consist of candidate genes or may be identified through genome-wide pathway analysis (GWPA). Pathway analysis in somatic illnesses (e.g., breast cancer, type 2 diabetes) has demonstrated that functionally related genes can collectively influence susceptibility for disease even if individual genetic loci within the pathway do not reach significance (Ramanan et al., 2012). One study (Aebi et al., 2016) employed a pathway analysis using neurotransmission pathways for serotonin, dopamine, and oxytocin to identify the genetic underpinnings of the irritable subtype of ODD. None of the pathways investigated in the study was significantly associated with ODD subtypes; however, pathway analysis remains a promising approach for investigating complex traits.

In contrast to candidate gene studies and pathway-analysis, GWAS require no prior knowledge or hypotheses regarding the etiology of irritability. Therefore, this type of study holds promise in identifying causal genes or even intergenic regions that have not been previously suspected (Stranger, Stahl, & Raj, 2011). GWAS test for association of each SNP with irritability in large samples of individuals. Three GWAS to date have been conducted on irritability within clinical populations (i.e., irritable subtype of ODD and irritable mania BD). In their multipronged investigation into the molecular genetics of ODD subtypes in a clinical sample of children and adolescents with ADHD (N = 750), Aebi and colleagues (2016) conducted a GWAS that did not result in genome-wide significant findings. However, a literature review revealed that 28 of the top-ranked 53 genes from the GWAS were involved in encoding proteins involved in β-catenin signaling and regulation of neurite outgrowth. A GWAS of irritable temperament in BD patients (N = 1,263; Greenwood, Akiskal, Akiskal, Bipolar Genome Study Consortium, & Kelsoe, 2012) found two genome-wide significant SNPs on chromosome 1. These SNPs are located in the *INTS7* and *DTL* genes involved in processing small nuclear RNAs and regulation of DNA replication, respectively. The results of another GWAS in a population of bipolar patients (N = 1,001; Greenwood, Kelsoe, & Bipolar Genome Study Consortium, 2013) suggest that irritable mania stems from a set of genes distinct from that of elated mania. Although not reaching genome-wide significance, 33 SNPs in a region on chromosome 13 differed between irritable and elated study participants. This location is a "gene desert" between genes *SITRK1* and *SLITRK6*, which functions in neurodevelopment to suppress neurite outgrowth. GWAS of irritability in an epidemiologic pediatric population would represent an important advance in efforts to identify genes associated with irritability. Future GWAS of irritability should take care to ensure adequate sample sizes based on a number of parameters, such as trait prevalence, case-control ratio in the study design, and effect size of the genetic variant (Hong & Park, 2012). Furthermore, GWAS could identify important biologically plausible candidate genes for focused follow-up analysis (e.g., pathway analysis and candidate gene analysis).

Another type of GWAS follow-up study is the development of *polygenic risk scores* (PRS), which index risk for a phenotype based on genome-wide significant hits. Risk scores can then be used to predict the phenotype or related phenotypes in other samples; however, the predictive validity of PRSs is constrained by the accuracy with which individual scores are weighted, among other factors. Riglin and colleagues (2017) developed a PRS based on alleles that were associated with schizophrenia case-status in an analysis using data from the Psychiatric Genetic Consortium (Riglin et al., 2017). The researchers found an association between the polygenic risk score for schizophrenia and irritability at age 7 (defined by temper tantrums reported in the Strengths and Difficulties Questionnaire; Goodman, 1997); however, this association did not hold after adjusting for social class and child sex. Thus, it cannot be concluded that irritability at age 7 indexes genetic liability for the development of schizophrenia.

GWAS has largely replaced older gene-finding methods such as *linkage analysis*, variations of which were undertaken in two molecular genetic studies of irritability. Although GWAS has greater power to detect associations with common genetic variants, linkage analysis can detect effects of both rare and common variants (Greenwood et al., 2013). Linkage analysis locates genomic regions that are co-inherited in families with the phenotype of interest (Bush & Haines, 2010). The primary output of a linkage analysis is the logarithm of odds (LOD) score, which estimates the likelihood that two genes (the "disease" gene and a marker gene) are located close together on the chromosome and, therefore, are inherited together (National Institutes of Health, 2017). LOD scores of 3 or higher are generally understood to indicate that the genes are located close to one another on the chromosome. One linkage study (Faraone, Su, & Tsuang, 2004) found a peak LOD score for an irritable dimension of BD (one of five domains of signs and symptoms associated with BD identified in a factor analysis: depression, psychosis, sleep disturbance, psychomotor acceleration, and irritability) of 1.47 on chromosome 5; however, this is not high enough to be statistically significant. Greenwood and colleagues (2013) also performed a linkage analysis in a population of BD patients, this time defining the phenotype as the irritable temperament of the TEMPS questionnaire. They reported a LOD score of 4.45 for irritability on chromosome 6q24, which the authors note is located within in the *GRM1*, a gene that plays a role in synaptic plasticity, learning, and memory (Greenwood et al., 2013). As with other genetic studies, replication of this finding would be an important next step to confirm that a true susceptibility locus has been identified (Bush & Haines, 2010).

In sum, consistent with the genetics of many internalizing and externalizing traits and phenotypes, a number of different genes have been found to be associated with irritability. However, with no replication of findings across or even within molecular genetic methodologies, we are left with no conclusive identification of genes that may be implicated in pediatric irritability in either healthy or clinical populations. We suspect that, as with the majority of complex traits studied in humans and model organisms, many loci contribute to variance in irritability (Stranger et al., 2011). Furthermore, GWAS of any complex traits thus far have identified variants with modest effects (odds ratio [OR] <2) (Stranger et al., 2011). Because of modest effects, GWAS sample sizes may need to be larger than those of the studies that have been performed to date. For example, Hong and Park (2012) suggest close to 2,000 participants for GWAS variant effect sizes of OR of 1.3–1.6, among other design considerations, to identify genes implicated in irritability. There may not be "a gene for" irritability, but rather, the phenotype is likely to be the result of multiple genes acting and interacting with the environment.

Conclusion and Future Directions

One of the evident take-home messages of this chapter is the lack of genetic studies specifically devoted to the study of irritability. This is not surprising, given the transdiagnostic nature of irritability and its expression as part of a number of differing psychiatric phenotypes. One suggested future approach is to take a Research Domain Criteria (RDoC) approach to the study of irritable mood (i.e., regardless of psychiatric phenotype). Studies dedicated to the irritability construct would undoubtedly include multiple, state-of-the-art measures including self-report, parent and/or teacher report, behavioral measurement (see Chapter 3), neural circuitry (see Chapter 9), and genetics. Relatedly, a current hindrance of the irritability literature is lack of use of well-validated irritability measures. As part of an irritability-focused workshop hosted by the National Institutes of Mental Health in 2014, effort was dedicated to the development of a common working definition of irritability to be used by the research community. Consistent use of a common working definition and psychometrically sounds measures will undeniably serve clinical research.

There also is a lack of multimethod (e.g., self-report, behavioral, genetic, functional magnetic resonance imaging) longitudinal assessments within the same individual, which is necessary to gain a developmental understanding of the emergence of irritable mood from young ages through childhood and into adulthood. The majority of the research on irritability has relied largely on single mode measures of irritability, typically a parent and/or child self-report or symptom endorsement from a clinical interview, measured cross-sectionally. It may be possible to generate additional leverage in genetic studies by measuring a number of different components of irritability including, but not limited to, physiology, behavioral patterns, biomarkers, and neurocircuitry. Longitudinal measurements will allow researchers to better understand both intra- and inter-individual variance across time, which will advance prognostic models, while the multimethod approach may reveal similar or distinct genetic influences between differing method types.

Another theme emerging in this chapter is that irritable mood appears to be moderately heritable and is influenced by unique environmental events, but not by common familial environment. If the influence of a common shared environment is small (e.g., 10% of the variance or less), then most, if not all, of the cited twin studies suffered from low statistical power to detect this influence. If the effects of a common shared environment are fairly large effects (e.g., 25% of the variance or more), then most reviewed studies were powered well enough to identify its influence to the manifestation of irritability (Visscher, Gordon, & Neal, 2008). Thus, it is possible that there are small effects of the common shared environment that were not detectable by most studies. Finally, the reviewed molecular genetic studies focused solely on genetic variants associated with irritable mood, with no other genomic markers being considered (e.g., gene expression, DNA methylation, proteomics). It may be that epigenetics (i.e., DNA/chromatin modifications that can influence gene expression but not sequence) play an important role in irritable mood expression. For example, if robust environmental risk factors (e.g., parenting, peer victimization) predict irritable mood, then epigenetics may be a key candidate mechanism through which environmental stress exerts its effect on genetic risk for irritability.

BG studies also indicate a role for unique environmental factors in the expression of irritable mood. Youth are exposed to a range of social–environmental contexts (e.g., school, neighborhoods). Emerging evidence suggests that environmental factors play a role in irritability (Barker & Salekin, 2012; Lipscomb et al., 2011), thereby supporting the integration of well-defined measures of social-environment factors into studies of irritable mood. The findings of BG studies also strongly support the search for genes involved in the etiology of irritability. Efforts to detect genetic risk loci for irritable mood will certainly be challenging, but identification of irritability's genetic structure is critical to developing targets for novel pharmacological therapies aimed at reducing the burden associated with this mood deficit. Moreover, identification of genetic and environmental factors and their interaction (i.e., *gene × environment interaction*) also may inform the treatment of irritability from a psychosocial perspective. For example, a new, innovative treatment aimed at improving various cognitive functions including face-emotion processing, cognitive flexibility, response inhibition, and frustration tolerance was recently developed to alleviate deficits related to mood-related dysfunction in youth (Dickstein, Cushman, Kim, Weissman, & Wegbreit, 2015). In summary, genetic studies, ranging from genetically-informed investigations to the study of genetic variants/variation, will inform our understanding and treatment of irritable mood.

References

1. Aebi, M., van Donkelaar, M. M., Poelmans, G., Buitelaar, J. K., Sonuga-Barke, E. J., Stringaris, A., . . .van Hulzen, K. J. (2016). Gene-set and multivariate genome-wide association analysis of oppositional defiant behavior subtypes in attention deficit/hyperactivity disorder. *American Journal of Medical Genetics Part B: Neuropsychiatric Genetics, 171,* 573–588.
2. American Psychiatry Association (APA). (2013). *Diagnostic and statistical manual of mental disorders* (5th ed.). Arlington, VA: American Psychiatric Publishing.
3. Barker, E. D., Salekin, R. T. (2012). Irritable oppositional defiance and callous unemotional traits: Is the association partially explained by peer victimization? *Journal of Child Psychology and Psychiatry, 53,* 1167–1175.
4. Borkowska, A., Bieliński, M., Szczęsny, W., Szwed, K., Tomaszewska, M., Kałwa, A.,...Tretyn, A. (2015). Effect of the 5-HTTLPR polymorphism on affective temperament, depression and body mass index in obesity. *Journal of Affective Disorders, 184,* 193–197.
5. Brotman, M. A., Kassem, L., Reising, M. M., Guyer, A. E., Dickstein, D. P., Rich, B. A., . . . Leibenluft, E. (2007). Parental diagnoses in youth with narrow phenotype bipolar disorder or severe mood dysregulation. *American Journal of Psychiatry, 164,* 1238–1241.
6. Bush, W. S., & Haines, J. (2010). Overview of linkage analysis in complex traits. *Current Protocols in Human Genetics, 64,* 1.9.1–1.9.18.
7. Buss, A. H., & Durkee, A. (1957). An inventory for assessing different types of hostility. *Journal of Consulting and Clinical Psychology, 21,* 343–349.
8. Buss, A. H., & Plomin, R. (1984). *Temperament: Early developing personality traits.* Hillside, NJ: Lawrence Erlbaum Associates.
9. Calati, R., Porcelli, S., Giegling, I., Hartmann, A. M., Möller, H. J., De Ronchi, D., . . . Rujescu, D. (2011). Catechol-o-methyltransferase gene modulation on suicidal behavior and personality traits: Review, meta-analysis and association study. *Journal of Psychiatric Research, 45,* 309–321.
10. Carmine, A., Chheda, M. G., Jönsson, E. G., Sedvall, G. C., Farde, L., Gustavsson, J. P., . . . Olson, L. (2003). Two NOTCH4 polymorphisms and their relation to schizophrenia susceptibility and different personality traits. *Psychiatric Genetics, 13,* 23–28.
11. Chang, K. D., Steiner, H., & Ketter, T. A. (2000). Psychiatric phenomenology of child and adolescent bipolar offspring, *Journal of the American Academy of Child and Adolescent Psychiatry, 39,* 453–460.
12. Coccaro, E. F., Bergeman, C. S., Kavoussi, R. J., & Seroczynski, A. D. (1997). Heritability of aggression and irritability: A twin study of the Buss-Durkee Aggression Scales in adult male subjects. *Biological Psychiatry, 41,* 273–284.
13. Coccaro, E. F., Bergeman, C. S., & McClearn, G. E. (1993). Heritability of irritable impulsiveness: A study of twins reared together and apart. *Psychiatry Research, 48,* 229–242.
14. Comings, D. E., Johnson, J. P., Gonzalez, N. S., Huss, M., Saucier, G., & McGue, M. (2000). Association between the adrenergic alpha 2A receptor gene (ADRA2A)

and measures of irritability, hostility, impulsivity and memory in normal subjects. *Psychiatric Genetics*, *10*, 39–42.

15. Damberg, M., Berggård, C., Mattila-Evenden, M., Rylander, G., Forslund, K., Garpenstrand, H., . . . Jönsson, E. G. (2003). Transcription factor AP-2β genotype associated with anxiety-related personality traits in women. *Neuropsychobiology*, *48*, 169–175.

16. Dickstein, D. P., Cushman, G. K., Kim, K. L., Weissman, A. B., & Wegbreit, E. (2015). Cognitive remediation: Potential novel brain-based treatment for bipolar disorder in children and adolescents. *CNS Spectrums*, *20*, 382–390.

17. Everett, G. M. (1977). Changes in brain dopamine levels and aggressive behavior with aging in 2 mouse strains. *Cellular and Molecular Life Sciences*, *33*, 645–646.

18. Faraone, S. V., Su, J., & Tsuang, M. T. (2004). A genome-wide scan of symptom dimensions in bipolar disorder pedigrees of adult probands. *Journal of Affective Disorders*, *82*, S71–S78.

19. Fristad, M. A., Wolfson, H., Algorta, G. P., Youngstrom, E. A., Arnold, L. E., Birmaher, B., . . . LAMS Group. (2016). Disruptive mood dysregulation disorder and bipolar disorder not otherwise specified: Fraternal or identical twins?. *Journal of Child and Adolescent Psychopharmacology*, *26*, 138–146.

20. Gietl, A., Giegling, I., Hartmann, A. M., Schneider, B., Schnabel, A., Maurer, K., . . . Rujescu, D. (2007). ABCG1 gene variants in suicidal behavior and aggression-related traits. *European Neuropsychopharmacology*, *17*, 410–416.

21. Goldsmith, H. H., & Gottesman, I. I. (1981). Origins of variation in behavioral style: A longitudinal study of temperament in young twins. *Child Development*, *52*, 91–103.

22. Gonda, X., Rihmer, Z., Zsombok, T., Bagdy, G., Akiskal, K. K., & Akiskal, H. S. (2006). The 5HTTLPR polymorphism of the serotonin transporter gene is associated with affective temperaments as measured by TEMPS-A. *Journal of Affective Disorders*, *91*, 125–131.

23. Goodman, R. (1997). The Strengths and Difficulties Questionnaire: A research note. *Journal of Child Psychology and Psychiatry*, *38*, 581–586.

24. Greenwood, T. A., Akiskal, H. S., Akiskal, K. K., Bipolar Genome Study (BiGS), & Kelsoe, J. R. (2012). Genome-wide association study of temperament in bipolar disorder reveals significant associations with three novel Loci. *Biological Psychiatry*, *72*, 303–310.

25. Greenwood, T. A., Badner, J. A., Byerley, W., Keck, P. E., McElroy, S. L., Remick, R. A., . . . Kelsoe, J. R. (2013). Heritability and genome-wide SNP linkage analysis of temperament in bipolar disorder. *Journal of Affective Disorders*, *150*, 1031–1040.

26. Greenwood, T. A., Kelsoe, J. R., & Bipolar Genome Study (BiGS) Consortium. (2013). Genome-wide association study of irritable vs. elated mania suggests genetic differences between clinical subtypes of bipolar disorder. *PLoS One*, *8*, e53804.

27. Hong, E. P., & Park, J. W. (2012). Sample size and statistical power calculation in genetic association studies. *Genomics & Informatics*, *10*, 117–122.

28. Institute of Medicine (US) Committee on Assessing Interactions Among Social, Behavioral, and Genetic Factors in Health (2006). Animal models. In Hernandez, L. M., & Blazer, D. G. (Eds.), *Genes, behavior, and the social environment: Moving beyond the nature/nurture debate*. Washington, DC: National Academies Press (US). Available from: https://www.ncbi.nlm.nih.gov/books/NBK19914/

29. Johansson, A. G., Nikamo, P., Schalling, M., & Landén, M. (2011). AKR1C4 gene variant associated with low euthymic serum progesterone and a history of mood irritability in males with bipolar disorder. *Journal of Affective Disorders, 133*, 346–351.

30. Kang, J. I., Namkoong, K., & Kim, S. J. (2008). The association of 5-HTTLPR and DRD4 VNTR polymorphisms with affective temperamental traits in healthy volunteers. *Journal of Affective Disorders, 109*, 157–163.

31. Kendler, K. S., Neale, M. C., Kessler, R. C., Heath, A. C., & Eaves, L. J. (1993). A test of the equal-environment assumption in twin studies of psychiatric illness. *Behavior Genetics, 23*, 21–27.

32. Kraemer, G. W., Moore, C. F., Newman, T. K., Barr, C. S., & Schneider, M. L. (2008). Moderate level fetal alcohol exposure and serotonin transporter gene promoter polymorphism affect neonatal temperament and limbic-hypothalamic-pituitary-adrenal axis regulation in monkeys. *Biological Psychiatry, 63*, 317–324.

33. Kuny, A. V., Althoff, R. R., Copeland, W., Barteis, M., Beijsterveidt, V., Baer, J., & Hudziak, J. J. (2013). Separating the domains of oppositional behavior: Comparing latent models of the Conners' Oppositional Subscale. *Journal of the American Academy of Child and Adolescent Psychiatry, 52*, 172–183.

34. Lieblich, I., & Driscoll, P. (1983). Genetic relation between the performance in a two-way avoidance task and increased emotionality following septal lesions. *Brain Research, 263*, 113–117.

35. Lipscomb, S. T., Leve, L. D., Harold, G. T., Neiderhiser, J. M., Shaw, D. S., Ge, X., & Reiss, D. (2011). Trajectories of parenting and child negative emotionality during infancy and toddlerhood: A longitudinal analysis. *Child Development, 82*, 1661–1675.

36. Mikolajewski, A. J., Taylor, J., & Iacono, W. G. (2017). Oppositional defiant disorder dimensions: Genetic influences and risk for later psychopathology. *Journal of Child Psychology and Psychiatry, 58*, 702–710.

37. Mineur, Y. S., Prasol, D. J., Belzung, C., & Crusio, W. E. (2003). Agonistic behavior and unpredictable chronic mild stress in mice. *Behavior Genetics, 33*, 513–519.

38. National Institutes of Health (NIH). National Human Genome Research Institute. *LOD Score*. Talking Glossary of Genetic Terms. Retrieved October 16, 2017, from https://www.genome.gov/glossary/

39. Neale, M. C., & Cardon, L. R. (1992). *Methodology for genetic studies of twins and families*. Dordrecht, Netherlands: Kluwer Academic Publishers.

40. Perich, T., Frankland, A., Roberts, G., Levy, F., Lenroot, R., & Mitchell, P. B. (2016). Disruptive mood dysregulation disorder, severe mood dysregulation and chronic irritability in youth at high familial risk of bipolar disorder. *Australian & New Zealand Journal of Psychiatry, 53*, 408–416.

41. Perlis, R. H., Purcell, S., Fagerness, J., Cusin, C., Yamaki, L., Fava, M., & Smoller, J. W. (2007). Clinical and genetic dissection of anger expression and CREB1 polymorphisms in major depressive disorder. *Biological Psychiatry, 62*, 536–540.

42. Ramanan, V. K., Shen, L., Moore, J. H., & Saykin, A. J. (2012). Pathway analysis of genomic data: Concepts, methods, and prospects for future development. *Trends in Genetics, 28*, 323–332.

43. Rice, F., Sellers, R., Hammerton, G., Eyre, O., Bevan-Jones, R., Thapar, A. K., . . . Thapar, A. (2017). Antecendants of new-onset major depressive disorder in children and adolescents at high familial risk. *JAMA Psychiatry, 74*, 153–160.

44. Riglin, L., Collishaw, S., Richards, A., Thapar, A. K., Maughan, B., O'Donovan, M. C., & Thapar, A. (2017). Schizophrenia risk alleles and neurodevelopmental outcomes in childhood: A population-based cohort study. *Lancet Psychiatry, 4*, 57–62.

45. Roberson-Nay, R., Leibenluft, E., Brotman, M. A., Myers, J., Larsson, H., Lichtenstein, P., & Kendler, K. S. (2015). Longitudinal stability of genetic and environmental influences on irritability: From childhood to young adulthood. *American Journal of Psychiatry, 172*, 657–664.

46. Rybakowski, J. K., Dmitrzak-Weglarz, M., Dembinska-Krajewska, D., Hauser, J., Akiskal, K. K., & Akiskal, H. H. (2014). Polymorphism of circadian clock genes and temperamental dimensions of the TEMPS-A in bipolar disorder. *Journal of Affective Disorders, 159*, 80–84.

47. Savage, J., Verhulst, B., Copeland, W., Althoff, R. R., Lichtenstein, P., & Roberson-Nay, R. (2015). A genetically informed study of the longitudinal relation between irritability and anxious/depressed symptoms. *Journal of the American Academy of Child and Adolescent Psychiatry, 54*, 377–384.

48. Simmons, D. (2008). The use of animal models in studying genetic disease: Transgenesis and induced mutation. *Nature Education, 1*, 70.

49. Stranger, B. E., Stahl, E. A., & Raj, T. (2011). Progress and promise of genome-wide association studies for human complex trait genetics. *Genetics, 187*, 367–383.

50. Stringaris, A., Zavos, H., Leibenluft, E., Maughan, B., & Eley, T. (2012). Adolescent irritability: Phenotypic associations and genetic links with depressed mood. *American Journal of Psychiatry, 169*, 47–54.

51. Suchankova, P., Pettersson, R., Nordenström, K., Holm, G., & Ekman, A. (2012). Personality traits and the R668Q polymorphism located in the MMP-9 gene. *Behavioural Brain Research, 228*, 232–235.

52. Tabor, H. K., Risch, N. J., & Myers, R. M. (2002). Opinion: Candidate-gene approaches for studying complex genetic traits: Practical considerations. *Nature Reviews. Genetics, 3*, 391.

53. Tsutsumi, T., Terao, T., Hatanaka, K., Goto, S., Hoaki, N., & Wang, Y. (2011). Association between affective temperaments and brain-derived neurotrophic factor, glycogen synthase kinase 3β and Wnt signaling pathway gene polymorphisms in healthy subjects. *Journal of Affective Disorders, 131*, 353–357.

54. Visscher, P. M., Gordon, S., & Neal, M. C. (2008). Power of the classical twin design revisited: II detection of common environmental variance. *Twin Research and Human Genetics, 11*, 48–54.

55. Westberg, L., Melke, J., Landén, M., Nilsson, S., Baghaei, F., Rosmond, R., . . . Eriksson, E. (2003). Association between a dinucleotide repeat polymorphism of the estrogen receptor alpha gene and personality traits in women. *Molecular Psychiatry, 8*, 118.

9

Neural Findings in Pediatric Irritability

Emily Hirsch and Leslie Hulvershorn

We begin this chapter by reviewing theoretical models of irritability and experimental approaches that have been used to study neural mechanisms of pediatric irritability, with a focus on normal versus dysfunctional reward and threat processing. We then critically review task-based neuroimaging research that has been conducted on typically developing youth, children with significant chronic irritability, and children with disorders associated with elevated irritability such as disruptive behavior disorders (DBD), attention-deficit/hyperactivity disorder (ADHD), autism, and mood disorders. Finally, we review structural and functional connectivity methods that have been used to examine irritability-related pathology in children and adolescents.

Conceptual Models of Irritability

Recent literature has converged on the notion that irritability can be broadly defined as the propensity to exhibit anger relative to peers (Brotman, Kircanski, & Leibenluft, 2017; Leibenluft, 2017). As shown in Figure 9.1, there are two primary conceptual models regarding the relationship between irritability and anger. First, irritability can be conceptualized as a form of *chronic anger with low frustration tolerance*. Frustration can be operationalized from a neuroscientific perspective as frustrative non-reward (FNR); FNR is a normative state experienced by an organism when it fails to obtain a reward that it has learned to expect, characterized by increased motor activity and aggression (Amsel, 1958). Irritable individuals have an aberrant FNR with a low threshold for and overreaction to blocked goal attainment (Amsel, 1958; Berkowitz, 1989). Such responses to non-reward also involve dopaminergic prediction errors, signals that encode the difference between expected and received outcome (Schultz & Dickinson, 2000). As a result, the extreme responses to frustration that children with chronic irritability exhibit might

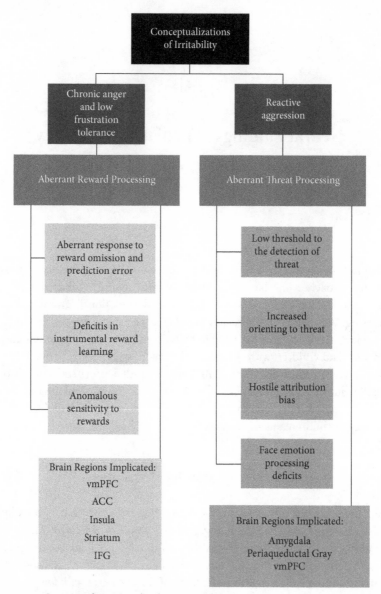

FIGURE 9.1 *Conceptualizations of pediatric irritability.*

vmPFC, ventromedial prefrontal cortex; ACC, anterior cingulate cortex; IFG, inferior frontal gyrus.

reflect deficits in these dopaminergic circuits (Adleman et al., 2011). Evidence for this comes from studies demonstrating that irritable youth show abnormal reward processing (Berkowitz, 1989; Luman, Sergeant, Knol, & Oosterlaan, 2010; Perlman et al., 2015) and behavioral deficits in reward learning (Blair, 2010). To assess this, tasks typically measure sensitivity to reward receipt and omission by including an initial phase of reward learning, followed by a second phase during which the reward is withheld (Rich et al., 2007; Ryan & Watson, 1968). Irritability can also be understood through the lens of *instrumental learning*, which is the process through which organisms learn behaviors in order to obtain reward or avoid punishment (Costa, Tran, Turchi, & Averbeck, 2015). Normative development requires the use of instrumental learning about rewards and threats to facilitate appropriate adaptation to environmental stimuli. *Response reversal learning tasks* rely on initial instrumental learning and measure one's ability to detect change and then modify behavior based on changing reward contingencies (Blair, Colledge, & Mitchell, 2001; Dickstein et al., 2010; Fellows & Farah, 2003). Children with irritability often exhibit deficits on such associative learning tasks (Adleman et al., 2011; Dickstein et al., 2007). Response reversal learning also depends on intact executive functioning, which has been implicated more broadly in emotion regulation (Wakschlag et al., 2018). As a result, some studies have examined executive functioning in relation to pediatric irritability (Li, Grabell, Wakschlag, Huppert, & Perlman, 2017). Irritability-related behavioral deficits in reward processing and learning have been associated with disruptions in regions including the ventromedial prefrontal cortex (vmPFC), insula, anterior cingulate cortex (ACC), striatum, and inferior frontal gyrus (IFG) (Leibenluft, 2017).

Second, irritability can manifest with *reactive aggression* associated with dysfunctional threat and emotion processing (Panksepp, 2006). In this model, approach responses are utilized in contexts that are perceived as threatening. In line with this view, researchers suggest that individuals with irritability have a low threshold for the detection of threat, at times seeing relatively benign or ambiguous behavior as threatening, thus causing them to respond with maladaptive aggression (Brotman, Kircanski, Stringaris, Pine, & Leibenluft, 2017). Associated behavioral deficits include attention orienting to threat assessed by tasks such as the dot probe (Bar-Haim, Lamy, Pergamin, Bakermans-Kranenburg, & Van Ijzendoorn, 2007; Fox, Russo, & Dutton, 2002; Hommer et al., 2014; Kircanski et al., 2018; Salum et al., 2017; Schippell, Vasey, Cravens-Brown, & Bretveld, 2003), as well as difficulties with face emotion processing (Brotman, Kircanski, & Leibenluft, 2017; Leibenluft, 2017). There are several versions of face emotion paradigms, including conscious (unmasked) stimuli that can be presented explicitly (Tseng et al., 2015), in which subjects are asked to focus on the facial emotion (Hariri, Bookheimer, & Mazziotta, 2000; McClure et al., 2005), or implicitly, in which participants are asked to focus on some other aspect of the face (Lieberman et al., 2007). Similarly, studies have also used video and auditory stimuli to induce emotional experiences (De Silva, Miyasato, & Nakatsu, 1997; Karim & Perlman, 2017; Robins, Hunyadi, & Schultz, 2009). Children with chronic irritability have also been shown to demonstrate a hostile attribution bias (Horsley, de Castro, & Van der Schoot, 2010), which is the tendency to interpret ambiguous or neutral social stimuli as threatening (Dodge, 1980). The brain regions implicated in these deficits in threat and face emotion processing include the amygdala, periaqueductal gray, and ventromedial PFC (Blair, 2016; Coker-Appiah et al., 2013).

In the following sections, we will review the task-based neuroimaging data supporting these conceptual hypotheses in healthy children and those with chronic irritability. We include studies of children with disruptive behavior disorders as these children typically exhibit significant irritability even if not reported directly. We follow these discussions with studies of anatomical and functional connectivity that further inform neuropathological models of pediatric irritability.

Irritability in Normative Development

Typically developing children normatively experience some degree of irritability as their increasing interests result in behaviors that often conflict with the wishes of their caregivers, leading to blocked goals (Wakschlag et al., 2012, 2018). For example, Wakschlag et al. (2012) reported that more than 83% of preschoolers had temper outbursts and 8.6% had them daily. However, most preschool children do not have frequent, long-lasting, and severely dysregulated tantrums (Wakschlag et al., 2018; Wiggins et al., 2018). Examination of the neurobiological bases of normative irritability across development is important so that pathological levels of irritability can be understood. Researchers have examined the neural basis for irritability across childhood and adolescence, as well as in comparison to healthy adults.

REWARD PROCESSING AND FRUSTRATION

Perlman and Pelphrey (2011) compared affective regulation in typically developing children (ages 5–11) and adults ($n = 45$; typically developing children = 20, adults = 25) during an emotional go/no-go task, which was designed to induce frustration due to loss of rewards, followed by a fearful face probe. They reported that, during recovery from a frustrating event, amygdala activation increased in adults but decreased in children. In addition, in children, ACC activity immediately preceded left amygdala activation, but only during episodes in which participants were expected to regulate emotion. This implicates amygdala/ACC circuitry in the development of affective self-regulation in response to frustration in children compared to adults. Other studies have differentiated the role of medial and lateral PFC in frustration processing in young children. Perlman, Luna, Hein, and Huppert (2014) used functional near-infrared spectroscopy (fNIRS) to measure prefrontal correlates of frustration in children aged 3–5 ($n = 17$) during a frustration task where a desired and expected prize was lost. They found that when the children were winning the desired prize, they displayed increased medial prefrontal cortex (mPFC) activity, suggesting that the mPFC has a defined role in the receipt of rewards. However, when the children experienced frustration, they showed greater lateral PFC activity than healthy comparisons. Moreover, parent ratings of children's frustration were positively related to increased activation of the lateral PFC during frustration. The results suggest that typically developing children who exhibit low frustration tolerance may require greater activation of the lateral PFC during frustrating situations in order to sufficiently modulate their responses.

Although they also utilized fNIRS and the same frustration task as Perlman et al. (2014), Grabell et al. (2018) did not find that those with greater levels of irritability exhibited a stronger lateral PFC response. Rather, they found evidence for an inverted U function that characterized the relationship between frustration and lateral PFC activation in children aged 3–7 (n = 92). Specifically, they found that children who reported mild frustration had greater lateral PFC activation than those who reported no or high frustration. This suggests that nonimpaired children who experience moderate levels of irritability have lateral PFC support that is well-developed. However, lateral PFC activation in those with impairing levels of irritability appeared to either be underactive or the impairing levels of irritability overwhelmed and interfered with the activation of the lateral PFC. Thus, the researchers postulated that those with high levels of irritability and an underactive lateral PFC may be at greatest risk for developing a psychiatric disorder.

Dougherty et al. (2018) examined the effects of preschool irritability on reward-related neural processing by investigating children (n = 46) with irritability during the preschool period (ages 3–5) and again 2 years later (ages 6–9). Psychological assessments were completed at both time points, and a functional magnetic resonance imaging (fMRI) scan utilizing a reward processing task was completed during the second assessment. When controlling for concurrent irritability, they found that children with higher levels of preschool irritability demonstrated alterations in right amygdala connectivity with the insula and inferior parietal lobe during reward processing. In addition, they exhibited altered connectivity between the left ventral striatum and lingual gyrus, postcentral gyrus, superior parietal lobe, and culmen. When controlling for preschool irritability, those with more severe concurrent irritability exhibited similar aberrant patterns of left and right amygdala connectivity with the superior frontal gyrus (SFG), as well as between the left ventral striatum with precuneus and culmen, suggesting similar but distinct neural signatures of irritability in preschool versus grade school irritability.

Overall, frustration paradigms in typically developing children highlight the role of the PFC and, more specifically, the ACC and lateral PFC in modulating irritability when encountering frustrating events. Appropriate levels of activation of these regions appear to be correlated with emotion regulation.

THREAT AND EMOTION PROCESSING

Functional MRI studies have also examined the neural correlates of irritability using threat and emotion processing paradigms in typically developing children. Karim and Perlman (2017) examined the role of irritable temperament in the neurodevelopmental maturation of affective reactivity in children aged 4–12

($n = 30$) and adults ($n = 21$) using film clips that showed positive and negative emotional content. Compared to adults, children exhibited greater activation in the amygdala, hippocampus, thalamus, visual cortex, and fusiform gyrus while observing the negative clips and in the hippocampus, thalamus, caudate, ACC, and orbitofrontal cortex (OFC) while observing positive emotional content. Importantly, they also found that activation of the SFG and subcortical regions while watching negative content increased with development in children with high irritable temperament scores, while activation decreased with age in those children with low irritability scores. The study highlighted that multiple cortical and subcortical regions are activated differently in youth compared to adults when viewing negative and positive emotional content and is dependent on the degree of irritable temperament.

While the previous studies examined activation of both cortical and subcortical structures, Gaffrey, Barch, and Luby (2016) specifically investigated amygdala reactivity to emotional stimuli by examining preschool children ($n = 31$) twice, a year apart, and compared those who had elevated depressive symptoms and negativity scores and those who did not. During an fMRI scan, the children viewed neutral, happy, sad, and fearful faces interleaved with fixation crosses. While there were no clear findings of face emotion type and amygdala activity, there was a positive relationship between negativity scores and right amygdala activity during sad face viewing. Increased amygdala activation in response to sad faces significantly predicted higher negativity scores for these children when seen 1 year later, suggesting an early trait marker for negative and irritable emotions and again highlighting the role of the amygdala in affect regulation.

Overall, studies utilizing paradigms assessing threat and face emotion processing in typically developing children highlight the same corticolimbic circuitry involved in emotion processing and regulation as in adults. However, when irritability is quantified, children, adolescents, and adults appear to differ in activation across the circuit.

COGNITIVE FLEXIBILITY

One study examined the relationship between irritability and executive functioning in typically developing children by focusing on the neural mechanisms underlying cognitive flexibility, or the ability to mentally switch between demands. Li et al. (2017) used fNIRS along with a dimensional card sort task to examine the neural correlates of cognitive flexibility and its relationship to irritability in a nonclinical sample of preschoolers ($n = 46$). As in other studies investigating cognitive flexibility (Moriguchi & Hiraki, 2011), activation of the left dorsolateral prefrontal cortex (dlPFC) was associated with cognitive flexibility. Children with higher irritability scores showed greater activation of the dlPFC bilaterally but performed the task as well as children who did not score high on irritability, suggesting that these children may be utilizing different cognitive strategies, possibly requiring greater activation, in an attempt to manage their irritability and frustration.

In sum, the literature on irritability across typical development underscores the relationship between the top-down role of the cortex (e.g., PFC and ACC) and the amygdala. Of note, the striatum also emerged as a central node in irritability-relevant circuits and is also implicated in clinically meaningful levels of irritability (Dougherty et al., 2018). In addition, studies that investigated a broader age range indicate a differential neural response across development. Studies assessing irritability in typically developing children suggest the potential for biomarkers that could be validated with additional research. Only one neuroimaging study to date examined the role of executive functioning in irritability. Thus, the cognitive basis of irritability warrants further attention, as deficits in executive functioning have been shown to lead to impairment in children's regulation of negative emotions. Furthermore, the recent finding that suggested a nonlinear association between irritability and frustration regulation may represent a shift from the typically linear conceptualization.

Irritability in Psychiatric Populations

Irritability is present in many psychiatric disorders and is a core symptom in several. Therefore, to better understand the nature of these disorders and to know whether irritability represents the same or different underlying neural signatures, researchers have compared children presenting with prominent irritability across a range of psychiatric conditions to typically developing children. The majority of studies examining the neural basis for pediatric irritability have been conducted in youth with severe mood dysregulation (SMD). This literature emerged from an attempt to elucidate whether chronic and severe irritability was a developmental presentation of bipolar disorder (BD). Leibenluft and colleagues operationalized SMD as a syndrome characterized by chronic and severe irritability (Leibenluft, 2011). SMD formed the basis for disruptive mood dysregulation disorder (DMDD) in the fifth edition of the *Diagnostic and Statistical Manual of Mental Disorders* (DSM-5; American Psychiatric Association, 2013). We will start each section with that work and then report on findings from other pediatric populations.

REWARD AND FRUSTRATION PROCESSING

A great deal of what is known about the brain mechanisms underlying pediatric irritability comes from studies of SMD and BD. Rich et al. (2011) used magnetoencephalography to examine neuronal activity following negative versus positive feedback during an attentional task involving blocked goal attainment in youth with BD (n = 20), SMD (n = 20), and typically developing children (n = 20). They found that, compared to those with SMD and typically developing children, those with BD exhibited greater SFG activation and decreased insula activation following negative feedback. In addition, compared to typically developing children, those with SMD showed greater activation of the ACC and medial frontal gyrus (MFG) in response to negative feedback and reduced activation of these regions in response to positive feedback. Because the ACC and MFG are implicated in evaluation and regulation of emotional conflict, including automatic self-evaluation, self-monitoring of emotional state, and facilitation of response selection, these findings suggest that, compared to typically developing children, those with SMD have responses that are more strongly dictated by negative information and less influenced by positive information. The researchers concluded that heightened attention to negative emotional information, though evident in both BD and SMD youth, is mediated by different frontal regions.

Deveney et al. (2013) compared neural activity of those with SMD ($n = 19$) to typically developing children ($n = 23$) during a cued-attention task completed under non-frustrating and frustrating conditions, with negative and positive feedback. They found that, during the frustration condition, youth with SMD exhibited deactivation of the left amygdala, the left and right striatum, the parietal cortex, and the posterior cingulate on negative feedback trials compared to typically developing children (between groups) and positive feedback trials (within groups). In contrast, typically developing children did not differ in activation between positive and negative feedback trials. Also, neural response to positive feedback during frustration did not differ between typically developing children and those with SMD. Tseng et al. (2017) conducted a similar study examining neural mechanisms of irritability in youth with a range of psychiatric disorders during the same cued-attention task. They found that across diagnoses (DMDD, ADHD, anxiety disorders), higher irritability was related to greater activation in the cingulate gyrus, SFG, dlPFC, and precentral gyrus when the youth had to perform an attentional task after receiving negative (i.e., rigged) versus positive feedback. The researchers concluded that frustration disrupts neural function in frontal circuits mediating attention and response selection in highly irritable children.

Bebko et al. (2014) compared a group of behaviorally and emotionally dysregulated youth aged 10–17 who were referred for a study on manic symptoms ($n = 85$) to typically developing children ($n = 20$) during a reward paradigm that consisted of win, loss, and control conditions. They found that of all diagnostic categories examined (including BD, cyclothymic disorder and BD not otherwise specified, oppositional defiant disorder [ODD], conduct disorder [CD], and disruptive behavior disorders not otherwise specified [DBDs]), only those with disruptive behavior disorders showed disorder-specific abnormalities in reward circuitry. Specifically, those with DBDs exhibited lower left ventrolateral PFC activity to win conditions compared to those without. This finding suggests that those with disruptive behavior may evaluate rewarding contexts as less salient than those without disruptive behavior, which in turn may be associated with reduced reward sensitivity and result in socially inappropriate behaviors characteristic of DBD. However, regardless of diagnosis, all youth with behavioral and emotional dysregulation exhibited activated bilateral dorsal ACC to win and loss conditions relative to typically developing children. Moreover, relative to typically developing children, these youth exhibited greater bilateral ventrolateral PFC activation to win conditions and right ventrolateral PFC activation to loss conditions, suggesting that they evaluated both conditions as salient. The authors also reported that, regardless of diagnosis, greater left anterolateral mPFC activity during win conditions was associated with higher scores of emotional and behavioral dysregulation. This suggests that activity in this region may be a biomarker of behavioral and emotional dysregulation and heightened reward sensitivity in rewarding contexts across these diagnostic groups.

Unlike Bebko et al. (2014) who examined general behavioral and emotional dysregulation, Perlman et al. (2015) focused on irritability by comparing school-age children seeking treatment for severe irritability ($n = 26$) with typically developing children ($n = 28$) during an fMRI study utilizing a frustrative non-reward paradigm similar to the one described earlier (Perlman et al., 2014). The children were diagnosed with a variety of psychiatric disorders including BD, depression, anxiety, ADHD, ODD, and conduct disorder. They found that, compared to typically developing children, those with irritability displayed higher activation of the ACC and middle frontal gyrus during reward conditions, which may reflect alterations in reward expectancy that persist after a frustrating incident. Alternatively, irritable participants may have found it particularly rewarding when advances were made toward a desired goal. Moreover, during the frustration tasks, those with high levels of irritability exhibited less activation of the ACC and middle frontal gyrus and greater activation of the posterior cingulate compared with typically developing children. In addition, parent report of irritability was dimensionally related to decreased activation of the ACC and striatum during frustration. The authors postulated that failure to suppress posterior cingulate activity in those with irritability may be associated with the intrusion of internal mentation during task performance and might suggest dysregulation in controlling the balance between an internal and external attentional focus. Interestingly, the authors found no amygdala involvement during frustrating situations in children with irritability. The authors concluded that there is deviation in reward and emotional function in children with irritability; the ACC might be particularly sensitive to the experience of blocked goals, and the reactivity to blocked goals may help distinguish normative from abnormal emotional processing.

To conclude, the literature on reward processing in irritable youth across diagnoses is limited, but several studies indicate that, regardless of psychiatric diagnosis, those with irritability demonstrate perturbations in various prefrontal regions and the ACC, which are areas that mediate reward learning, and in the striatum, which is involved in reward, as well as prediction error.

THREAT AND FACIAL EMOTION PROCESSING

Studies of Irritable Youth

IMPLICIT AND EXPLICIT FACE EMOTION TASKS

Studies of irritable youth have utilized a range of different facial paradigms to assess threat and emotion processing. Facial stimuli have been used more generally (e.g., implicit vs. explicit facial emotion processing). Because face-emotion processing is an important feature of social cognition and is deficient in several disorders, Brotman et al. (2010) compared amygdala response during an explicit face-viewing task (emotional and non-emotional ratings of neutral faces) to compare youth with BD (n = 43), ADHD (n = 18), SMD (n = 29), and typically developing children (n = 37). They found that when rating levels of subjective fear relative to the other three groups, those with non-irritable ADHD demonstrated left amygdala hyperactivity. In contrast, relative to the other three groups, those with SMD demonstrated amygdala hypoactivity; those with BD did not differ significantly from typically developing children in amygdala activation. In contrast, Thomas et al. (2012) looked at this population using a paradigm that combined implicit and explicit emotion face-viewing in which the faces morphed from neutral-to-happy or neutral-to-angry and found amygdala hypoactivation in both youth with BD (n = 19) and SMD (n =15) compared to typically developing children (n = 23) when faces morphed to anger. Wiggins et al. (2016) examined neural mechanisms mediating irritability that differ between those with BD (n = 24) and DMDD (n = 25) using an explicit face emotion labeling paradigm. They found that irritability was correlated with amygdala activity across all intensities for all emotions in those with DMDD, but irritability was only correlated with amygdala activity for fearful faces in those with BD. Moreover, they found that, in the ventral visual stream, associations between neural activity and irritability were found more consistently in those with DMDD than in BD, especially in response to ambiguous angry faces. Specifically, there were associations between neural activity and irritability for those with DMDD but not for those with BD in the amygdala, superior temporal sulcus, frontal pole, and lingual gyrus. In addition, they found divergent alterations in neural responses associated with irritability in those with DMDD compared with BD when subjects correctly labeled subtle faces, not the overt faces often used in face tasks; this may indicate that subtle, ambiguous social stimuli are necessary to capture differences in neural correlates, possibly because these faces are more difficult to identify. Finally, they failed to replicate findings of hypoactivation in the left amygdala to neutral faces in DMDD (Brotman et al., 2010). However, it must be noted that the task demands were different across these studies.

Thomas et al. (2013) conducted a similar study using an implicit face-emotion processing paradigm in which subjects identified the gender of fearful, angry, and neutral faces. They found that youth with SMD (n = 19) and BD (n = 19) both demonstrated amygdala hyperactivity versus typically developing children (n = 15) across all three emotional expressions. However, youth with SMD differed from the other two groups in showing deactivation in response to fearful expressions in the posterior cingulate cortex (PCC), inferior parietal lobe/precuneus, and posterior insula. In contrast, youth with BD differed from the other two groups in showing deactivation in response to angry expressions in those same regions. They also differed from those with SMD but not typically developing children in showing ACC deactivation in response to angry faces. Findings suggest that implicit face emotion processing in those with BD and SMD may elicit similar amygdala dysfunction but unique neural dysfunction in information integration and monitoring regions.

AWARE AND NONAWARE FACE EMOTION TASKS

Studies have also directly compared the neural correlates of aware (e.g., consciously processed) versus nonaware (e.g., stimulus presentation too fast for conscious processing) face-emotion processing between healthy controls and irritable youth. First, Thomas et al. (2014) compared youth with BD ($n = 20$), SMD ($n = 18$), and typically developing children ($n = 22$). They found that controls had greater occipital activation for aware versus nonaware, while youth with BD and SMD had greater occipital activation for nonaware versus aware. In addition, youth with BD had greater activity versus typically developing children in the precentral gyrus in response to happy faces and versus youth with SMD in response to neutral and no-face stimuli. Youth with BD also had greater activation versus those with SMD in the superior temporal gyrus for neutral stimuli and MFG for fear and neutral faces. In response to angry faces, those with SMD showed greater activity versus typically developing children in the superior temporal gyrus, posterior cingulate, and middle occipital gyrus. In response to angry faces, those with SMD showed greater activity than those with BD in the middle occipital gyrus. Tseng et al. (2015) replicated the Thomas et al. (2014) study on neural correlates of face emotion processing above and below awareness level using an independent sample of youth with SMD ($n = 17$) compared with typically developing children ($n = 20$) but removed fearful faces from their paradigm. They found that, relative to typically developing children, those with SMD exhibited greater vmPFC activation during processing of masked faces, regardless of emotion. In addition, they found that typically developing children, but not those with SMD, showed differential vmPFC activation between the two awareness conditions. Moreover, relative to typically developing children, those with SMD exhibited increased activation in the parahippocampal gyrus (PHG) and superior temporal gyrus when processing masked and unmasked angry faces. In addition, relative to typically developing children, those with SMD showed decreased activation in the insula, PHG, and thalamus when processing masked and unmasked happy faces. Thus, the researchers concluded that perturbed activation in emotion processing areas (e.g., insula, PHG, superior temporal gyrus, and thalamus) reflecting hypersensitivity toward negative emotions and hyposensitivity toward positive emotions may be important in the etiology and maintenance of irritability, aggression, and depressive symptoms in SMD; furthermore, vmPFC dysfunction may mediate overreactivity to face emotions associated with irritability.

Based on findings that children with chronic irritability have deficits in labeling facial expressions, Stoddard et al. (2016) examined neural mechanisms of irritability through a treatment study of these deficits. Specifically, they investigated whether an active balance-point training in youth with DMDD (n = 10), which would treat their tendency to judge ambiguous facial expressions as angry, would be associated with reduced irritability and associated brain changes during an implicit face-emotion processing task. Findings showed that open interpretation bias training was associated with reduced irritability and, possibly, altered brain function in the lateral OFC and amygdala in response to subtle expressions of happiness relative to anger.

THREAT PROCESSING TASKS

Studies investigating threat processing across diagnostic categories highlight a relationship between anxiety and irritability in that both have a heightened orientation to threat (Bar-Haim et al., 2007; Salum et al., 2017). Threat processing studies reveal that anxiety also results in atypical corticolimbic networks in irritable youth. Stoddard et al. (2017) examined shared and unique effects of irritability and anxiety on neural responses (psychophysiological interaction and task-based activation) to facial emotions in youth aged 8–17 with a range of psychiatric disorders (DMDD = 37, Anxiety = 32, ADHD = 24; typically developing children = 22). Results showed interactive, rather than additive, effects of anxiety and irritability on functional connectivity when participants process social threat. Specifically, they found that, during implicit processing of emotional, specifically intensely angry, faces, high levels of irritability and anxiety were associated with decreased amygdala-medial prefrontal cortex connectivity, and low levels of irritability and high levels of anxiety were associated with increased amygdala-medial prefrontal cortex connectivity. These findings suggest that decreased amygdala–medial prefrontal cortex connectivity may mediate emotion dysregulation when very anxious and irritable youth process threat-related faces. Moreover, co-occurring anxiety seems to modulate amygdala–medial prefrontal cortex connectivity in irritable youth, suggesting that youth with high levels of irritability and anxiety represent a meaningful subgroup in terms of brain function. In contrast, when examining regional activation, the researchers found that irritability predicted increased neural activity in response to angry/or happy relative to fearful faces in the ventral visual stream and pulvinar. Activation in this ventral visual circuitry suggests a mechanism through which signals of social approach (i.e., happy and angry expressions) may capture attention in irritable youth. Of note, the researchers did not detect associations between irritability-associated neural responses and psychiatric diagnosis.

Like Stoddard et al. (2017), Kircanski et al. (2018) also examined shared and unique effects of irritability and anxiety on neural responses in youth with a range of psychiatric disorders, including typically developing children (n = 56), DMDD (n = 54), ADHD (n = 37), and anxiety disorders (n = 50). However, Kircanski et al. (2018) focused on threat processing via a dot-probe attentional task that assessed the impact of a threat cue (angry vs. neutral face) on neural activation, as well as functional connectivity. They found that, when viewing angry versus neutral faces, higher negative affectivity was associated with increased activation in the thalamus, but when the probe followed the neutral versus angry faces, higher irritability was associated with increased activation in the left amygdala, bilateral caudate, inferior parietal lobule, right insula, bilateral dlPFC, and left vmPFC. In addition, they found that higher anxiety was associated with decreased connectivity of the amygdala to the thalamus, bilateral cingulate, and left precentral gyrus. These findings suggest that individual differences in neural activation were largely driven by irritability, whereas differences in neural connectivity were driven by anxiety.

Studies of Aggressive Youth

Finally, several studies have examined the neural correlates of aggression, which often co-occur with irritability, particularly in ODD and CD. For example, compared to typically developing children (n = 14), adolescents with aggressive CD (n = 13) showed marked deactivation of the ACC when viewing negatively valenced faces, suggesting a failure of top-down cognitive control (Sterzer, Stadler, Krebs, Kleinschmidt, & Poustka (2005). A negative correlation was found between level of aggressiveness and left amygdala activation, which may reflect an impaired ability to recognize affective information in social contexts. Using a similar paradigm and patient population but looking more specifically at particular temperamental styles, Stadler et al. (2007) also found that, compared to typically developing children (n = 14), individuals with CD had reduced activation of the right ACC when seeing negatively valenced pictures; they noted that the temperamental dimension of novelty seeking, as opposed to aggression or attention, was the best predictor of reduced ACC response to negative pictures, suggesting that this may be due to poor cognitive control strategies.

Two recent studies focused specifically on the reactive aggression subtype in youth with DBD. White et al. (2015) examined the neural basis of reactive aggression utilizing an ultimatum game in youth with disruptive behavior disorders (n = 56; DBD = 30, typically developing children = 26), half of whom also had comorbid ADHD. They found that those with low levels of callous and unemotional (CU) traits showed exaggerated basic threat circuitry (periaqueductal gray/amygdala) activation as a function of level of retaliation, suggesting that atypical ventromedial PFC–amygdala connectivity is critically involved in reactive aggression in youth with disruptive behavior disorders. However, this study did not examine irritability directly. More recently, Bubenzer-Busch et al. (2016) compared children with ADHD with and without comorbid disruptive behavior disorders (n = 18) and typically developing children (n = 18) using a modified version of the Point Subtraction Aggression game, a paradigm designed to elicit reactive aggression. They found that while typically developing controls showed higher ACC activation for highly aggressive responses, this level of activation in youth with ADHD/DBD was already reached for low levels of reactive aggressive behavior. Additionally, those with ADHD/DBD showed diminished activation of the ventral ACC for highly aggressive responses.

In summary, the majority of research in this section focused on processing facial emotions, including threatening faces, during MRI scanning. These studies generally distinguished youth with irritability from controls across a range of brain regions, encompassing cortical, limbic, and visual circuits (i.e., amygdala, occipital cortex, posterior insula, mPFC, PCC). Such varied findings are not surprising given the complexity of facial and emotional processing. Of note, activation differed in youth with episodic versus chronic irritability in several studies. Finally, both face and non-face tasks were also successfully used to elicit the neural correlates of reactive aggression such as alterations in the amygdala, ACC, and PFC, which were similar to those associated with irritability, suggesting an association between these constructs.

BRAIN STRUCTURE AND CONNECTIVITY IN IRRITABLE YOUTH

While task-based studies, by their nature, focus on one area of interest, such as reward or face emotion processing, structural connectivity and intrinsic functional connectivity (iFC) allow for broader exploration of circuits that may be involved in one or both of these processes. Neuroanatomy studies suggest that children with chronic irritability exhibit smaller gray matter volumes in the presupplementatry motor area, dlPFC, and the insula compared to healthy peers (Adleman et al., 2012). In contrast, Seymour et al. (2017) found localized volume *expansion* in the right globus pallidus, putamen, and right amygdala that was significantly correlated with emotion dysregulation in boys with ADHD (n = 218; ADHD = 109, typically developing children = 109). In fact, they postulated that this localized expansion may represent a biomarker for emotion dysregulation in boys with ADHD.

Pagliaccio, Pine, Barch, Luby, and Leibenluft (2018) examined the developmental trajectories of irritability among preschoolers (n = 271) oversampled for depressive symptoms by investigating youth starting at age 3–5 years and conducting three annual neuroimaging waves beginning at 7–12 years of age. They found that those who exhibited consistently elevated irritability over time showed thicker cortex in the left superior frontal and the right inferior parietal lobe. Henderson et al. (2013) used diffusion tensor imaging (DTI) to examine white matter microstructure in adolescents with major depressive disorder (MDD; n = 17) and typically developing children (n = 16) and specifically examined irritability and anhedonia in MDD. They found that irritability was associated with decreased integrity in the sagittal stratum, anterior corona radiata, and tracts leading to the prefrontal and temporal/occipital cortices.

Stoddard et al. (2015) evaluated functional connectivity using resting state fMRI in children with BD ($n = 14$), SMD ($n = 19$), and typically developing children ($n = 20$) and found that those with BD differed from typically developing children and SMD youth in iFC between the left basolateral amygdala and the medial prefrontal cortex, posterior cingulate, and precuneus. Specifically, those with BD showed hyperconnectivity between the amygdala and these regions. Roy et al. (2018) examined iFC of the anterior midcingulate cortex (aMCC) in young children who demonstrated a feature of irritability—severe temper outbursts ($n = 20$)—85% of whom had ADHD, and compared them to children with ADHD without severe temper outbursts ($n = 18$) and to typically developing children ($n = 18$). They found that, compared to those with ADHD without temper outbursts and to typically developing children, those with severe temper outbursts demonstrated reduced iFC between the aMCC and surrounding regions of the ACC, and increased iFC between the aMCC and precuneus. The precuneus is a core region of the default network, which plays a role in social emotion regulation, suggesting that the increased connectivity between the aMCC and the precuneus in those with severe temper outbursts may reflect a greater reliance on others to help regulate strong emotions. Alternatively, hyperconnectivity with the precuneus may prevent the aMCC from effectively regulating negative affect.

There is also evidence of associations between iFC and emotional lability in ADHD. For example, Posner et al. (2013) investigated affective circuits including the ventral striatum, subgenual and orbitofrontal cortices, the amygdala, and hippocampus. Compared to typically developing children ($n = 20$), children with ADHD ($n = 22$) showed reduced iFC between the ventral striatum and the orbitofrontal cortex. Children with ADHD also demonstrated an inverse correlation between connectivity in the emotional regulation circuit and levels of emotional lability, such that, as emotional lability increased, the connectivity between the ventral striatum and left orbitofrontal cortex decreased. Hulvershorn et al. (2014) also investigated emotional lability in youth with ADHD. Specifically, they examined the relationship between iFC of amygdala circuits and emotion regulation deficits in ADHD ($n = 82$; ADHD = 63, typically developing children = 19). They found that, for children with ADHD, higher emotional lability scores were associated with greater functional connectivity between bilateral amygdala and mPFC regions, suggesting that elevated positive amygdala-prefrontal cortex connectivity is associated with difficulty in regulating the expression of negative emotions. High emotional lability scores were also negatively associated with functional connectivity between the amygdala and bilateral insula/superior temporal gyrus, suggesting that a failure in emotional perception and related action may partly underlie observed emotion dysregulation in ADHD. These patterns of amygdala–cortical functional connectivity did not differ between ADHD children with low emotional lability and typically developing controls.

Bennett, Somandapalli, Di Martino, and Roy (2017) found that emotional lability in youth with autism spectrum disorder (ASD; N = 58) was associated with iFC between the middle frontal gyrus and bilateral dorsal anterior insula. Also, emotional lability was associated with iFC between posterior insula and associative visual cortex. However, they did not find significant relationships between amygdala iFC and emotional lability, as in other studies described earlier.

Conclusion

During the past decade, an increasing number of researchers have begun to disentangle the neural correlates of pediatric irritability, including typically developing and clinical samples. The most common approaches have examined brain activation during threat and reward processing and, more recently, functional connectivity. Studies that utilize frustrative non-reward paradigms have reported dysfunction in the amygdala, striatum, and PFC. They also highlight the critical involvement of the ACC and changes in activation tracking with reward expectancies, which suggests a possible mechanism which could explain why irritable children are so sensitive to reward and, conversely, non-reward. From the facial emotion/threat processing literature, most studies suggest that children with irritability are more likely to perceive ambiguous and neutral faces as threatening and that threat bias is associated with dysfunction in the amygdala and vmPFC. These studies report disruptions in PFC-amygdala connectivity during threat tasks and in resting state connectivity of the amygdala-putamen.

Pediatric irritability has unquestionably been best studied in SMD and BD. In these disorders, the findings on social emotion processing depend in part on the nature of the facial paradigm, whether subjects were presented with neutral, angry, or fearful faces; if emotional priming is presented; and how ambiguous the presentation is. Because the studies use different tasks, it is difficult to make direct comparisons. However, overall, it appears that despite some clinical overlap, SMD and BD have distinct neural signatures in the amygdala and brain areas that have inhibitory control over the amygdala (ACC and IFG), as well as over areas that are involved in face processing and identification (MFG, insula, superior temporal gyrus, parahippocampal gyrus, ventral visual stream). See Figure 9.2. These finding suggest that activation and connectivity of neural circuits differ substantially between samples with chronic (i.e., SMD/DMDD) versus episodic (i.e., BD) irritability. Some of the noteworthy differences include reduced gray matter volume in the PFC in those with SMD/DMDD, increased activation of the SFG in those with BD in response to negative feedback, and decreased ACC and PFC activation in those with BD. In addition, amygdala activation was inconsistent during face emotion tasks across studies.

Given the putative association between irritability and reactive aggression, studies examining DBDs can also inform us about neural circuits that may underlie pediatric

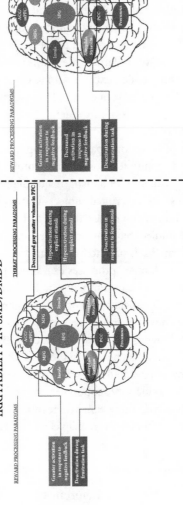

FIGURE 9.2 *Differential neuroimaging findings in severe mood dysregulation (SMD)/disruptive mood dysregulation disorder (DMDD) versus bipolar disorder.*

irritability. These investigations point to the role of the periaqueductal gray and amygdala in the exaggerated threat response in childhood disruptive behavior disorders. The ACC, which has strong connections to the amygdala and hypothalamus, also appears to play a role in controlling emotional processes in these populations. It also suggests that, in highly aggressive individuals, the ACC's ability to monitor and control emotional responses is overwhelmed, resulting in more severe behaviors, although additional studies are needed to confirm these preliminary observations.

Limitations and Future Directions

Pediatric neuroimaging studies have inherent limitations. First, the specification of brain–behavior substrates underlying particular clinical syndromes is still evolving. Although it would be optimal for neural abnormalities to be correlated with traits (e.g., irritability) in large-scale studies across a population, these data generally exist only for smaller, extreme-group comparisons. Furthermore, these smaller groups are limited by including only those children who can remain still during the scan, as high levels of movement bias the data. Second, findings from various studies are difficult to integrate because methodologies vary widely with respect to the type of behavioral paradigm employed. Third, despite the prominence of irritability in multiple disorders, few studies have focused on examining the neural basis of irritability in autism, major depression, or anxiety disorders. Finally, while many studies recruited subjects who were medication naïve, several included patients who were on medications, which is to be expected when severely impaired youth are studied, but may impact results.

In sum, research methods used to investigate the neural bases of pediatric irritability vary widely, with many processes examined, paradigms used, and regions of interest investigated. As a result, pediatric irritability and the relevant neural markers have become heterogeneous constructs. Genetic mechanisms associated with neural findings have yet to be investigated. Aside from larger sample sizes with longitudinal follow-up to help determine predictors of eventual disorders, innovative approaches are also needed in the field. To better understand the heterogeneity in the literature, the field may need to utilize machine learning and bioinformatics approaches to identify subpopulations and neural activation associated with various aspects of irritability. Finally, the future may hold treatment trials that include neuroimaging components to help elucidate neural changes brought on by interventions.

References

Adleman, N. E., Fromm, S. J., Razdan, V., Kayser, R., Dickstein, D. P., Brotman, M. A., . . . Leibenluft, E. (2012). Cross-sectional and longitudinal abnormalities in brain structure in children with severe mood dysregulation or bipolar disorder. *Journal of Child Psychology and Psychiatry, 53*(11), 1149–1156. doi:10.1111/j.1469-7610.2012.02568.x

Adleman, N. E., Kayser, R., Dickstein, D., Blair, R. J. R., Pine, D., & Leibenluft, E. (2011). Neural correlates of reversal learning in severe mood dysregulation and pediatric bipolar disorder. *Journal of the American Academy of Child & Adolescent Psychiatry, 50*(11), 1173–1185. e1172. doi:10.1016/j.jaac.2011.07.011

American Psychiatric Association (APA). (2013). *Diagnostic and statistical manual of mental disorders* (5th edition). Washington, CD: American Psychiatric Publishing.

Amsel, A. (1958). The role of frustrative nonreward in noncontinuous reward situations. *Psychological Bulletin, 55*(2), 102–119. doi:10.1037/h0043125

Bar-Haim, Y., Lamy, D., Pergamin, L., Bakermans-Kranenburg, M. J., & Van Ijzendoorn, M. H. (2007). Threat-related attentional bias in anxious and nonanxious individuals: A meta-analytic study. *Psychological Bulletin, 133*(1), 1–24. doi:10.1037/0033-2909.133.1.1

Bebko, G., Bertocci, M. A., Fournier, J. C., Hinze, A. K., Bonar, L., Almeida, J. R., . . . Travis, M. (2014). Parsing dimensional vs diagnostic category–related patterns of reward circuitry function in behaviorally and emotionally dysregulated youth in the longitudinal assessment of manic symptoms study. *JAMA Psychiatry, 71*(1), 71–80. doi:10.1001/jamapsychiatry.2013.2870

Bennett, R., Somandapalli, K., Di Martino, A., & Roy, A. (2017). The neural correlates of emotional lability in children with ASD. *Brain Connectivity, 7*(5), 281–288. doi:10.1089/brain.2016.0472

Berkowitz, L. (1989). Frustration-aggression hypothesis: Examination and reformulation. *Psychological Bulletin, 106*(1), 59–73.

Blair, R. (2010). Psychopathy, frustration, and reactive aggression: The role of ventromedial prefrontal cortex. *British Journal of Psychology, 101*(3), 383–399. doi:10.1348/000712609X418480

Blair, R., Colledge, E., & Mitchell, D. (2001). Somatic markers and response reversal: Is there orbitofrontal cortex dysfunction in boys with psychopathic tendencies? *Journal of Abnormal Child Psychology, 29*(6), 499–511.

Blair, R. J. (2016). The neurobiology of impulsive aggression. *Journal of Child and Adolescent Psychopharmacology, 26*(1), 4–9.

Brotman, M. A., Kircanski, K., & Leibenluft, E. (2017). Irritability in children and adolescents. *Annual Review of Clinical Psychology, 13*, 317–341. doi:10.1146/annurev-clinpsy-032816-044941

Brotman, M. A., Kircanski, K., Stringaris, A., Pine, D. S., & Leibenluft, E. (2017). Irritability in youths: A translational model. *American Journal of Psychiatry, 174*(6), 520–532. doi:10.1176/appi.ajp.2016.16070839

Brotman, M. A., Rich, B. A., Guyer, A. E., Lunsford, J. R., Horsey, S. E., Reising, M. M., . . . Pine, D. S. (2010). Amygdala activation during emotion processing of neutral faces in children with severe mood dysregulation versus ADHD or bipolar disorder. *American Journal of Psychiatry, 167*(1), 61–69. doi:10.1176/appi.ajp.2009.09010043

Bubenzer-Busch, S., Herpertz-Dahlmann, B., Kuzmanovic, B., Gaber, T., Helmbold, K., Ullisch, M. G., . . . Zepf, F. (2016). Neural correlates of reactive aggression in children with attention deficit/hyperactivity disorder and comorbid disruptive behaviour disorders. *Acta Psychiatrica Scandinavica, 133*(4), 310–323. doi:10.1111/acps.12475

Coker-Appiah, D. S., White, S. F., Clanton, R., Yang, J., Martin, A., & Blair, R. (2013). Looming animate and inanimate threats: The response of the amygdala and periaqueductal gray. *Social Neuroscience, 8*(6), 621–630. doi:10.1080/17470919.2013.839480

Costa, V. D., Tran, V. L., Turchi, J., & Averbeck, B. B. (2015). Reversal learning and dopamine: A bayesian perspective. *Journal of Neuroscience, 35*(6), 2407–2416. doi:10.1523/JNEUROSCI.1989-14.2015

De Silva, L. C., Miyasato, T., & Nakatsu, R. (1997). *Facial emotion recognition using multimodal information.* Paper presented at the International Conference on Information, Communications and Signal Processing (ICICS), 1997.

Deveney, C. M., Connolly, M. E., Haring, C. T., Bones, B. L., Reynolds, R. C., Kim, P., . . . Leibenluft, E. (2013). Neural mechanisms of frustration in chronically irritable children. *American Journal of Psychiatry, 170*(10), 1186–1194. doi:10.1176/appi.ajp.2013.12070917

Dickstein, D., Finger, E., Brotman, M., Rich, B., Pine, D., Blair, J., & Leibenluft, E. (2010). Impaired probabilistic reversal learning in youths with mood and anxiety disorders. *Psychological Medicine, 40*(7), 1089–1100. doi:10.1017/S0033291709991462

Dickstein, D. P., Nelson, E. E., McClure, E. B., Grimley, M. E., Knopf, L., Brotman, M. A., . . . Leibenluft, E. (2007). Cognitive flexibility in phenotypes of pediatric bipolar disorder. *Journal of the American Academy of Child & Adolescent Psychiatry, 46*(3), 341–355. doi:10.1097/chi.0b013e31802d0b3d

Dodge, K. A. (1980). Social cognition and children's aggressive behavior. *Child Development, 51*(1), 162–170.

Dougherty, L., Schwartz, K. T., Kryza-Lacombe, M., Weisberg, J., Spechler, P. A., & Wiggins, J. L. (2018). Preschool and school-age irritability predict reward-related brain function. *Journal of the American Academy of Child & Adolescent Psychiatry.* doi:10.1016/j.jaac.2018.03.012

Fellows, L. K., & Farah, M. J. (2003). Ventromedial frontal cortex mediates affective shifting in humans: Evidence from a reversal learning paradigm. *Brain, 126*(8), 1830–1837. doi:10.1093/brain/awg180

Fox, E., Russo, R., & Dutton, K. (2002). Attentional bias for threat: Evidence for delayed disengagement from emotional faces. *Cognition & Emotion, 16*(3), 355–379. doi:10.1080/02699930143000527

Gaffrey, M. S., Barch, D. M., & Luby, J. L. (2016). Amygdala reactivity to sad faces in preschool children: An early neural marker of persistent negative affect. *Developmental Cognitive Neuroscience, 17*, 94–100. doi:10.1016/j.dcn.2015.12.015

Grabell, A. S., Li, Y., Barker, J. W., Wakschlag, L. S., Huppert, T. J., & Perlman, S. B. (2018). Evidence of non-linear associations between frustration-related prefrontal cortex activation and the normal: Abnormal spectrum of irritability in young children. *Journal of Abnormal Child Psychology, 46*(1), 137–147. doi:10.1007/s10802-017-0286-5

Hariri, A. R., Bookheimer, S. Y., & Mazziotta, J. C. (2000). Modulating emotional responses: Effects of a neocortical network on the limbic system. *Neuroreport, 11*(1), 43–48.

Henderson, S. E., Johnson, A. R., Vallejo, A. I., Katz, L., Wong, E., & Gabbay, V. (2013). A preliminary study of white matter in adolescent depression: Relationships with illness severity, anhedonia, and irritability. *Frontiers in Psychiatry, 4*, 152. doi:10.3389/fpsyt.2013.00152

Hommer, R. E., Meyer, A., Stoddard, J., Connolly, M. E., Mogg, K., Bradley, B. P., . . . Brotman, M. A. (2014). Attention bias to threat faces in severe mood dysregulation. *Depression and Anxiety, 31*(7), 559–565. doi:10.1002/da.22145

Horsley, T. A., de Castro, B. O., & Van der Schoot, M. (2010). In the eye of the beholder: Eye-tracking assessment of social information processing in aggressive behavior. *Journal of Abnormal Child Psychology, 38*(5), 587–599. doi:10.1007/s10802-009-9361-x

Hulvershorn, L. A., Mennes, M., Castellanos, F. X., Di Martino, A., Milham, M. P., Hummer, T. A., & Roy, A. K. (2014). Abnormal amygdala functional connectivity associated with emotional lability in children with attention-deficit/hyperactivity disorder. *Journal of the American Academy of Child & Adolescent Psychiatry, 53*(3), 351–361. e351. doi:10.1016/j.jaac.2013.11.012

Karim, H. T., & Perlman, S. B. (2017). Neurodevelopmental maturation as a function of irritable temperament. *Human Brain Mapping, 38*(10), 5307–5321.

Kircanski, K., White, L. K., Tseng, W.-L., Wiggins, J. L., Frank, H. R., Sequeira, S., . . . Stringaris, A. (2018). A latent variable approach to differentiating neural mechanisms of irritability and anxiety in youth. *JAMA Psychiatry*. doi:10.1001/jamapsychiatry.2018.0468

Leibenluft, E. (2011). Severe mood dysregulation, irritability, and the diagnostic boundaries of bipolar disorder in youths. *American Journal of Psychiatry, 168*(2), 129–142. doi:10.1176/appi.ajp.2010.10050766

Leibenluft, E. (2017). Pediatric irritability: A systems neuroscience approach. *Trends in Cognitive Sciences, 21*(4), 277–289. doi:10.1016/j.tics.2017.02.002

Li, Y., Grabell, A. S., Wakschlag, L. S., Huppert, T. J., & Perlman, S. B. (2017). The neural substrates of cognitive flexibility are related to individual differences in preschool irritability: A fNIRS investigation. *Developmental Cognitive Neuroscience, 25*, 138–144. doi:10.1016/j.dcn.2016.07.002

Lieberman, M. D., Eisenberger, N. I., Crockett, M. J., Tom, S. M., Pfeifer, J. H., & Way, B. M. (2007). Putting feelings into words. *Psychological Science, 18*(5), 421–428.

Luman, M., Sergeant, J. A., Knol, D. L., & Oosterlaan, J. (2010). Impaired decision making in oppositional defiant disorder related to altered psychophysiological responses to reinforcement. *Biological Psychiatry, 68*(4), 337–344. doi:10.1016/j.biopsych.2009.12.037

McClure, E. B., Treland, J. E., Snow, J., Schmajuk, M., Dickstein, D. P., Towbin, K. E., . . . Leibenluft, E. (2005). Deficits in social cognition and response flexibility in pediatric bipolar disorder. *American Journal of Psychiatry, 162*(9), 1644–1651. doi:10.1176/appi.ajp.162.9.1644

Moriguchi, Y., & Hiraki, K. (2011). Longitudinal development of prefrontal function during early childhood. *Developmental Cognitive Neuroscience, 1*(2), 153–162. doi:10.1016/j.dcn.2010.12.004

Pagliaccio, D., Pine, D. S., Barch, D. M., Luby, J. L., & Leibenluft, E. (2018). Irritability trajectories, cortical thickness, and clinical outcomes in a sample enriched for preschool depression. *Journal of the American Academy of Child & Adolescent Psychiatry, 57*(5), 336–342 doi:10.1016/j.jaac.2018.02.010

Panksepp, J. (2006). Emotional endophenotypes in evolutionary psychiatry. *Progress in Neuro-Psychopharmacology and Biological Psychiatry, 30*(5), 774–784. doi:10.1016/j.pnpbp.2006.01.004

Perlman, S. B., Jones, B. M., Wakschlag, L. S., Axelson, D., Birmaher, B., & Phillips, M. L. (2015). Neural substrates of child irritability in typically developing and

psychiatric populations. *Developmental Cognitive Neuroscience, 14,* 71–80. doi:10.1016/
j.dcn.2015.07.003

Perlman, S. B., Luna, B., Hein, T. C., & Huppert, T. J. (2014). Fnirs evidence of prefrontal
regulation of frustration in early childhood. *Neuroimage, 85,* 326–334. doi:10.1016/
j.neuroimage.2013.04.057

Perlman, S. B., & Pelphrey, K. A. (2011). Developing connections for affective regulation: Age-related changes in emotional brain connectivity. *Journal of Experimental Child
Psychology, 108*(3), 607–620. doi:10.1016/j.jecp.2010.08.006

Posner, J., Rauh, V., Gruber, A., Gat, I., Wang, Z., & Peterson, B. S. (2013). Dissociable attentional and affective circuits in medication-naive children with attention-deficit/
hyperactivity disorder. *Psychiatry Research: Neuroimaging, 213*(1), 24–30. doi:10.1016/
j.pscychresns.2013.01.004

Rich, B. A., Carver, F. W., Holroyd, T., Rosen, H. R., Mendoza, J. K., Cornwell, B.
R., . . . Leibenluft, E. (2011). Different neural pathways to negative affect in youth with pediatric bipolar disorder and severe mood dysregulation. *Journal of Psychiatric Research,
45*(10), 1283–1294. doi:10.1016/j.jpsychires.2011.04.006

Rich, B. A., Schmajuk, M., Perez-Edgar, K. E., Fox, N. A., Pine, D. S., & Leibenluft, E. (2007).
Different psychophysiological and behavioral responses elicited by frustration in pediatric bipolar disorder and severe mood dysregulation. *American Journal of Psychiatry,
164*(2), 309–317. doi:10.1176/ajp.2007.164.2.309

Robins, D. L., Hunyadi, E., & Schultz, R. T. (2009). Superior temporal activation in response to dynamic audio-visual emotional cues. *Brain and Cognition, 69*(2), 269–278.
doi:10.1016/j.bandc.2008.08.007

Roy, A. K., Bennett, R., Posner, J., Hulvershorn, L., Castellanos, F. X., & Klein, R. G. (2018).
Altered intrinsic functional connectivity of the cingulate cortex in children with se-
vere temper outbursts. *Development and Psychopathology, 30*(2), 571–579. doi:10.1017/
S0954579417001080

Ryan, T. J., & Watson, P. (1968). Frustrative nonreward theory applied to children's behavior.
Psychological Bulletin, 69(2), 111–125.

Salum, G. A., Mogg, K., Bradley, B. P., Stringaris, A., Gadelha, A., Pan, P. M., . . . Pine, D.
S. (2017). Association between irritability and bias in attention orienting to threat in
children and adolescents. *Journal of Child Psychology and Psychiatry, 58*(5), 595–602.
doi:10.1111/jcpp.12659

Schippell, P. L., Vasey, M. W., Cravens-Brown, L. M., & Bretveld, R. A. (2003). Suppressed
attention to rejection, ridicule, and failure cues: A unique correlate of reactive but not
proactive aggression in youth. *Journal of Clinical Child and Adolescent Psychology, 32*(1),
40–55. doi:10.1207/S15374424JCCP3201_05

Schultz, W., & Dickinson, A. (2000). Neuronal coding of prediction errors. *Annual Review
of Neuroscience, 23*(1), 473–500. doi:10.1146/annurev.neuro.23.1.473

Seymour, K. E., Tang, X., Crocetti, D., Mostofsky, S. H., Miller, M. I., & Rosch, K. S. (2017).
Anomalous subcortical morphology in boys, but not girls, with ADHD compared to
typically developing controls and correlates with emotion dysregulation. *Psychiatry
Research: Neuroimaging, 261,* 20–28. doi:10.1016/j.pscychresns.2017.01.002

Stadler, C., Sterzer, P., Schmeck, K., Krebs, A., Kleinschmidt, A., & Poustka, F. (2007).
Reduced anterior cingulate activation in aggressive children and adolescents during

affective stimulation: Association with temperament traits. *Journal of Psychiatric Research,* 41(5), 410–417. doi:10.1016/j.jpsychires.2006.01.006

Sterzer, P., Stadler, C., Krebs, A., Kleinschmidt, A., & Poustka, F. (2005). Abnormal neural responses to emotional visual stimuli in adolescents with conduct disorder. *Biological Psychiatry,* 57(1), 7–15. doi:10.1016/j.biopsych.2004.10.008

Stoddard, J., Hsu, D., Reynolds, R. C., Brotman, M. A., Ernst, M., Pine, D. S., . . . Dickstein, D. P. (2015). Aberrant amygdala intrinsic functional connectivity distinguishes youths with bipolar disorder from those with severe mood dysregulation. *Psychiatry Research: Neuroimaging,* 231(2), 120–125. doi:10.1016/j.pscychresns.2014.11.006

Stoddard, J., Sharif-Askary, B., Harkins, E. A., Frank, H. R., Brotman, M. A., Penton-Voak, I. S., . . . Pine, D. S. (2016). An open pilot study of training hostile interpretation bias to treat disruptive mood dysregulation disorder. *Journal of Child and Adolescent Psychopharmacology,* 26(1), 49–57. doi:10.1089/cap.2015.0100

Stoddard, J., Tseng, W.-L., Kim, P., Chen, G., Yi, J., Donahue, L., . . . Leibenluft, E. (2017). Association of irritability and anxiety with the neural mechanisms of implicit face emotion processing in youths with psychopathology. *JAMA Psychiatry,* 74(1), 95–103. doi:10.1001/jamapsychiatry.2016.3282

Thomas, L. A., Brotman, M. A., Bones, B. L., Chen, G., Rosen, B. H., Pine, D. S., & Leibenluft, E. (2014). Neural circuitry of masked emotional face processing in youth with bipolar disorder, severe mood dysregulation, and healthy volunteers. *Developmental Cognitive Neuroscience,* 8, 110–120. doi:10.1016/j.dcn.2013.09.007

Thomas, L. A., Brotman, M. A., Muhrer, E. J., Rosen, B. H., Bones, B. L., Reynolds, R. C., . . . Leibenluft, E. (2012). Parametric modulation of neural activity by emotion in youth with bipolar disorder, youth with severe mood dysregulation, and healthy volunteers. *Archives of General Psychiatry,* 69(12), 1257–1266. doi:10.1001/archgenpsychiatry.2012.913

Thomas, L. A., Kim, P., Bones, B. L., Hinton, K. E., Milch, H. S., Reynolds, R. C., . . . Pine, D. S. (2013). Elevated amygdala responses to emotional faces in youths with chronic irritability or bipolar disorder. *NeuroImage: Clinical,* 2, 637–645. doi:10.1016/j.nicl.2013.04.007

Tseng, W.-L., Deveney, C., Brotman, M., Stoddard, J., Moroney, E., Machlin, L., . . . Pine, D. (2017). 37-neural mechanisms of frustration and irritability across diagnoses. *Biological Psychiatry,* 81(10), S16.

Tseng, W.-L., Thomas, L. A., Harkins, E., Pine, D. S., Leibenluft, E., & Brotman, M. A. (2015). Neural correlates of masked and unmasked face emotion processing in youth with severe mood dysregulation. *Social Cognitive and Affective Neuroscience,* 11(1), 78–88. doi:10.1093/scan/nsv087

Wakschlag, L. S., Choi, S. W., Carter, A. S., Hullsiek, H., Burns, J., McCarthy, K., . . . Briggs-Gowan, M. J. (2012). Defining the developmental parameters of temper loss in early childhood: Implications for developmental psychopathology. *Journal of Child Psychology and Psychiatry,* 53(11), 1099–1108. doi:10.1111/j.1469-7610.2012.02595.x

Wakschlag, L. S., Perlman, S. B., Blair, J., Leibenluft, E., Briggs-Gowan, M. J., & Pine, D. S. (2018). The neurodevelopmental basis of early childhood disruptive behavior: Irritable and callous phenotypes as exemplars. *American Journal of Psychiatry,* 175(2), 114–130. doi:10.1176/appi.ajp.2017.17010045

White, S. F., VanTieghem, M., Brislin, S. J., Sypher, I., Sinclair, S., Pine, D. S., . . . Blair, R. J. R. (2015). Neural correlates of the propensity for retaliatory behavior in youths with disruptive behavior disorders. *American Journal of Psychiatry, 173*(3), 282–290. doi:10.1176/appi.ajp.2015.15020250

Wiggins, J. L., Briggs-Gowan, M. J., Estabrook, R., Brotman, M. A., Pine, D. S., Leibenluft, E., & Wakschlag, L. S. (2018). Identifying clinically significant irritability in early childhood. *Journal of the American Academy of Child & Adolescent Psychiatry, 57*(3), 191–199 e192. doi:10.1016/j.jaac.2017.12.008

Wiggins, J. L., Brotman, M. A., Adleman, N. E., Kim, P., Oakes, A. H., Reynolds, R. C., . . . Leibenluft, E. (2016). Neural correlates of irritability in disruptive mood dysregulation and bipolar disorders. *American Journal of Psychiatry, 173*(7), 722–730. doi:10.1176/appi.ajp.2015.15060833

Clinical Presentation

10

Irritability and Disruptive Behavior Disorders
Joel Stoddard, Valerie Scelsa, and Soonjo Hwang

Chronic irritability stands at the crossroads between disruptive behavior and emotional dysregulation. Defined as a decreased threshold to respond to provocation with anger and temper outbursts, it has long been considered an important feature of emotionally driven, disruptive behavior (Buss & Durkee, 1957; Caprara et al., 1985). As such, psychological, neuroscientific, and sociological investigations of aggression have provided a basis for more recent, clinically focused investigations of pediatric chronic irritability (Leibenluft & Stoddard, 2013). The recognition of irritability as an affective feature of disruptive behavioral problems has been a major advance in clinical science and has already inspired new clinical approaches. In this chapter, we review irritability in the context of disruptive behaviors.

We begin with a review of two transdiagnostic constructs that inform our understanding of the phenomenological and clinical relationships between irritability and disruptive behavior: aggression and temper loss. We follow this section with further evidence on how research on irritability has begun to transform our understanding of major disruptive behavioral diagnoses—oppositional defiant disorder (ODD), attention deficit/hyperactivity disorder (ADHD), and conduct disorder (CD). Throughout, we orient readers to important constructs, such as reactive aggression, and discuss their relationship to irritability. We end the review with an overview of the development of treatments for irritability rooted in the long-standing work on disruptive behaviors.

Aggression

Aggression is broadly defined as any behavior intended to harm an individual who does not want to be harmed. It is associated with all major disruptive behavior disorders (Tremblay, 2010; Waschbusch et al., 2002, 2004). It may be a manifestation of severe irritability, typically in response to a frustrating or threatening event in the context of poor emotional regulation (Avenevoli, Blader, & Leibenluft, 2015; Leibenluft, 2017; Leibenluft & Stoddard, 2013). Aggression can be differentiated from nonaggressive expressions of irritability, such as angry affect, defiance, property destruction, and self-injury. In this section, we first describe the relationship between irritability and aggression. Then, we focus on a specific type of aggression, reactive aggression, which has a particularly strong association with irritability.

Early work in personality traits provides some clue to the association between irritability and a tendency toward aggression. Trait aggression has consistently been associated with trait irritability ($r = 0.3$–0.7 in one meta-analysis) (Bettencourt, Talley, Benjamin, & Valentine, 2006). In this work, both trait aggression and trait irritability have typically been measured using similar items testing a proclivity to negative emotions, possibly accounting for the overlap (Bettencourt et al., 2006). Investigations into the relationship between chronic irritability and aggression in youth with disruptive behavioral problems are lacking, with one notable exception. One large, prospective study (Generation R, $N = 6{,}209$) (Bolhuis et al., 2017) examined associations among all disruptive behavioral symptoms as measured by parent-report on the Child Behavior Checklist (Achenbach & Rescorla, 2014) for youth at 6 and 10 years of age. This study found that irritability and aggression formed distinct but associated dimensions best explaining disruptive behavior in youth (Bolhuis et al., 2017). By distinct, we mean that irritability items correlate more with each other than with aggressive items and vice versa. In this study, authors also replicated this type of separation between irritability and aggression in two other large samples. Furthermore, the dimensions were stable over time: from age 6 to 10 years, irritability best predicted irritability and aggression best predicted aggression. Despite showing some distinction, aggression and irritability were also found to be associated dimensions of disruptive behavior in the Generation R study. For example, they had a strong cross-sectional association in 10-year-old children (adjusted $r = 0.59$). The authors concluded that both irritability and aggression should be considered as major dimensions when evaluating disruptive behavior in middle childhood.

There are many ways to characterize aggression, including by its means (e.g., physical, verbal, or relational), its goals (to address a threat or obtain something), or even its display (overt or covert). A review of the typology of aggression is beyond the scope of this chapter. However, a particularly relevant classification of aggression for pediatric irritability is the distinction between proactive and reactive aggression (Dodge, Lochman, Harnish, Bates, & Pettit, 1997; Kempes, Matthys, de Vries, & van Engeland, 2005; Raine et al., 2006). Reactive aggression is a response to a perceived, aversive provocation (e.g., frustration, insult, or threat). Thus, it is usually an improvised, impulsive, and ill-planned action. In reactive aggression, there is no clear reward anticipated or goals to achieve, other than to remove an immediately frustrating object, escape punishment, or as an act of self-defense (Berkowitz, 1993). On the other hand, proactive aggression is premeditated, goal-oriented aggressive behavior. It is also called *instrumental aggression*, meaning the use of aggression as a tool, or instrument, to obtain material, domination, or pleasure. In particular, reactive aggression is relevant to irritability because of their conceptual associations; indeed, work on reactive aggression has led to several broad hypotheses and theories, which inspire current investigations of the pathophysiology and treatment of irritability.

It may immediately strike the reader that reactive aggression has a definition very close to that of irritability. Both describe a response to specific types of aversive provocation (frustration, threat, insult, etc.). A conceptual distinction between the two is that reactive aggression describes harmful behavior, while irritability describes an increased intensity and frequency of an emotional state (i.e., anger), which may or may not be accompanied by emotionally driven outbursts; these outbursts, in turn, may or may not be characterized by aggression. Almost no work has empirically tested the association between reactive aggression and irritability except for one study of youth with cyclothymia, where the two were found to be distinct (Van Meter et al., 2016). Nonetheless, given the paucity of research into pediatric irritability, researchers have drawn inferences from studies on reactive aggression, and so we review the extant research here.

Developmental research on reactive aggression has begun to map out its associations from toddlerhood to adulthood. Reactive aggression is associated with history of maltreatment, early onset of behavioral and emotional problems, peer victimization, ADHD-symptoms, and psychosocial adjustment difficulties (Card & Little, 2006). In childhood and adolescence, a tendency toward reactive aggression is associated with lower self-esteem, lower emotional awareness, and higher levels of depression and delinquency (Rieffe et al., 2016). In childhood, a tendency toward reactive aggression is typically preceded by negative emotionality (Vitaro, Barker, Boivin, Brendgen, & Tremblay, 2006) and sensitivity to anger/frustration (Xu, Farver, & Zhang, 2009). A 10-year longitudinal study by Fite, Raine, Stouthamer-Loeber, Loeber, and Pardini (2009) found that adolescent reactive aggression was associated with negative emotionality, especially anxiety, as well as substance use in adulthood. Some of these associations are similar to those of irritability (e.g., the relationship between reactive aggression and negative emotionality). Other associations have yet to be tested. For example, the association between peer victimization and rejection is well established in reactive aggression but has yet to be investigated in irritability. Furthermore, studies examining shared and unique associations between reactive aggression and irritability have yet to be done. Such studies will have high clinical utility because both reactive aggression and irritability have been identified as major dimensions of disruptive behavior. Furthermore, we need to understand what factors distinguish irritable youth who differ in their use of reactive aggression.

Several major hypotheses on reactive aggression have informed irritability research. A prominent one is the frustration-aggression hypothesis (Dollard, Miller, Doob, Mowrer, & Sears, 1939). Specifically, frustration describes the emotional and behavioral response to the absence of an expected reward (Berkowitz, 1989;

Miller, 1941). A frustrating stimulus is well-defined and straightforward to induce, making it possible to do experimental studies which can determine cause–effect relationships. Researchers have successfully used frustrating stimuli to investigate neural mechanisms of the frustration response in pediatric irritability, illuminating irritability-associated aberrant responses to frustration in systems underlying reward processing and emotional regulation (Brotman, Kircanski, Stringaris, Pine, & Leibenluft, 2017). See Chapters 3 and 8 for more details about this work.

Another set of hypotheses that influenced irritability research were those proposed by Dodge (1980) to explain social dysfunction in youth with a tendency toward reactive aggression (Camodeca, 2005; Hwang, Kim, Koh, Bishop, & Leventhal, 2017; Lansford, Malone, Dodge, Pettit, & Bates, 2010; van Reemst, Fischer, & Zwirs, 2016; Ziv, 2012). Together, these hypotheses comprise *social information processing theory* (Crick & Dodge, 1994). Briefly, this theory predicts that reactively aggressive youth preferentially attend to social threat cues, are biased toward interpreting ambiguous cues as reflecting hostile intent (hostile interpretation bias), have impaired flexibility in choosing appropriate behavior, and have a limited repertoire of behavioral responses. This theory has influenced research into pediatric irritability. Consistent with the theory's predictions for reactively aggressive youth, investigations of irritable youth have demonstrated that they have an attentional bias toward social threat (Hommer et al., 2013; Salum et al., 2017), hostile interpretation bias (Stoddard et al., 2016), and inflexibility in response (Adleman et al., 2011; Dickstein et al., 2007; Li, Grabell, Wakschlag, Huppert, & Perlman, 2017). As a result, trials of treatments that aim to reduce irritability by specifically targeting social information processing are under way (NCT02531893; NCT01965184).

A final set of influential hypotheses that address the developmental origins of reactive aggression may have implications for pediatric irritability research. An influential "social learning" hypothesis suggests that reactive aggression is learned from others who demonstrate it as an effective means of dealing with provocation (Bandura, 1978). Some support for this hypothesis may be found in the associations between reactive aggression and childhood maltreatment (Augsburger, Dohrmann, Schauer, & Elbert, 2017) and exposure to violent media and aggression (Craig & Brad, 2001). Alternatively, another hypothesis recognizes an inborn capacity for aggression that reduces with the development of language and emotional regulation (Tremblay, 2010). This hypothesis is consistent with trajectory studies showing that a tendency toward and severity of reactive aggression is highest for almost everyone very early in life and reduces with development (Ezpeleta, Granero, de la Osa, Trepat, & Domènech, 2016; Wiggins, Mitchell, Stringaris, & Leibenluft, 2014). Thus, rather than learning to aggress or respond irritably, most people appear to learn to inhibit socially inappropriate strategies, such as aggression, to achieve goals or manage provocation. It has been suggested that impairment in one's ability to learn such inhibition is a mechanism for pathologic irritability (Leibenluft & Stoddard, 2013; Wakschlag et al., 2017). Data suggest that irritability has moderate heritability (~0.4; see Chapter 7), suggesting the importance of considering both environmental and inborn factors in its development. Future work investigating these factors may be informed by these two developmental hypotheses of reactive aggression.

We have reviewed the relationship between aggression and irritability, two prominent transdiagnostic dimensions of disruptive behavior. In particular, we reviewed close associations between irritability and reactive aggression. The study of reactive aggression has been a rich source of inspiration for research on irritability and may continue to inform such work.

Temper Loss

Temper loss is a recently established construct in young children that represents a readily observable symptom of irritability, the tantrum. This construct was developed to describe and formally measure a particularly disruptive aspect of preschool irritability (Dougherty et al., 2013; Wakschlag et al., 2012). Other investigational constructs also represent this explosive, often disruptive, behavior associated with irritability, including phasic irritability (Copeland, Brotman, & Costello, 2015) or outbursts (American Psychiatric Association [APA], 2013). However, we focus on temper loss here because of its origin in a prospective longitudinal study designed to validate measures and investigate both normative and clinically significant aspects of disruptive behavior across development, the Multidimensional Assessment of Preschoolers Study (MAPS) (Wakschlag et al., 2012). In addition, the initial construction of the MAPS parent-report temper loss scale (the MAPS-DB) uses state-of-the-art psychometrics incorporating a computational model of decision-making (Wakschlag et al., 2012). Temper loss in preschool is strongly associated with aggression ($r = .79$ in $N = 1,490$) (Wakschlag et al., 2012). Though temper loss is common in preschoolers, parameters describing the onset, frequency, duration, and length of tantrums can be clinically meaningful (Wakschlag et al., 2012; Wiggins et al., 2018). Future work will clarify the clinical utility of the temper loss construct and its relationship to other measures representing irritability or its components.

DSM-5 Disorders Defined by Disruptive Behavior

OPPOSITIONAL DEFIANT DISORDER

The lifetime prevalence of ODD is about 10.2% and is slightly more common in boys over a lifetime (11.2%) than girls (9.2%) (Nock, Kazdin, Hiripi, & Kessler, 2007). ODD is rarely diagnosed on its own; approximately 92% of individuals who are diagnosed ODD will have at least one other mental illness in their lifetime (Harvey, Breaux, & Lugo-Candelas, 2016; Nock et al., 2007). The most common comorbid diagnoses are ADHD (19%-40%) and CD (10-42%) (Angold, Costello, & Erkanli, 1999; Lavigne et al., 2001; Nock et al., 2007).

The *Diagnostic and Statistical Manual of Mental Disorders*, Fifth Edition (DSM-5) divides the eight ODD symptoms into three categories: angry/irritable, argumentative/defiant, and vindictiveness (a single symptom, spitefulness). Of the three, empirical evidence consistently supports at least two dimensions: angry/irritable (usually called irritable) and argumentative/defiant (frequently called headstrong) (Burke, Hipwell, & Loeber, 2010; Herzhoff & Tackett, 2016). Irritable symptoms include frequent temper tantrums, anger, and being easily annoyed. Headstrong symptoms involve arguing with adults and actively disobeying rules set by authority figures. Irritable and headstrong dimensions of ODD are separable but not independent, as evidenced by their high correlation ($r = .78$) (Stringaris & Goodman, 2009a) and formal tests for independence in confirmatory factor analyses (Burke et al., 2014). Like the relationship between irritability and aggression that we described earlier, irritability and headstrong symptoms are distinguishable, but usually co-occur in individuals. So, irritable and headstrong symptoms may be considered prominent dimensions along which youth with ODD vary (Bolhuis et al., 2017).

In children diagnosed with ODD, irritable and headstrong symptoms occur at the same rate (Bolhuis et al., 2017; Gadow & Drabick, 2012). Boys and girls seem equally likely to exhibit irritable ODD symptoms (Herzhoff & Tackett, 2016; Stringaris, Maughan, & Goodman, 2010). Across childhood and adolescence, irritable symptoms suggest a worse course of ODD. In a sample of 417 preschoolers who met criteria for ODD, irritability trajectories were either decreasing, increasing, or high persistent. High-persistent irritability predicted more comorbid diagnoses, greater difficulties with peers, and worse overall functioning (Ezpeleta et al., 2016). Similarly, in children with ODD, irritable symptoms, but not headstrong symptoms, are associated cross-sectionally with increased severity of internalizing symptoms and conduct problems (Aebi, Barra, et al., 2016; Drabick & Gadow, 2012). There is also evidence that the irritable dimension of ODD is related to suicidality and self-harm behaviors among adolescents (Aebi, Barra, et al., 2016; Muratori, Pisano, Milone, & Masi, 2017).

Recent investigations have identified relationships among risk factors for irritable and headstrong dimensions of ODD. Maternal depression and anxiety have been linked to ODD, especially irritable symptoms (Antúnez, de la Osa, Granero, & Ezpeleta, 2016; Whelan, Leibenluft, Stringaris, & Barker, 2015). Ineffective parenting behaviors, such a coerciveness, were found to be related to both irritable and headstrong symptoms, although the relationship was stronger for headstrong symptoms (Aebi, van Donkelaar, et al., 2016). In addition to parental considerations, peer factors also put individuals at risk. In a recent study of 706 school-age children, both irritable and headstrong symptoms were related to teacher-reported relational victimization and peer rejection. However, only irritability was associated with physical victimization (Evans, Pederson, Fite,

Blossom, & Cooley, 2016). Genetically, twin data show a stronger genetic correlation between irritability and internalizing disorders than between irritability and delinquency, a pattern that is reversed for headstrong symptoms (Mikolajewski, Taylor, & Iacono, 2017; Stringaris, Zavos, Leibenluft, Maughan, & Eley, 2012). In particular, genetics play a larger role in explaining the relationship between irritable symptoms and future depression than do nonshared environmental factors (Savage et al., 2015; Stringaris et al., 2012).

In sum, irritability and headstrong symptoms are distinct, though closely associated, dimensions of ODD with unique predictive validity. Work on the irritable aspect of ODD illuminates its affective nature, with clear prognostic implications.

DISRUPTIVE MOOD DYSREGULATION DISORDER

Disruptive mood dysregulation disorder (DMDD) occurs in about 1–3% of youth (Brotman et al., 2006; Copeland, Angold, Costello, & Egger, 2013) and is defined by chronic, severe irritability, explicitly incorporating both temper outbursts and irritable mood between outbursts. While DMDD is classified as a mood disorder and reviewed in Chapter 11, it is important to include here due to the overlap in symptoms, namely irritability, with ODD. According to DSM-5 rules, one cannot diagnosis comorbid ODD and DMDD because, if both are present, only DMDD can be diagnosed (APA, 2013). The framers of DMDD intended it to represent the top 15% of ODD in terms of irritability severity, consistent with investigations demonstrating that the two cannot be discriminated based on irritable symptoms alone (Mayes, Waxmonsky, Calhoun, & Bixler, 2016). Others have argued that DMDD should not be a free-standing diagnosis to represent chronic irritability, but ODD should have a specifier, *with chronic irritability* (Evans et al., 2017). In any case, both approaches emphasize the importance of denoting the presence of pathologic, severe, chronic irritability. However, the two ways of constructing these symptoms into mental disorders clearly emphasize different aspects of severe, chronic irritability. The construction of DMDD emphasizes that it is a form of affective psychopathology; the construction of ODD emphasizes its close associations with disruptive behavior. We do not take a position here. However, with regards to the aim of this chapter and consistent with associations between irritability and dimensions of disruptive behavior, it is important to note that clinically significant, disruptive behaviors, such as aggression, rule violations, and headstrong symptoms, are common in youth with DMDD (Axelson et al., 2012; Blader et al., 2016; Martin et al., 2017; Tufan et al., 2016).

ATTENTION DEFICIT HYPERACTIVITY DISORDER

ADHD occurs in about 5% of youth (Polanczyk, Willcutt, Salum, Kieling, & Rohde, 2014). Though not a defining feature of ADHD, irritability has long been recognized as common in youth with ADHD (Lange, Reichl, Lange, Tucha, &

Tucha, 2010; Pylypow, Quinn, Duncan, & Balbuena, 2017; Stringaris & Goodman, 2009b). Conversely, ADHD symptoms are common in youth with irritability (Wakschlag et al., 2015). To explain the association between ADHD and irritability, Shaw, Stringaris, Nigg, and Leibenluft (2014) postulate that ADHD-associated neural dysfunction impedes a child's ability to regulate his or her own emotions, thus leading to irritability.

Not only are there strong bidirectional associations between irritability and ADHD, but emerging evidence also suggests that an irritable subgroup may be recognizable in those with ADHD. Membership in this group may have important nosologic, treatment, and prognostic implications (Karalunas et al., 2014; Kircanski et al., 2017; Pylypow et al., 2017). Karalunas et al. (2014) used an empirical clustering method to find that 40% of $N = 247$ school-age youth with ADHD were defined by higher levels of irritability than the rest of the sample. Relative to the other two subgroups (minimal symptoms and impulsive/surgent), membership in the irritable ADHD subgroup was associated with increased physiologic reactivity, amygdala disconnectivity to prefrontal and insular cortex, and worse clinical outcomes at 1-year follow-up. Notably, this subgroup was more than twice as likely as the other two ADHD subgroups to develop a new DSM-5 disorder in the follow-up period. Two other studies provide some convergent evidence because they empirically detect irritable-ADHD subgroups in independent samples (Kircanski et al., 2017; Pylypow et al., 2017).

In sum, ADHD is a disruptive behavior disorder which is associated with irritability, but its clinical significance in the context of ADHD is an area of active investigation. For those with ADHD who experience clinically significant irritability, it may be an important indicator of more severe psychopathology.

CONDUCT DISORDER

CD is defined as a persistent pattern of violating the basic rights of others and violating social norms. This is manifested as aggression toward people and animals, destruction of property, deceitfulness or theft, or serious violation of rules. About 4% of children and adolescents have a diagnosis of CD (APA, 2013). It is a remarkably broad construct, capturing a wide group of individuals who engage in a variety of antisocial behaviors, with prognosis most closely linked to the severity of their symptoms (Burke, Loeber, & Birmaher, 2002; Loeber, Burke, Lahey, Winters, & Zera, 2000).

Two major features have been associated with a more severe course of CD: earlier age of onset and callous unemotional traits (Blair, Leibenluft, & Pine, 2014; Loeber et al., 2000). High callous-unemotional traits are indicated in youth with CD by the limited prosocial emotions specifier in DSM-5 (APA, 2013). Callous-unemotional traits are a major dimension of disruptive behavior (Frick, 1995), which, like irritability, is evident early in life and may have substantial clinical predictive power (Wakschlag et al., 2017). Callous-unemotional traits consist of a lack of empathy, disregard for the rights of others, lack of remorse or guilt, shallow and/or deficient affect, and lack of concern about performance (academically and in relations with peer and family) (Frick, 1995; White & Frick, 2010). Unlike irritability in ADHD and ODD, investigations of irritability in children and adolescents with CD, with or without callous-unemotional traits, have yet to be done.

Treatment

Promising pharmacological and psychological treatments for irritability have arisen from prior work on disruptive and affective behavioral disorders. Transdiagnostic treatment approaches to irritability are covered in Chapters 12 and 13. Here, we focus on a few nuances related to disruptive behavioral disorders.

Of psychopharmacologic treatments, only two enjoy US Food and Drug Administration approval for child or adolescent irritability: risperidone and aripiprazole. These are approved for irritability in the context of an autism spectrum disorder only. Two other dopamine antagonists, chlorpromazine and haloperidol, also have approval in children for emergency treatment of "severe disruptive behavior." However, our understanding of the effects of antipsychotics on irritability in the context of disruptive behavioral disorders is limited because randomized controlled trials of antipsychotics targeting irritability as the primary outcome measure have yet to be done (Loy, Merry, Hetrick, & Stasiak, 2012; van Schalkwyk et al., 2017). A major clinical concern with antipsychotics is their low tolerability and risk of long-term metabolic and motor side effects.

Stimulants are the most promising pharmacologic option to treat irritability in the context of disruptive behaviors. These were noted to reduce reactive aggression and disruptive behavior in youth with ADHD during the landmark Multimodal Treatment of ADHD (MTA) study (Jensen, 1999; Molina et al., 2009). Secondary analysis of the MTA demonstrates that stimulants improved irritability (medium effect, *Cohen's d* =.63) more than did behavioral management (small effect, $d = 0.42$), although a combination stimulant/behavioral treatment was superior to either alone (large effect, $d = 0.82$) (de la Cruz et al., 2015). These results are consistent with a number of studies demonstrating that stimulants such as methylphenidate reduce aggression (Klein et al., 1997; Pappadopulos et al., 2006). This has typically been seen in the context of treatment studies of ADHD, which also demonstrate the often observed clinically problematic phenomenon of "drop off," where rebound irritability is encountered during stimulant withdrawal (Jensen et al., 1999; Sinzig et al., 2007; Waschbusch, Carrey, Willoughby, King, & Andrade, 2007).

Several psychotherapies have some preliminary evidence of improving irritability or DMDD symptoms, which, like disruptive behaviors, are associated with emotion dysregulation. Dialectical behavior therapy (DBT) was originally developed as a treatment for emotion dysregulation for individuals with borderline personality disorder, but it has also been effective at treating a number of conditions for which emotional dysregulation is a prominent feature (Linehan et al., 2002; Lynch, Morse, Mendelson, & Robins, 2003; Neacsiu, Eberle, Kramer, Wiesmann, & Linehan, 2014). A recently reported, randomized clinical trial of DBT to treat DMDD showed greater symptom improvement in the DBT group than the treatment as usual (TAU) group in the primary outcome measure, the Clinical Global Impression Scales (CGI-I) (Perepletchikova et al., 2017). CGI-I positive response was 19 of 21 in the DBT group and 10 of 22 in the TAU group (p = .002). Another novel therapy for DMDD also targets emotion dysregulation through interpersonal therapy (IPT-MBD). In a preliminary randomized trial, it resulted in CGI-I (p = .04) rated improvement in DMDD for those in IPT-MBD (n = 10) versus TAU (n = 9) (Miller et al., 2018). Finally, in youth with ADHD and severe mood dysregulation (a research precursor to DMDD), there is preliminary evidence that children in a group-based therapy targeting emotion dysregulation (AIM; n = 31) had transient improvement in parent-reported irritability symptoms versus community care (n = 25) (Waxmonsky et al., 2016).

An investigational psychological treatment specifically targeting emotion dysregulation, family function, and multiple social information processing biases related to reactive aggression is underway (Sukhodolsky, Smith, McCauley, Ibrahim, & Piasecka, 2016). This intervention combines promising practices in cognitive behavioral therapy and parent management training to specifically target primary outcomes measures of aggression and disruptive behavior (NCT 01965184). However, the authors propose that this intervention may also reduce irritability because it targets mechanisms (which we reviewed earlier) that likely contribute to both pathologic irritability and aggression (Sukhodolsky et al., 2016).

A third psychotherapy under study has a greater mechanistic focus, employing reinforcement learning techniques such as exposure to target frustration sensitivity in irritable youth (Kircanski, Clayton, Leibenluft, & Brotman, 2018). The narrower focus allows a complementary computational modeling imaging protocol to test specific neural mechanisms (Brotman et al., 2017).

Finally, two cognitive retraining methods are being investigated for the treatment of irritability. These involve computer-assisted rote training to correct maladaptive cognitive biases. Both target social information processing biases reviewed in the aggression section earlier. The first targets hostile interpretation bias, or the tendency to judge ambiguous social cues as having hostile intent (Stoddard et al., 2016). The second targets an attentional bias that favors encoding threatening facial cues (NCT03238118).

Conclusion

Irritability is a key component of disruptive behavior disorders, along with headstrong behaviors and aggression. While these components commonly co-occur in youth with disruptive behavioral disorders, they are important to differentiate because they are related to different outcomes. For example, irritability is associated with a more severe course and worse prognosis in children diagnosed with ADHD or ODD. Promising mechanism-based treatments for irritability in youth with disruptive behavioral disorders incorporate lessons from affective disorder treatments and those targeting social information processing for aggression.

At this point, the irritable dimension of disruptive behavioral disorders has been well established. However, there is much more work needed to establish the predictive utility of irritability and its moderators for both scientific and clinical use. Future work will certainly require optimized, robust measures of irritability; seek to identify associations with the largest magnitude; and incorporate biological measures. As exemplified by the MAPS study, this requires measurement development and prospective longitudinal design.

References

Achenbach, T. M., & Rescorla, L. A. (2014). The Achenbach system of empirically based assessment (ASEBA) for ages 1.5 to 18 years. In Maruish, M. E. (Ed.), *The use of psychological testing for treatment planning and outcomes assessment, 2* (pp. 179–213). New York: Routledge.

Adleman, N. E., Kayser, R., Dickstein, D., Blair, R. J., Pine, D., & Leibenluft, E. (2011). Neural correlates of reversal learning in severe mood dysregulation and pediatric bipolar disorder. *Journal of the American Academy of Child and Adolescent Psychiatry, 50*(11), 1173–1185.

Aebi, M., Barra, S., Bessler, C., Steinhausen, H. C., Walitza, S., & Plattner, B. (2016). Oppositional defiant disorder dimensions and subtypes among detained male adolescent offenders. *Journal of Child Psychology and Psychiatry, 57*(6), 729–736.

Aebi, M., van Donkelaar, M. M., Poelmans, G., Buitelaar, J. K., Sonuga-Barke, E. J., Stringaris, A., . . . van Hulzen, K. J. (2016). Gene-set and multivariate genome-wide association analysis of oppositional defiant behavior subtypes in attention-deficit/hyperactivity disorder. *American Journal of Medical Genetics Part B: Neuropsychiatric Genetics, 171*(5), 573–588.

Angold, A., Costello, E. J., & Erkanli, A. (1999). Comorbidity. *Journal of Child Psychology and Psychiatry, 40*(1), 57–87.

Antúnez, Z., de la Osa, N., Granero, R., & Ezpeleta, L. (2016). Parental psychopathology levels as a moderator of temperament and oppositional defiant disorder symptoms in preschoolers. *Journal of Child and Family Studies, 25*(10), 3124–3135.

American Psychiatric Association (APA). (2013). *Diagnostic and Statistical Manual of Mental Disorders* (5th edition). Washington, DC: American Psychiatric Association.

Augsburger, M., Dohrmann, K., Schauer, M., & Elbert, T. (2017). Relations between traumatic stress, dimensions of impulsivity, and reactive and appetitive aggression in individuals with refugee status. *Psychological Trauma: Theory, Research, Practice and Policy, 9*(S1), 137–144.

Avenevoli, S., Blader, J. C., & Leibenluft, E. (2015). Irritability in youth: An update. *Journal of the American Academy of Child and Adolescent Psychiatry, 54*(11), 881–883.

Axelson, D., Findling, R. L., Fristad, M. A., Kowatch, R. A., Youngstrom, E. A., Horwitz, S. M., . . . Birmaher, B. (2012). Examining the proposed disruptive mood dysregulation disorder diagnosis in children in the Longitudinal Assessment of Manic Symptoms Study. *Journal of Clinical Psychiatry, 73*(10), 1342–1350.

Bandura, A. (1978). Social learning theory of aggression. *Journal of Communication, 28*(3), 12–29.

Berkowitz, L. (1989). Frustration-aggression hypothesis: Examination and reformulation. *Psychological Bulletin, 106*(1), 59–73.

Berkowitz, L. (1993). *Aggression: Its causes, consequences, and control*: New York: McGraw-Hill Book Company.

Bettencourt, B. A., Talley, A., Benjamin, A. J., & Valentine, J. (2006). Personality and aggressive behavior under provoking and neutral conditions: A meta-analytic review. *Psychological Bulletin, 132*(5), 751–777.

Blader, J. C., Pliszka, S. R., Kafantaris, V., Sauder, C., Posner, J., Foley, C. A., . . . Margulies, D. M. (2016). Prevalence and treatment outcomes of persistent negative mood among children with attention-deficit/hyperactivity disorder and aggressive behavior. *Journal of Child and Adolescent Psychopharmacology, 26*(2), 164–173.

Blair, R. J., Leibenluft, E., & Pine, D. S. (2014). Conduct disorder and callous-unemotional traits in youth. *New England Journal of Medicine, 371*(23), 2207–2216.

Bolhuis, K., Lubke, G. H., van der Ende, J., Bartels, M., van Beijsterveldt, C. E., Lichtenstein, P., . . . Verhulst, F. C. (2017). Disentangling heterogeneity of childhood disruptive behavior problems into dimensions and subgroups. *Journal of the American Academy of Child and Adolescent Psychiatry, 56*(6), 678–686.

Brotman, M. A., Kircanski, K., Stringaris, A., Pine, D. S., & Leibenluft, E. (2017). Irritability in youths: A translational model. *American Journal of Psychiatry*, appi-ajp.

Brotman, M. A., Schmajuk, M., Rich, B. A., Dickstein, D. P., Guyer, A. E., Costello, E. J., . . . Leibenluft, E. (2006). Prevalence, clinical correlates, and longitudinal course of severe mood dysregulation in children. *Biological Psychiatry, 60*(9), 991–997.

Burke, J. D., Boylan, K., Rowe, R., Duku, E., Stepp, S. D., Hipwell, A. E., & Waldman, I. D. (2014). Identifying the irritability dimension of ODD: Application of a modified bifactor model across five large community samples of children. *Journal of Abnormal Psychology, 123*(4), 841.

Burke, J. D., Hipwell, A. E., & Loeber, R. (2010). Dimensions of oppositional defiant disorder as predictors of depression and conduct disorder in preadolescent girls. *Journal of the American Academy of Child and Adolescent Psychiatry, 49*(5), 484–492.

Burke, J. D., Loeber, R., & Birmaher, B. (2002). Oppositional defiant disorder and conduct disorder: A review of the past 10 years, part II. *Journal of the American Academy of Child and Adolescent Psychiatry, 41*(11), 1275–1293.

Buss, A. H., & Durkee, A. (1957). An inventory for assessing different kinds of hostility. *Journal of Consulting Psychology, 21*(4), 343–349.

Camodeca, M., & Goossens, F. A. (2005). Aggression, social cognitions, anger and sadness in bullies and victims. *Journal of Child Psychology and Psychiatry, 46*(2), 186–197.

Caprara, G. V., Cinanni, V., D'Imperio, G., Passerini, S., Renzi, P., & Travaglia, G. (1985). Indicators of impulsive aggression: Present status of research on irritability and emotional susceptibility scales. *Personality and Individual Differences, 6*(6), 665–674.

Card, N. A., & Little, T. D. (2006). Proactive and reactive aggression in childhood and adolescence: A meta-analysis of differential relations with psychosocial adjustment. *International Journal of Behavioral Development, 30*(5), 466–480.

Copeland, W. E., Angold, A., Costello, E. J., & Egger, H. (2013). Prevalence, comorbidity, and correlates of DSM-5 proposed disruptive mood dysregulation disorder. *American Journal of Psychiatry, 170*(2), 173–179.

Copeland, W. E., Brotman, M. A., & Costello, E. J. (2015). Normative irritability in youth: Developmental findings from the Great Smoky Mountains Study. *Journal of the American Academy of Child and Adolescent Psychiatry, 54*(8), 635–642.

Craig, A. A., & Brad, J. B. (2001). Effects of violent video games on aggressive behavior, aggressive cognition, aggressive affect, physiological arousal, and prosocial behavior: A meta-analytic review of the scientific literature. *Psychological Science, 12*(5), 353–359.

Crick, N. R., & Dodge, K. A. (1994). A review and reformulation of social information-processing mechanisms in children's social adjustment. *Psychological Bulletin, 115*(1), 74–101.

de la Cruz, L. F., Simonoff, E., McGough, J. J., Halperin, J. M., Arnold, L. E., & Stringaris, A. (2015). Treatment of children with attention-deficit/hyperactivity disorder (ADHD) and irritability: Results from the Multimodal Treatment Study of Children with ADHD (MTA). *Journal of the American Academy of Child and Adolescent Psychiatry, 54*(1), 62–70.

Dickstein, D. P., Nelson, E. E., McClure, E. B., Grimley, M. E., Knopf, L., Brotman, M. A., . . . Leibenluft, E. (2007). Cognitive flexibility in phenotypes of pediatric bipolar disorder. *Journal of the American Academy of Child and Adolescent Psychiatry, 46*(3), 341–355.

Dodge, K. A. (1980). Social cognition and children's aggressive behavior. *Child Development, 51*(1), 162–170.

Dodge, K. A., Lochman, J. E., Harnish, J. D., Bates, J. E., & Pettit, G. S. (1997). Reactive and proactive aggression in school children and psychiatrically impaired chronically assaultive youth. *Journal of Abnormal Psychology, 106*(1), 37–51.

Dollard, J., Miller, N. E., Doob, L. W., Mowrer, O. H., & Sears, R. R. (1939). *Frustration and Aggression*: New Haven, CT: Yale University Press.

Dougherty, L. R., Smith, V. C., Bufferd, S. J., Stringaris, A., Leibenluft, E., Carlson, G. A., & Klein, D. N. (2013). Preschool irritability: Longitudinal associations with psychiatric disorders at age 6 and parental psychopathology. *Journal of the American Academy of Child and Adolescent Psychiatry, 52*(12), 1304–1313.

Drabick, D. A., & Gadow, K. D. (2012). Deconstructing oppositional defiant disorder: Clinic-based evidence for an anger/irritability phenotype. *Journal of the American Academy of Child and Adolescent Psychiatry, 51*(4), 384–393.

Evans, S. C., Burke, J. D., Roberts, M. C., Fite, P. J., Lochman, J. E., de la Peña, F. R., & Reed, G. M. (2017). Irritability in child and adolescent psychopathology: An integrative review for ICD-11. *Clinical Psychology Review, 53*, 29–45.

Evans, S. C., Pederson, C. A., Fite, P. J., Blossom, J. B., & Cooley, J. L. (2016). Teacher-reported irritable and defiant dimensions of oppositional defiant disorder: Social, behavioral, and academic correlates. *School Mental Health, 8*(2), 292–304.

Ezpeleta, L., Granero, R., de la Osa, N., Trepat, E., & Domènech, J. M. (2016). Trajectories of oppositional defiant disorder irritability symptoms in preschool children. *Journal of Abnormal Child Psychology, 44*(1), 115–128.

Fite, P. J., Raine, A., Stouthamer-Loeber, M., Loeber, R., & Pardini, D. A. (2009). Reactive and proactive aggression in adolescent males: Examining differential outcomes 10 years later in early adulthood. *Criminal Justice and Behavior, 37*(2), 141–157.

Frick, P. J. (1995). Callous-unemotional traits and conduct problems: A two-factor model of psychopathy in children. *Issues in Criminological and Legal Psychology, 24,* 47–51.

Gadow, K. D., & Drabick, D. A. (2012). Anger and irritability symptoms among youth with ODD: Cross-informant versus source-exclusive syndromes. *Journal of abnormal child psychology, 40*(7), 1073–1085.

Harvey, E. A., Breaux, R. P., & Lugo-Candelas, C. I. (2016). Early development of comorbidity between symptoms of attention-deficit/hyperactivity disorder (ADHD) and oppositional defiant disorder (ODD). *Journal of Abnormal Psychology, 125*(2), 154.

Herzhoff, K., & Tackett, J. L. (2016). Subfactors of oppositional defiant disorder: Converging evidence from structural and latent class analyses. *Journal of Child Psychology and Psychiatry, 57*(1), 18–29.

Hommer, R. E., Meyer, A., Stoddard, J., Connolly, M. E., Mogg, K., Bradley, B. P., . . . Brotman, M. A. (2013). Attention bias to threat faces in severe mood dysregulation. *Depression and Anxiety, 31*(7), 559–565.

Hwang, S., Kim, Y. S., Koh, Y. J., Bishop, S., & Leventhal, B. L. (2017). Discrepancy in perception of bullying experiences and later internalizing and externalizing behavior: A prospective study. *Aggressive Behavior, 43*(5), 493–502.

Jensen, P. S. (1999). A 14-month randomized clinical trial of treatment strategies for attention-deficit/hyperactivity disorder. *Archives General Psychiatry, 56*(12), 1073–1086.

Karalunas, S. L., Fair, D., Musser, E. D., Aykes, K., Iyer, S. P., & Nigg, J. T. (2014). Subtyping attention-deficit/hyperactivity disorder using temperament dimensions: Toward biologically based nosologic criteria. *JAMA Psychiatry, 71*(9), 1015–1024.

Kempes, M., Matthys, W., de Vries, H., & van Engeland, H. (2005). Reactive and proactive aggression in children: A review of theory, findings and the relevance for child and adolescent psychiatry. *European Child and Adolescent Psychiatry, 14*(1), 11–19.

Kircanski, K., Clayton, M. E., Leibenluft, E., & Brotman, M. A. (2018). Psychosocial treatment of irritability in youth. *Current Treatment Options in Psychiatry, 5*(1), 129–140.

Kircanski, K., Zhang, S., Stringaris, A., Wiggins, J. L., Towbin, K. E., Pine, D. S., . . . Brotman, M. A. (2017). Empirically derived patterns of psychiatric symptoms in youth: A latent profile analysis. *Journal of Affective Disorders, 216,* 109–116.

Klein, R. G., Abikoff, H., Klass, E., Ganeles, D., Seese, L. M., & Pollack, S. (1997). Clinical efficacy of methylphenidate in conduct disorder with and without attention deficit hyperactivity disorder. *Archives of General Psychiatry, 54*(12), 1073–1080.

Lange, K. W., Reichl, S., Lange, K. M., Tucha, L., & Tucha, O. (2010). The history of attention deficit hyperactivity disorder. *Attention Deficit and Hyperactivity Disorders, 2*(4), 241–255.

Lansford, J. E., Malone, P. S., Dodge, K. A., Pettit, G. S., & Bates, J. E. (2010). Developmental cascades of peer rejection, social information processing biases, and aggression during middle childhood. *Development and Psychopathology, 22*(3), 593–602.

Lavigne, J. V., Cicchetti, C., Gibbons, R. D., Binns, H. J., Larsen, L., & DeVito, C. (2001). Oppositional defiant disorder with onset in preschool years: Longitudinal stability and pathways to other disorders. *Journal of the American Academy of Child and Adolescent Psychiatry, 40*(12), 1393–1400.

Leibenluft, E. (2017). Pediatric irritability: A systems neuroscience approach. *Trends in Cognitive Science. 21*(4), 277–289.

Leibenluft, E., & Stoddard, J. (2013). The developmental psychopathology of irritability. *Development and Psychopathology, 25*(4pt2), 1473–1487.

Li, Y., Grabell, A. S., Wakschlag, L. S., Huppert, T. J., & Perlman, S. B. (2017). The neural substrates of cognitive flexibility are related to individual differences in preschool irritability: A fNIRS investigation. *Developmental Cognitive Neuroscience, 25*, 138–144.

Linehan, M. M., Dimeff, L. A., Reynolds, S. K., Comtois, K. A., Welch, S. S., Heagerty, P., & Kivlahan, D. R. (2002). Dialectical behavior therapy versus comprehensive validation therapy plus 12-step for the treatment of opioid dependent women meeting criteria for borderline personality disorder. *Drug and Alcohol Dependence, 67*(1), 13–26.

Loeber, R., Burke, J. D., Lahey, B. B., Winters, A., & Zera, M. (2000). Oppositional defiant and conduct disorder: A review of the past 10 years, part I. *Journal of the American Academy of Child and Adolescent Psychiatry, 39*(12), 1468–1484.

Loy, J. H., Merry, S. N., Hetrick, S. E., & Stasiak, K. (2012). Atypical antipsychotics for disruptive behaviour disorders in children and youths. *Cochrane Database Syst Rev, 9*, CD008559.

Lynch, T. R., Morse, J. Q., Mendelson, T., & Robins, C. J. (2003). Dialectical behavior therapy for depressed older adults: A randomized pilot study. *American Journal of Geriatric Psychiatry, 11*(1), 33–45.

Martin, S. E., Hunt, J. I., Mernick, L. R., DeMarco, M., Hunter, H. L., Coutinho, M. T., & Boekamp, J. R. (2017). Temper loss and persistent irritability in preschoolers: Implications for diagnosing disruptive mood dysregulation disorder in early childhood. *Child Psychiatry and Human Development, 48*(3), 498–508.

Mayes, S. D., Waxmonsky, J. D., Calhoun, S. L., & Bixler, E. O. (2016). Disruptive mood dysregulation disorder symptoms and association with oppositional defiant and other disorders in a general population child sample. *Journal of Child and Adolescent Psychopharmacology, 26*(2), 101–106.

Mikolajewski, A. J., Taylor, J., & Iacono, W. G. (2017). Oppositional defiant disorder dimensions: Genetic influences and risk for later psychopathology. *Journal of Child Psychology and Psychiatry, 58*(6), 702–710.

Miller, L., Hlastala, S. A., Mufson, L., Leibenluft, E., Yenokyan, G., & Riddle, M. (2018). Interpersonal psychotherapy for mood and behavior dysregulation: Pilot randomized trial. *Depression and Anxiety.* doi:10.1002/da.22761

Miller, N. E. (1941). The frustration-aggression hypothesis. *Psychological Review, 48*(4), 337–342.

Molina, B. S. G., Hinshaw, S. P., Swanson, J. M., Arnold, L. E., Vitiello, B., Jensen, P. S., . . . Houck, P. R. (2009). The MTA at 8 years: Prospective follow-up of children treated for combined-type ADHD in a multisite study. *Journal of the American Academy of Child and Adolescent Psychiatry, 48*(5), 484–500.

Muratori, P., Pisano, S., Milone, A., & Masi, G. (2017). Is emotional dysregulation a risk indicator for auto-aggression behaviors in adolescents with oppositional defiant disorder? *Journal of Affective Disorders, 208*, 110–112.

Neacsiu, A. D., Eberle, J. W., Kramer, R., Wiesmann, T., & Linehan, M. M. (2014). Dialectical behavior therapy skills for transdiagnostic emotion dysregulation: A pilot randomized controlled trial. *Behaviour Research and Therapy, 59*, 40–51.

Nock, M. K., Kazdin, A. E., Hiripi, E., & Kessler, R. C. (2007). Lifetime prevalence, correlates, and persistence of oppositional defiant disorder: Results from the National Comorbidity Survey Replication. *Journal Child Psychology and Psychiatry, 48*(7), 703–713.

Pappadopulos, E., Woolston, S., Chait, A., Perkins, M., Connor, D. F., & Jensen, P. S. (2006). Pharmacotherapy of aggression in children and adolescents: Efficacy and effect size. *Journal of the Canadian Academy of Child and Adolescent Psychiatry, 15*(1), 27–39.

Perepletchikova, F., Nathanson, D., Axelrod, S. R., Merrill, C., Walker, A., Grossman, M., . . . Flye, B. (2017). Randomized clinical trial of dialectical behavior therapy for preadolescent children with disruptive mood dysregulation disorder: Feasibility and outcomes. *Journal of the American Academy of Child and Adolescent Psychiatry, 56*(10), 832–840.

Polanczyk, G. V., Willcutt, E. G., Salum, G. A., Kieling, C., & Rohde, L. A. (2014). ADHD prevalence estimates across three decades: An updated systematic review and meta-regression analysis. *International Journal of Epidemiology, 43*(2), 434–442.

Pylypow, J., Quinn, D., Duncan, D., & Balbuena, L. (2017). A measure of emotional regulation and irritability in children and adolescents: The Clinical Evaluation of Emotional Regulation-9. *Journal of Attention Disorders.* https://doi.org/10.1177/1087054717737162

Raine, A., Dodge, K., Loeber, R., Gatzke-Kopp, L., Lynam, D., Reynolds, C., . . . Liu, J. (2006). The Reactive-Proactive Aggression Questionnaire: Differential correlates of reactive and proactive aggression in adolescent boys. *Aggressive Behavior, 32*(2), 159–171.

Rieffe, C., Broekhof, E., Kouwenberg, M., Faber, J., Tsutsui, M. M., & Guroglu, B. (2016). Disentangling proactive and reactive aggression in children using self-report. *European Journal of Developmental Psychology, 13*(4), 439–451.

Salum, G. A., Mogg, K., Bradley, B. P., Stringaris, A., Gadelha, A., Pan, P. M., . . . Pine, D. S. (2017). Association between irritability and bias in attention orienting to threat in children and adolescents. *Journal of Child Psychology and Psychiatry, 58*(5), 595–602.

Savage, J., Verhulst, B., Copeland, W., Althoff, R. R., Lichtenstein, P., & Roberson-Nay, R. (2015). A genetically informed study of the longitudinal relation between irritability and anxious/depressed symptoms. *Journal of the American Academy of Child and Adolescent Psychiatry, 54*(5), 377–384.

Shaw, P., Stringaris, A., Nigg, J., & Leibenluft, E. (2014). Emotion dysregulation in attention deficit hyperactivity disorder. *American Journal Psychiatry, 171*(3), 276–293.

Sinzig, J., Dopfner, M., Lehmkuhl, G., Uebel, H., Schmeck, K., Poustka, F., . . . Fischer, R. (2007). Long-acting methylphenidate has an effect on aggressive behavior in children with attention-deficit/hyperactivity disorder. *Journal of Child and Adolescent Psychopharmacology, 17*(4), 421–432.

Stoddard, J., Sharif-Askary, B., Harkins, E. A., Frank, H. R., Brotman, M. A., Penton-Voak, I. S., . . . Leibenluft, E. (2016). An open pilot study of training hostile interpretation bias to treat disruptive mood dysregulation disorder. *Journal of Child and Adolescent Psychopharmacology, 26*(1), 49–57.

Stringaris, A., & Goodman, R. (2009a). Longitudinal outcome of youth oppositionality: Irritable, headstrong, and hurtful behaviors have distinctive predictions. *Journal of the American Academy of Child and Adolescent Psychiatry, 48*(4), 404–412.

Stringaris, A., & Goodman, R. (2009b). Mood lability and psychopathology in youth. *Psychological Medicine, 39*(8), 1237–1245.

Stringaris, A., Maughan, B., & Goodman, R. (2010). What's in a disruptive disorder? Temperamental antecedents of oppositional defiant disorder: Findings from the Avon longitudinal study. *Journal of the American Academy of Child and Adolescent Psychiatry, 49*(5), 474–483.

Stringaris, A., Zavos, H., Leibenluft, E., Maughan, B., & Eley, T. C. (2012). Adolescent irritability: Phenotypic associations and genetic links with depressed mood. *American Journal of Psychiatry, 169*(1), 47–54.

Sukhodolsky, D. G., Smith, S. D., McCauley, S. A., Ibrahim, K., & Piasecka, J. B. (2016). Behavioral interventions for anger, irritability, and aggression in children and adolescents. *Journal of Child and Adolescent Psychopharmacology, 26*(1), 58–64.

Tremblay, R. E. (2010). Developmental origins of disruptive behaviour problems: The "original sin" hypothesis, epigenetics and their consequences for prevention. *Journal of Child Psychology and Psychiatry, 51*(4), 341–367.

Tufan, E., Topal, Z., Demir, N., Taskiran, S., Savci, U., Cansiz, M. A., & Semerci, B. (2016). Sociodemographic and clinical features of disruptive mood dysregulation disorder: A chart review. *Journal of Child and Adolescent Psychopharmacology, 26*(2), 94–100.

Van Meter, A., Youngstrom, E., Freeman, A., Feeny, N., Youngstrom, J. K., & Findling, R. L. (2016). Impact of irritability and impulsive aggressive behavior on impairment and social functioning in youth with cyclothymic disorder. *Journal of Child and Adolescent Psychopharmacology, 26*(1), 26–37.

van Reemst, L., Fischer, T. F., & Zwirs, B. W. (2016). Social information processing mechanisms and victimization: A literature review. *Trauma, Violence, and Abuse, 17*(1), 3–25.

van Schalkwyk, G. I., Lewis, A. S., Beyer, C., Johnson, J., van Rensburg, S., & Bloch, M. H. (2017). Efficacy of antipsychotics for irritability and aggression in children: A meta-analysis. *Expert Rev Neurother, 17*(10), 1045–1053.

Vitaro, F., Barker, E. D., Boivin, M., Brendgen, M., & Tremblay, R. E. (2006). Do early difficult temperament and harsh parenting differentially predict reactive and proactive aggression? *Journal of Abnormal Child Psychology, 34*(5), 681–691.

Wakschlag, L. S., Choi, S. W., Carter, A. S., Hullsiek, H., Burns, J., McCarthy, K., . . . Briggs-Gowan, M. J. (2012). Defining the developmental parameters of temper loss in early childhood: Implications for developmental psychopathology. *Journal of Child Psychology and Psychiatry, 53*(11), 1099–1108.

Wakschlag, L. S., Estabrook, R., Petitclerc, A., Henry, D., Burns, J. L., Perlman, S. B., . . . Briggs-Gowan, M. L. (2015). Clinical implications of a dimensional approach: The normal-abnormal spectrum of early irritability. *Journal of the American Academy of Child and Adolescent Psychiatry, 54*(8), 626–634.

Wakschlag, L. S., Henry, D. B., Tolan, P. H., Carter, A. S., Burns, J. L., & Briggs-Gowan, M. J. (2012). Putting theory to the test: Modeling a multidimensional, developmentally-based approach to preschool disruptive behavior. *Journal of the American Academy of Child and Adolescent Psychiatry, 51*(6), 593–604.

Wakschlag, L. S., Perlman, S. B., Blair, R. J., Leibenluft, E., Briggs-Gowan, M. J., & Pine, D. S. (2017). The neurodevelopmental basis of early childhood disruptive behavior: Irritable and callous phenotypes as exemplars. *American Journal of Psychiatry, 175*(2), 114–130.

Waschbusch, D. A., Carrey, N. J., Willoughby, M. T., King, S., & Andrade, B. F. (2007). Effects of methylphenidate and behavior modification on the social and academic behavior of children with disruptive behavior disorders: The moderating role of callous/ unemotional traits. *Journal of Clinical Child and Adolescent Psychology, 36*(4), 629–644.

Waschbusch, D. A., Pelham, W. E., Jennings, J. R., Greiner, A. R., Tarter, R. E., & Moss, H. B. (2002). Reactive aggression in boys with disruptive behavior disorders: Behavior, physiology, and affect. *Journal of Abnormal Child Psychology, 30*(6), 641–656.

Waschbusch, D. A., Porter, S., Carrey, N., Kazmi, S. O., Roach, K. A., & D'Amico, D. A. (2004). Investigation of the heterogeneity of disruptive behaviour in elementary-age children. *Canadian Journal of Behavioural Science/Revue Canadienne des Sciences du Comportement, 36*(2), 97.

Waxmonsky, J. G., Waschbusch, D. A., Belin, P., Li, T., Babocsai, L., Humphery, H., . . . Mazzant, J. R. (2016). A randomized clinical trial of an integrative group therapy for children with severe mood dysregulation. *Journal of the American Academy of Child and Adolescent Psychiatry, 55*(3), 196–207.

Whelan, Y. M., Leibenluft, E., Stringaris, A., & Barker, E. D. (2015). Pathways from maternal depressive symptoms to adolescent depressive symptoms: The unique contribution of irritability symptoms. *Journal of Child Psychology and Psychiatry, 56*(10), 1092–1100.

White, S. F., & Frick, P. J. (2010). Callous-unemotional traits and their importance to causal models of severe antisocial behavior in youth. In R. T. Salekin & D. R. Lynam (Eds.), *Handbook of child and adolescent psychopathy* (pp. 135–155). New York: Guilford.

Wiggins, J. L., Briggs-Gowan, M. J., Estabrook, R., Brotman, M. A., Pine, D. S., Leibenluft, E., & Wakschlag, L. S. (2018). Identifying clinically significant irritability in early childhood. *Journal of the American Academy of Child and Adolescent Psychiatry, 57*(3), 191–199.

Wiggins, J. L., Mitchell, C., Stringaris, A., & Leibenluft, E. (2014). Developmental trajectories of irritability and bidirectional associations with maternal depression. *Journal of the American Academy of Child and Adolescent Psychiatry, 53*(11), 1191–1205.

Xu, Y., Farver, J. A. M., & Zhang, Z. (2009). Temperament, harsh and indulgent parenting, and Chinese children's proactive and reactive aggression. *Child Development, 80*(1), 244–258.

Ziv, Y. (2012). Exposure to violence, social information processing, and problem behavior in preschool children. *Aggressive Behavior, 38*(6), 429–441.

11

Irritability in Pediatric Psychopathology

AUTISM

Carla A. Mazefsky, Taylor N. Day, and Joshua Golt

Autism spectrum disorder (ASD) is defined based on the presence of differences in social interaction and communicative behaviors together with the presence of restrictive and repetitive behaviors (DSM-5; American Psychiatric Association [APA], 2013). At present, ASD can be reliably diagnosed by 18–24 months of age based on behavioral markers, despite significant heterogeneity in the phenotypic expression (Zwaigenbaum et al., 2015). The causes of ASD are largely unknown, although it is theorized that ASD results from an interaction between genetic and environmental factors (Goldani, Downs, Widjaja, Lawton, & Hendren, 2014).

ASD is often referred to as a "systems disorder" because it is rare that an individual with ASD does not have co-occurring medical and mental health disorders that extend beyond the diagnostic criteria. Irritability is one concern that is commonly associated with ASD, often warranting specific treatment (McGuire et al., 2016). In fact, as many as two-thirds of children seen in research clinics for youth with severe irritability and mood disorders, but without diagnosed ASD, exceed cutoffs indicative of ASD on at least one ASD screening questionnaire, and 8% exceed cutoffs across three questionnaires (Towbin, Pradella, Gorrindo, Pine, & Leibenluft, 2005). This suggests that irritability may even overshadow an underlying ASD diagnosis in verbal youth. Diagnostic overshadowing may be explained by findings that levels of irritability in high-functioning boys with ASD are comparable to boys identified with severe mood dysregulation who do not have ASD (Mikita et al., 2015). While one study found that irritability was present at a moderate degree or greater in at least 80% of youth with ASD (Mayes, Calhoun, Murray, Ahuja, & Smith, 2011), the exact prevalence of irritability in ASD is difficult to pinpoint, in part due to how it has been defined within ASD research.

Pure definitions of irritability emphasize mood disturbance characterized by persistent angry negative affect and outbursts or tantrums. While irritability may be a risk factor for problem behavior or mood disorders, irritability does not necessarily result in these additional problems (Leibenluft, 2011). In ASD, however, most studies of irritability have applied the term to capture presentations characterized by severe behavioral disturbance (Mikita et al., 2015). In fact, a recent practice pathway for irritability and problem behavior described them as "interchangeable" (McGuire et al., 2016). Furthermore, the majority of irritability studies in ASD have focused on psychopharmacological treatment of agitation in association with severe problem behaviors, such as aggression or self-injury.

Two lines of research in ASD that have a greater emphasis on emotional and mood disturbances may shed light on our understanding of irritability in ASD. First, irritability/frustration is included as one of two forms of negative affect in Rothbart and Bates's (1998) temperament model, and several studies have investigated early temperament profiles of youth with or at-risk for ASD. Second, irritability may reflect higher emotional reactivity and difficulty regulating emotional responses, referred to as impaired emotion regulation. The role of emotion regulation in ASD is now widely appreciated, and this growing body of research provides some insights into the common presence of high and chronic irritability in ASD (Mazefsky et al., 2013). Here, research on temperament and emotion regulation in ASD is discussed, with an emphasis on the developmental course of and risk factors for irritability specific to ASD, followed by a discussion of existing assessment and treatment options for irritability in ASD.

Developmental Course of Irritability in ASD

Children at high genetic risk for ASD (i.e., younger siblings of children diagnosed with ASD) demonstrate greater negative affect than control subjects without genetic risk for ASD at 12 and 24 months of age based on parent-report temperament measures (Garon et al., 2016). The presence of negative affect at 12 months positively predicted (1) increased negative affect and (2) decreased effortful control (i.e., emotion regulation) at 24 months. The latter pathway (2) predicted more ASD symptoms at 36 months of age in high-risk children only (Garon et al., 2016). Parental perceptions of negative emotionality and effortful control also differentiate toddlers diagnosed with ASD from typically developing toddlers (Macari, Koller, Campbell, & Chawarska, 2017). These findings suggest that irritability is often present before the full manifestation of ASD symptoms and may be an early indicator of ASD risk, consistent with Bryson et al.'s (2007) conclusions from a small series of case studies that found the emergence of ASD symptoms either preceded or coincided with irritability, emotional and behavioral regulation difficulties, and rigid behavior (e.g., disliking change).

By the preschool and school-age years, there are no longer group-level differences (ASD vs. typically developing peers) in negative affectivity based on behavioral observations (Jahromi, Meek, & Ober-Reynolds, 2012) or parent report on temperament measures (Konstantareas & Stewart, 2006). However, children with ASD continue to demonstrate differences in emotion regulation. For example, children with ASD demonstrate fewer adaptive emotion regulation strategies during frustrating tasks than do controls, and they often resign from the task or suppress frustration to control their emotional arousal (Jahromi et al., 2012; Konstantareas & Stewart, 2006; Samson, Hardan, Podell, Phillips, & Gross, 2015). This suggests that while children with ASD may not differ in their negative *reactions* from typically developing children, they employ more maladaptive regulation strategies to reduce their irritability and frustration. These findings from early childhood are consistent with a rapidly growing body of research that indicates a reliance on maladaptive or ineffective emotion regulation strategies in ASD across childhood and into adulthood (see Weiss, Riosa, Mazefsky, & Beaumont, 2017, for review). Therefore, impaired emotion regulation is one likely pathway contributing to the high occurrence of irritability in ASD.

ASD-Related Risk for Irritability

The prominence of irritability in ASD, starting early in development, has raised questions about how irritability is related to the ASD phenotype. Although studies suggest that negative emotionality and poor emotional control are independent of ASD symptoms (e.g., not merely a proxy for greater ASD severity; Macari et al., 2017), patterns of psychotropic medication prescriptions to target mood suggest that irritability is often conceptualized as related to the primary ASD diagnosis. For example, based on a recent large-scale study of youth with and without ASD, 17.83% of children with ASD are prescribed antidepressants and 9.07% are on mood stabilizers, compared to less than 2% of children without ASD for antidepressants and mood stabilizers combined (Madden et al., 2017). Interestingly, 79.4% of the ASD sample prescribed antidepressants did not have a diagnosed depression or anxiety disorder (Madden et al., 2017), suggesting that internalizing symptoms are likely conceptualized as related to ASD in these cases and do not rise to a level above and beyond the core deficits of ASD (Mazefsky et al., 2013). The pattern was similar for antipsychotic use, such that youth with ASD were markedly more likely to receive antipsychotics without a psychosis or disruptive mood disorder diagnosis compared to children without ASD, with an odds ratio of 59.40 (Madden et al., 2017). Although this may be explained by US Food and Drug Administration (FDA) approval of antipsychotics to treat irritability in ASD, it nonetheless suggests that prescribers are not conceptualizing the irritability as due to a co-occurring disorder (Madden et al., 2017; Marcus et al., 2009, McCracken et al., 2002).

Several ASD characteristics have been theorized to increase emotional reactivity and interfere with effective emotion regulation, thereby leading to irritability (see Mazefsky & White, 2014, for review). Some of the potential pathways are summarized in Figure 11.1. For example, a child may experience distress and physiological arousal due to a sensory stimulus in the environment that is perceived as aversive, have difficulty accurately identifying and communicating those feelings to others to request help, and then have poor problem-solving, resulting in escalating irritability. As an alternative example, a verbal adolescent may attempt to initiate with a peer, misperceive the peer's social cues or experience rejection, feel hostile or agitated, and then perseverate on the incident so that the irritability persists.

A recent study found that, of the core ASD symptoms, restricted and repetitive behaviors were most predictive of emotion dysregulation cross-sectionally (Samson et al., 2014). Causation cannot be assumed, however, and there are many potential explanations for the association between restricted behavior and irritability. It is conceivable that a child who is more irritable may engage in restricted and repetitive behaviors as a coping mechanism. On the other hand, cognitive inflexibility, a well-documented and common manifestation of repetitive behavior in ASD, may interfere with the modulation of negative emotions (White et al., 2014). For example, children with ASD may have difficulty recognizing that a solution is ineffective and that alternate strategies are needed, which can result in heightened irritability.

Although there has been little direct research on the biological factors that may increase risk for irritability in ASD, evidence from related fields of inquiry suggests that youth with ASD may be biologically predisposed to irritability. First, several studies have documented that parents and siblings of youth with ASD have substantially higher rates of mood disorders than the general population and families of children with other developmental disorders (Bolton, Pickles, Murphy, & Rutter, 1998; Mezzacappa et al., 2017; Piven et al., 1990; Smalley, McCracken, & Tanguay, 1995). Importantly, these studies found that the majority of parental mood disorders onset prior to the birth of the child with ASD. Furthermore, like

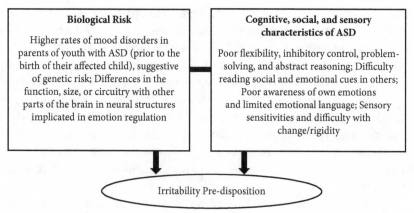

FIGURE 11.1 *Illustrative examples of autism spectrum disorder (ASD)-related risk factors for irritability.*

non-ASD populations, children with ASD who have a parent with a mood disorder history are more likely to have a mood disorder diagnosis themselves (Mazefsky, Folstein, & Lainhart, 2008). Finally, genome-wide studies support shared genetic contributions between ASD and bipolar disorder (Group of the Psychiatric Genomics Consortium, 2013). Likewise, there appears to be overlap between brain regions implicated in irritability (Vidal-Ribas, Brotman, Valdivieso, Leibenluft, & Stringaris, 2016) and ASD (Mazefsky et al., 2013) that may suggest some shared underlying risk. For example, substantial evidence indicates altered connectivity as a neural mechanism underlying ASD (Minshew & Williams, 2007), and a recent study found that altered amygdala-prefrontal cortex connectivity in youth with ASD was correlated with higher irritability (Kiefer et al., 2017), consistent with neural models of irritably outside of ASD (Leibenluft, 2017).

IRRITABILITY AND PSYCHIATRIC COMORBIDITY WITHIN ASD

Although irritability is often conceptualized as related to the ASD phenotype, youth with ASD are also significantly more likely to receive co-occurring psychiatric diagnoses characterized by high irritability. Using a structured psychiatric interview not specific to ASD, 56% of youth with ASD met DSM-IV criteria for major depressive disorder (MDD), 31% met criteria for bipolar disorder, and 73% met criteria for oppositional defiant disorder (ODD) (Joshi et al., 2010), all of which incorporate irritability as a core symptom (APA, 2000). However, considerably lower rates were found using an ASD-specific structured psychiatric interview that systematically takes ASD-related impairment into account (the Autism Comorbidity Interview [ACI]), including 10% for MDD, 3% for bipolar disorder, and 7% for ODD (Leyfer et al., 2006). This discrepancy is consistent with a study by Mazefsky et al. (2012), which found that approximately 60% of community-based diagnoses were not supported when assessed with the ACI. For example, in that modest sample, 14.3% of children with ASD were diagnosed with bipolar disorder by a community provider, but none of these diagnoses was supported by the ACI despite the presence of irritability (Mazefsky et al., 2012).

While irritability is more common than the other traditional symptoms of depression and anxiety in ASD (Mayes et al., 2011), irritability, along with labile mood, agitation, and aggression, frequently presents as part of the atypical manifestation of depression in youth with ASD (Magnuson & Constantino, 2011). Likewise, there is a link between anxiety and irritability in ASD, such that emotion dysregulation manifesting as irritability serves as a proximal risk factor for the development of anxious behavior (White et al., 2014). Overall, these findings suggest that irritability may influence the diagnosis of psychiatric disorders in ASD and that mood and behavioral disorders characterized by irritability are quite common in ASD. However, the frequent conceptualization of irritability as suggestive of a comorbid disorder may be an oversimplification and even at times lead to misdiagnosis.

The inconsistencies of psychiatric comorbidity rates and potential misdiagnoses may arise due to the complexity of differentiating irritability that may be related to the ASD phenotype from an additional comorbid disorder. Through an initiative of Autism Speaks, McGuire et al. (2016) developed a pathway for the evaluation and treatment of irritability and related behavioral problems in primary care settings. They argue that to attribute irritability to a psychiatric disorder other than ASD, it is essential to look for an acute onset or a worsening of severity (McGuire et al., 2016). Furthermore, although mood disorders may include atypical presentations in ASD (e.g., Magnuson & Constantino, 2011), it remains important to ensure that the primary defining characteristics of the comorbid disorder being considered are present. For example, although youth with ASD often present with greater irritability prior to diagnosis of bipolar disorder than their non-ASD peers, youth with ASD and rigorously confirmed bipolar disorder have symptom profiles like their non-ASD peers with bipolar disorder (Borue et al., 2016).

The differential diagnosis of ASD-related irritability and disruptive mood dysregulation disorder (DMDD) may be especially complex, with far less research to provide guidance given the relative infancy of this diagnostic category (APA, 2013). McGuire and colleagues (2016) state that DMDD should "rarely, if ever, be diagnosed in patients with ASD," because DSM-5 specifies that DMDD should not be diagnosed if core symptoms (irritability and severe temper outbursts) could be better explained by ASD. Mayes et al. (2017) found that the percentage of DMDD symptoms is high (i.e., 45%) in individuals with ASD, and the prevalence is very stable from preschool to adolescence. They posit that DMDD symptoms may emerge as a consequence of the core and chronic symptoms of ASD (Mayes et al., 2017), while others provide preliminary support for DMDD as a comorbidity of ASD (Pan & Yeh, 2016). Further complicating differential diagnosis, youth with severe mood disorders and irritability present with more ASD symptoms than do healthy youth (Pine et al., 2008; Towbin et al., 2005). Clearly, more research is needed on the intersection of ASD and DMDD to better understand its co-occurrence and how to best define the boundaries between the two disorders.

Assessment of Irritability in ASD

Regardless of whether irritability is conceptualized as part of the ASD phenotype or due to a comorbid disorder, it often requires treatment and, therefore, monitoring. In addition, universal screening for psychiatric comorbidity has been recommended as a component of routine care, given the prominence of emotional problems in ASD (Chandler et al., 2016). Although structured tasks have been utilized to understand frustration response (e.g., Jahromi et al., 2012) and self-report is commonly applied to assess emotion regulation strategy use among those with ASD without intellectual disability (e.g., Samson, Hardan, Lee, Phillips, & Gross, 2015), caregiver report has been the primary method of assessment for irritability. Caregiver report can be an appropriate method of data collection for individuals with cognitive or other limitations (Irwin et al., 2012). In addition, caregiver report may also be useful among cognitively able youth with ASD due to limitations in emotional insight and self-awareness (Griffin, Lombardo, & Auyeung, 2016). Although the majority of existing measures that have been used in ASD are caregiver-reported, it is recommended to obtain self-report and other perspectives, including behavioral observations, as part of a multimodal battery when possible.

The most widely used measure of irritability in ASD samples is the Aberrant Behavior Checklist (ABC; Aman & Singh, 1986), which is a measure of problem behaviors developed for children and adults with developmental disabilities. The ABC contains a 15-item Irritability Scale (ABC-I). The ABC-I has been the primary outcome measure for large multisite studies investigating the use of risperidone and aripiprazole in ASD (e.g., Marcus et al., 2009; McCracken et al., 2002; Owen et al., 2009). A recent factor analysis confirmed the original factor structure of the ABC-I, but also highlighted that the items with the highest factor loadings are actually indicators of behavioral problems (aggression and self-injurious behavior) rather than those specific to mood and tantrums (Kaat, Lecavalier, & Aman, 2014). Others have also noted that it seems to be a better measure of behavioral dysregulation than irritability per se (Mikita et al., 2015).

The Affective Reactivity Index (ARI) is a widely used self- and parent-report measure of irritability in non-ASD samples (ARI; Stringaris et al., 2012). It includes six items that assess irritability over the past 6 months as well as one item that asks about the degree of impairment. Its psychometric properties were recently evaluated in an unmedicated sample of 47 boys with high-functioning ASD (Mikita et al., 2015). Overall the findings supported its use in ASD, as evidenced by similar item-level performance to a non-ASD sample, with internal consistency of greater than .80 for both parent- and self-report and moderate correlations between parent- and self-report ($r =.55$) (Mikita et al., 2015). Future research with larger ASD samples, particularly studies that do not exclude medicated youth, are warranted.

The Emotion Dysregulation Inventory (EDI; Mazefsky, Day, et al., 2018, Mazefsky, Yu, et al., 2018) is a recently developed caregiver report measure that assesses observable indicators of emotion regulation in youth with ASD aged 6–20. The EDI was developed using the National Institutes of Health (NIH) PROMIS guidelines (nihpromis.net), and the final items were selected based on a combination of classical test theory and item response theory (IRT) analyses using data from a sample of 1,755 youth with ASD (Mazefsky, Yu, White, Siegel, & Pilkonis, 2018). The EDI queries how much of a problem certain behaviors have been over the past 7-day period and is rated on a 5-point Likert scale that probes severity and frequency in order to obtain an estimate of overall interference. The items were shown to have no differential item functioning based on verbal ability, intellectual ability, gender, or age, making it suitable for youth with ASD of varying

TABLE 11.1 Emotion dysregulation inventory (EDI) reactivity scale short form items

Has explosive outbursts
Hard to calm him/her down when mad or upset
Has extreme or intense emotional reactions
Has trouble calming him/herself down
Emotions go from 0 to 100 instantly
Cries or stays angry for 5 minutes or longer
Reactions are usually more severe than the situations calls for

functioning levels. The EDI includes a 24-item Reactivity bank, suitable for computerized adaptive testing, as well as a 7-item Reactivity short form (correlated .98 with the full item bank) that is most relevant to the assessment of irritability (see Table 11.1), as well as a 6-item Dysphoria scale. The Reactivity scale captures intense, rapidly escalating, sustained, and poorly regulated negative emotional reactions and has evidence of change-sensitivity.

Another important component of assessment for irritability is determining safety, particularly in highly irritable individuals with ASD. McGuire et al. (2016) proposed a treatment matrix that assesses the safety of the patient, including self-injury and suicidal behaviors, and those around him or her. Primary considerations are if the patient has been aggressive or caused tissue damage to him- or herself or others. If this is true, then the assessment asks if the family is in crisis and unable to manage behaviors; if so, transport to a psychiatric emergency department is recommended.

Treatment of Irritability in ASD: Evidence for Psychopharmacological Treatment

Use of pharmacological interventions should be considered for irritability in ASD if irritability is severe or if other problem behaviors are present (McGuire et al., 2016). Before initiating a psychotropic medication for irritability, there should be a full assessment of current behaviors and all possible contributing factors, such as potential underlying medical causes for irritability, as well as determining whether other indicated interventions have not helped. The only two medications with FDA approval for use in ASD, risperidone and aripiprazole, are indicated for the treatment of irritability (Siegel & Beaulieu, 2012). Interestingly, use of these medications to treat irritability is specific to ASD and is not approved by the FDA for this use in other populations.

An 8-week trial of aripiprazole to treat irritability in children and adolescents with ASD showed significantly greater improvement in ABC-I subscale scores compared to a placebo (Marcus et al., 2009; Owen et al., 2009). This double-blind study also found significant reduction in irritability based on clinician impression, with minimal adverse effects and generally good tolerance (Owen et al., 2009). McCracken et al. (2002) conducted an 8-week double-blind trial of risperidone in children with ASD and serious behavioral problems. Similar to findings of aripiprazole, there was a significant reduction in ABC-I scores in the risperidone group compared to placebo. This study also included an extension phase; during a 6-month period following the initial trial, 23 of the 34 children in the risperidone group maintained these outcomes. Some children discontinued the study because the risperidone was no longer effective on its own and others withdrew for various other reasons. While no serious adverse events were reported and no children exhibited extrapyramidal symptoms such as shaking, restlessness, slowness of movement, and irregular, jerky body movements, there was a significantly greater mean increase in weight in the risperidone group (2.7 ± 2.9 kg) than the placebo group (0.8 ± 2.2 kg) ($p < 0.001$). A systematic review done by Siegel and Beaulieu (2012) indicated that these antipsychotics are the only medications with "established evidence" for treating irritability. Notably, there are other psychopharmacological treatments that demonstrate promise, though many require more research (see Table 11.2). All of the following medications were tested to target irritability in ASD but resulted in "insufficient evidence" for use in children with ASD (Siegel & Beaulieu, 2012): divalproex sodium/valproic acid, lamotrigine, levetiracetam, clomipramine, and amantadine hydrochloride. Additionally, pentoxifylline,

TABLE 11.2 Drug type and level of evidence for the treatment of irritability in autism spectrum disorder (ASD)

Medication	Common Examples	Drug Class	Level of Evidence
Aripiprazole	Abilify	Antipsychotic	Established evidence
Risperidone	Risperdal	Antipsychotic	Established evidence
N-acetylcysteine	-	Glutamatergic modulator and an antioxidant	Preliminary evidence
Pentoxifylline	Trental, Pentoxil	Xanthine derivative	Preliminary evidence
STX209	Arbaclofen	Selective GABA-B agonist	Preliminary evidence
Amantadine hydrochloride	Symmetrel	Antiviral, dopamine promoter	Insufficient evidence
Clomipramine	Anafranil	Tricyclic antidepressant	Insufficient evidence
Divalproex sodium/ valproic acid	Depakote/Depakene	Mood stabilizer	Insufficient evidence
Lamotrigine	Lamictal	Mood stabilizer	Insufficient evidence
Levetiracetam	Keppra, Spritam	Mood stabilizer	Insufficient evidence

Modified from Siegel and Beaulieu (2012). They defined Established Evidence as "≥2 strong studies conducted in separate settings by research teams OR ≥4 adequate studies conducted in at least two separate settings by separate research teams," Preliminary Evidence as "≥1 adequate study," and Insufficient Evidence as "Conclusions cannot be drawn due to lack of quality research and/or mixed outcomes across several studies." N-acetylcysteine and STX209 were not included in the Siegel and Beaulieu (2012) review, but were considered promising in the Fung et al. (2016) meta-analysis, appearing to satisfy the described criteria for Preliminary Evidence.

which has immunologic and serotonergic effects, was found to significantly improve ABC-I scores in children when used in conjunction with risperidone (Akhondzadeh et al., 2010), but results were deemed "preliminary" (Siegel & Beaulieu, 2012).

In a recent meta-analysis of pharmacologic treatment of irritability in ASD (Fung et al., 2016), N-acetylcysteine was identified as another potential medication, demonstrating significant reductions in ABC-I scores (Hardan et al., 2012). Finally, STX209 (arbaclofen) improved ABC-I scores as well as ABC Lethargy and Social Withdrawal subscale scores and ASD symptom severity in children and teens with ASD (Erickson et al., 2014). Arbaclofen was tolerated somewhat well but commonly caused agitation and irritability, although those side effects were typically resolved with dose changes. While initial results may be promising, a larger placebo-controlled trial is necessary. In sum, there are an encouraging number of compounds with preliminary results for the treatment of irritability in ASD (in addition to evidence-based risperidone and aripiprazole) that are in need of further investigation.

It is important to recognize that studies of new compounds have been hindered by the lack of widely accepted diagnostic tools for comorbid psychopathology in ASD, and any assertions made from data collected on neurotypical individuals as to how they apply to an ASD sample are simply speculative (Siegel, 2012). As measures developed for and validated in individuals with ASD gain popularity, particularly ones that target the emotional rather than behavioral component of irritability (e.g., EDI), there may be additional opportunities to explore alternative psychopharmacologic treatments.

Treatment of Irritability in ASD: Evidence for Psychotherapy

In addition to recommendations for the assessment and psychopharmacological treatment of irritability, McGuire and colleagues (2016) also recommend strategies and therapeutic services for intervening on irritability and related problematic behaviors. These include (1) treating underlying medical conditions, such as gastrointestinal issues and sleep difficulties; (2) increasing functional communication through speech-language therapy; and (3) conducting a functional behavioral analysis and implementing positive behavioral supports, as indicated. The pathway also advocates for treating psychiatric comorbidities that may underlie the irritability when indicated. However, evidence-based psychosocial treatments that are appropriately tailored for individuals with ASD are somewhat limited.

Cognitive behavioral therapy (CBT) has demonstrated efficacy for treating anxiety in individuals with ASD (Vasa et al., 2014), but there is underwhelming evidence for addressing other comorbid psychopathology. One exception is the successful application of CBT to reduce anger in children with high-functioning ASD, which also increased parental perceptions of their efficacy in managing their children's anger outbursts (Sofronoff, Attwood, Hinton, & Levin, 2007). Additionally, a pilot study of CBT to treat emotion dysregulation in young children with ASD resulted in decreased lability/negativity and shorter outbursts (Scarpa & Reyes, 2011). Although both CBT-based treatments offer promise for the reduction of irritability in ASD, results are preliminary given that they have not been replicated and conclusions were based exclusively on parent report. Moreover, while advances have been made in transdiagnostic CBT interventions (e.g., Ehrenreich-May & Bilek, 2012), there is a dearth of work applying these to children with ASD.

Mindfulness as a treatment for individuals with ASD has promise for addressing a myriad of psychological difficulties, including mood disorders and irritability. Four studies in a recent systematic review (see Cachia, Anderson, & Moore, 2016) included adapted mindfulness interventions for children and/or adolescents with ASD. Collectively, these studies found reductions in anxiety, rumination, and aggression. A separate open-trial study focused on piloting a new transdiagnostic emotion regulation intervention targeting irritability via mindfulness for adolescents and young adults with ASD found preliminary support for its acceptability and feasibility, as well as preliminary evidence of large effect sizes for improvement in emotion regulation, irritability, depression, and overall functioning and symptom impairment (Conner, White, Beck, Golt, Smith, & Mazefsky, 2018). Although this is a promising direction for future research, larger randomized controlled trials are needed.

Conclusion

In sum, it is clear that irritability is a prominent problem among youth with ASD, but there are many aspects of our current understanding of irritability in ASD that remain limited. Although there is sufficient evidence that irritability presents early for many youth with ASD, the developmental course is not clear. It is likely that early temperamental characteristics and indicators of emotion regulation may predict which youth with ASD will continue to express high irritability throughout development. However, the existing literature primarily consists of cross-sectional or short-term longitudinal studies, thus limiting conclusions about the development and consequences of irritability in ASD.

Based on temperamental methodologies, it appears that irritability in individuals with ASD is better predicted by *if* and *how* children attempt to regulate their elevated negative emotional states rather than reactivity (negative affect) alone. Indeed, studies examining both emotional reactivity and regulation in children with ASD suggest that these facets are explained by a single factor in ASD (Mazefsky, Yu, et al., 2018), consistent with findings in the non-ASD literature (Zelkowitz & Cole, 2016). Therefore, the tendency to experience strong negative affect and difficulty regulating that affect likely co-occur temporally, and both aspects may contribute to irritability and would require treatment.

Psychopharmacological treatment of irritability in ASD is arguably further advanced than psychopharmacological management of core ASD symptoms, for which no FDA-approved medications exist (Siegel, 2012). However, as the majority of studies evaluating the use of atypical antipsychotics in ASD relied on the ABC-I, which emphasizes behavioral dysregulation, it may be important to evaluate these evidence-based and experimental medications with measures that more directly measure emotion. Psychometric evaluation of measures originally designed for non-ASD populations (e.g., ARI) as well as the development of new measures with proven validity and precision in ASD (e.g., EDI) may make this more feasible.

Treatment development efforts would also be enhanced by additional studies of the biological mechanisms underlying ASD. There is some evidence that a biologically based stress response is related to the occurrence of irritability in ASD (Mikita et al., 2015), but this is generally an underresearched area of inquiry. Identifying underlying biological mechanisms may provide new targets for treatment. While there are some promising psychotherapeutic approaches for higher functioning youth with ASD that utilize cognitive behavioral therapy or mindfulness, larger, randomized controlled trials are needed, especially in youth with more severe ASD symptomatology or comorbid intellectual disability.

Another area in need of clarification is how to conceptualize irritability's association with ASD. Research findings to date suggest that irritability and frustration may be components of the early phenotype of ASD, although it is important to note that there are likely individual differences (e.g., low negative affectivity also associated with early diagnoses of ASD; Garon et al., 2016). Therefore, it will be important to elucidate how irritability may contribute to risk for additional psychiatric and behavioral problems in ASD. There is a growing evidence base to suggest that impaired emotion regulation contributes to anxiety, depression, social problems, and aggression in ASD (Mazefsky, Borue, Day, & Minshew, 2014; Nader-Grosbois & Mazzone, 2014; Rieffe et al., 2011; Samson, Hardan, Lee, et al., 2015; White et al., 2014). Impaired emotional reactivity and regulation as a mechanism underlying psychiatric comorbidities in individuals with ASD is a promising theoretical conceptualization for which more research and, in particular, long-term longitudinal studies are needed (Mazefsky et al., 2013). Discerning the boundary between "typical" levels of irritability in ASD and irritability that is distinct from ASD and that thereby warrants a separate diagnosis is an important and complex clinical issue.

Despite the many ways in which having ASD may contribute to irritability and how common irritability is within the disorder, current diagnostic systems do not address irritability as part of the diagnostic criteria for ASD. This may partly lead to an overreliance on the use of comorbid psychiatric diagnoses to convey the related emotional treatment needs. However, if irritability, or the mechanisms that may give rise to irritability (e.g., emotion regulation, cognitive and behavioral characteristics of ASD) are considered core features of ASD, an additional diagnostic specifier such as "with emotion dysregulation" or "with irritability" may better highlight irritability as a key dimension upon which individuals with ASD vary (similar to language and intellectual impairment specifiers), and it would serve to clearly inform treatment needs while reserving the additional psychiatric diagnoses for those circumstances when there is true comorbidity (Mazefsky, 2015).

References

Akhondzadeh, S., Fallah, J., Mohammadi, M. R., Imani, R., Mohammadi, M., Salehi, B., . . . Forghani, S. (2010). Double-blind placebo-controlled trial of pentoxifylline added to risperidone: Effects on aberrant behavior in children with autism. *Progress in Neuro-Psychopharmacology and Biological Psychiatry, 34*(1), 32–36. https://doi.org/10.1016/j.pnpbp.2009.09.012

Aman, M. G., & Singh, N. N. (1986). *Aberrant Behavior Checklist manual.* New York: Slosson Educational Publications.

American Psychiatric Association (APA). (2000). *Diagnostic and Statistical Manual of Mental Disorders* (4th edition, Text Revision). Washington, DC: American Psychiatric Association.

American Psychiatric Association (APA). (2013). *The Diagnostic and Statistical Manual of Mental Disorders* (5th edition). Arlington, VA: American Psychiatric Association.

Bolton, P. F., Pickles, A., Murphy, M., & Rutter, M. (1998). Autism, affective and other psychiatric disorders: Patterns of familial. *Psychological Medicine, 28,* 385–395.

Borue, X., Mazefsky, C., Rooks, B. T., Strober, M., Keller, M. B., Hower, H., . . . Birmaher, B. (2016). Longitudinal course of bipolar disorder in youth with high-functioning autism spectrum disorder. *Journal of the American Academy of Child & Adolescent Psychiatry, 55*(12), 1064–1072.e6. https://doi.org/10.1016/j.jaac.2016.08.011

Bryson, S. E., Zwaigenbaum, L., Brian, J., Roberts, W., Szatmari, P., Rombough, V., & McDermott, C. (2007). A prospective case series of high-risk infants who developed autism. *Journal of Autism and Developmental Disorders, 37*(1), 12–24. https://doi.org/10.1007/s10803-006-0328-2

Cachia, R. L., Anderson, A., & Moore, D. W. (2016). Mindfulness in individuals with autism spectrum disorder: A systematic review and narrative analysis. *Review Journal of Autism and Developmental Disorders, 3*(2), 165–178. https://doi.org/10.1007/s40489-016-0074-0

Chandler, S., Howlin, P., Simonoff, E., O'Sullivan, T., Tseng, E., Kennedy, J., . . . Baird, G. (2016). Emotional and behavioural problems in young children with autism spectrum disorder. *Developmental Medicine and Child Neurology, 58*(2), 202–208. https://doi.org/10.1111/dmcn.12830

Conner, C. M., White, S. W., Beck, K. B., Golt, J., Smith, I. C., & Mazefsky, C. A. (2018). Improving Emotion Regulation Ability in Autism: The Emotion Awareness and Skills Enhancement (EASE) Program. *Autism: The International Journal of Research and Practice,* [Advance online publication]. https://doi.org/10.1177/1362361318810709

Ehrenreich-May, J., & Bilek, E. L. (2012). The development of a transdiagnostic, cognitive behavioral group intervention for childhood anxiety disorders and co-occurring depression symptoms. *Cognitive and Behavioral Practice, 19*(1), 41–55. https://doi.org/ 10.1016/j.cbpra.2011.02.003

Erickson, C. A., Veenstra-Vanderweele, J. M., Melmed, R. D., McCracken, J. T., Ginsberg, L. D., Sikich, L., . . . King, B. H. (2014). STX209 (arbaclofen) for autism spectrum disorders: An 8-week open-label study. *Journal of Autism and Developmental Disorders, 44*(4), 958–964. https://doi.org/10.1007/s10803-013-1963-z

Fung, L. K., Mahajan, R., Nozzolillo, A., Bernal, P., Krasner, A., Jo, B., . . . Hardan, A. Y. (2016). Pharmacologic treatment of severe irritability and problem behaviors in autism: A systematic review and meta-analysis. *Pediatrics, 137*(February), S124–S135. https://doi.org/10.1542/peds.2015-2851K

Garon, N., Zwaigenbaum, L., Bryson, S., Smith, I. M., Brian, J., Roncadin, C., . . . Roberts, W. (2016). Temperament and its association with autism symptoms in a high-risk population. *Journal of Abnormal Child Psychology, 44*(4), 757–769. https://doi.org/10.1007/ s10802-015-0064-1

Goldani, A. A. S., Downs, S. R., Widjaja, F., Lawton, B., & Hendren, R. L. (2014). Biomarkers in autism. *Frontiers in Psychiatry, 5*(100), 1–13. https://doi.org/10.3389/fpsyt.2014.00100

Griffin, C., Lombardo, M. V., & Auyeung, B. (2016). Alexithymia in children with and without autism spectrum disorders. *Autism Research, 9*(7), 773–780. https://doi.org/ 10.1002/aur.1569

Group of the Psychiatric Genomics Consortium (2013). Identification of risk loci with shared effects on five major psychiatric disorders: A genome-wide analysis. *The Lancet, 381*(9875), 1371–1379. https://doi.org/10.1016/S0140-6736(12)62129-1

Hardan, A. Y., Fung, L. K., Libove, R. A., Obukhanych, T. V, Nair, S., Herzenberg, L. A., . . . Tirouvanziam, R. (2012). A randomized controlled pilot trial of oral N-acetylcysteine in children with autism. *Biological Psychiatry, 71*(11), 956–961. https://doi. org/10.1016/j.biopsych.2012.01.014

Irwin, D. E., Gross, H. E., Stucky, B. D., Thissen, D., DeWitt, E., Lai, J., . . . DeWalt, D. A. (2012). Development of six PROMIS pediatrics proxy-report item banks. *Health and Quality of Life Outcomes, 10*(1), 22. https://doi.org/10.1186/1477-7525-10-22

Jahromi, L. B., Meek, S. E., & Ober-Reynolds, S. (2012). Emotion regulation in the context of frustration in children with high functioning autism and their typical peers. *Journal of Child Psychology and Psychiatry, 53*(12), 1250–1258. https://doi.org/10.1111/ j.1469-7610.2012.02560.x

Joshi, G., Petty, C., Wozniak, J., Henin, A., Fried, R., Galdo, M., . . . Biederman, J. (2010). The heavy burden of psychiatric comorbidity in youth with autism spectrum disorders: A large comparative study of a psychiatrically referred population. *Journal of Autism and Developmental Disorders, 40*(11), 1361–1370. https://doi.org/10.1007/ s10803-010-0996-9

Kaat, A. J., Lecavalier, L., & Aman, M. G. (2014). Validity of the aberrant behavior checklist in children with autism spectrum disorder. *Journal of Autism and Developmental Disorders, 44*(5), 1103–1116. https://doi.org/10.1007/s10803-013-1970-0

Kiefer, C., Kryza-Lacombe, M., Cole, K., Lord, C., Monk, C., & Lee Wiggins, J. (2017). Irritability and amygdala-ventral prefrontal cortex connectivity in children with high functioning autism spectrum disorder. *Biological Psychiatry, 81*(10), S53. https://doi.org/ 10.1016/j.biopsych.2017.02.138

Konstantareas, M. M., & Stewart, K. (2006). Affect regulation and temperament in children with autism spectrum disorder. *Journal of Autism and Developmental Disorders, 36*(2), 143–154. https://doi.org/10.1007/s10803-005-0051-4

Leibenluft, E. (2011). Severe mood dysregulation, irritability, and the diagnostic boundaries of bipolar disorder in youths. *American Journal of Psychiatry, 168*(2), 129–142. https://doi.org/10.1176/appi.ajp.2010.10050766

Leibenluft, E. (2017). Pediatric irritability: A systems neuroscience approach. *Trends in Cognitive Sciences, 21*(4), 277–289. https://doi.org/10.1016/j.tics.2017.02.002

Leyfer, O. T., Folstein, S. E., Bacalman, S., Davis, N. O., Dinh, E., Morgan, J., . . . Lainhart, J. E. (2006). Comorbid psychiatric disorders in children with autism: Interview development and rates of disorders. *Journal of Autism and Developmental Disorders, 36*(7), 849–861. https://doi.org/10.1007/s10803-006-0123-0

Macari, S. L., Koller, J., Campbell, D. J., & Chawarska, K. (2017). Temperamental markers in toddlers with autism spectrum disorder. *Journal of Child Psychology and Psychiatry and Allied Disciplines, 58*(7), 819–828. https://doi.org/10.1111/jcpp.12710

Madden, J. M., Lakoma, M. D., Lynch, F. L., Rusinak, D., Owen-Smith, A. A., Coleman, K. J., . . . Croen, L. A. (2017). Psychotropic medication use among insured children with autism spectrum disorder. *Journal of Autism and Developmental Disorders, 47*(1), 144–154. https://doi.org/10.1007/s10803-016-2946-7

Magnuson, K. M., & Constantino, J. N. (2011). Characterization of depression in children with autism spectrum disorders. *Journal of Developmental & Behavioral Pediatrics, 32*(4), 332–340. https://doi.org/10.1097/DBP.0b013e318213f56c

Marcus, R. N., Owen, R., Kamen, L., Manos, G., McQuade, R. D., Carson, W. H., & Aman, M. G. (2009). A placebo-controlled, fixed-dose study of aripiprazole in children and adolescents with irritability associated with autistic disorder. *Journal of the American Academy of Child & Adolescent Psychiatry, 48*(11), 1110–1119. https://doi.org/10.1097/CHI.0b013e3181b76658

Mayes, S. D., Calhoun, S. L., Murray, M. J., Ahuja, M., & Smith, L. A. (2011). Anxiety, depression, and irritability in children with autism relative to other neuropsychiatric disorders and typical development. *Research in Autism Spectrum Disorders, 5*(1), 474–485. https://doi.org/10.1016/j.rasd.2010.06.012

Mayes, S. D., Kokotovich, C., Mathiowetz, C., Baweja, R., Calhoun, S. L., & Waxmonsky, J. (2017). Disruptive mood dysregulation disorder symptoms by age in autism, ADHD, and general population samples. *Journal of Mental Health Research in Intellectual Disabilities, 10*(4), 345–359. https://doi.org/10.1080/19315864.2017.1338804

Mazefsky, C. A. (2015). Emotion regulation and emotional distress in ASD: Foundations and considerations for future research. *Journal of Autism and Developmental Disorders, 45*(11), 3405–3408. https://doi.org/10.1007/s10803-015-2602-7

Mazefsky, C. A., Borue, X., Day, T. N., & Minshew, N. J. (2014). Emotion regulation patterns in adolescents with high-functioning autism spectrum disorder: Comparison to typically developing adolescents and association with psychiatric symptoms. *Autism Research, 7*(3), 344–54. https://doi.org/10.1002/aur.1366

Mazefsky, C. A., Day, T. N., Siegel, M., White, S. W., Yu, L., & Pilkonis, P. A. (2018). Development of the Emotion Dysregulation Inventory: A PROMISing method for creating sensitive and unbiased questionnaires for autism spectrum disorder. *Journal of Autism and Developmental Disorder, 48*(11), 3736–3746 s. https://doi.org/10.1007/ s10803-016-2907-1

Mazefsky, C. A., Folstein, S. E., & Lainhart, J. E. (2008). Overrepresentation of mood and anxiety disorders in adults with autism and their first-degree relatives: What does it mean? *Autism Research, 1*(3), 193–197. https://doi.org/10.1002/aur.23

Mazefsky, C. A., Herrington, J., Siegel, M., Scarpa, A., Maddox, B. B., Scahill, L., & White, S. W. (2013). The role of emotion regulation in autism. *Journal of the American Academy of Child & Adolescent Psychiatry, 52*(7), 679–688. https://doi.org/10.1016/j.jaac.2013.05.006

Mazefsky, C. A., Oswald, D., Day, T. N., Eack, S. M., Minshew, N. J., & Lainhart, J. E. (2012). ASD, a psychiatric disorder, or both? Psychiatric diagnoses in adolescents with high-functioning ASD. *Journal of Clinical Child and Adolescent Psychology, 41*(4), 516–23.

Mazefsky, C. A., & White, S. W. (2014). Emotion regulation. *Child and Adolescent Psychiatric Clinics of North America, 23*(1), 15–24. https://doi.org/10.1016/j.chc.2013.07.002

Mazefsky, C. A., Yu, L., White, S., Siegel, M., & Pilkonis, P. (2018). The Emotion Dysregulation Inventory: Psychometric properties and item response theory calibration in an autism spectrum disorder sample. *Autism Research, 11*(6), 928–941. doi:10.1002/aur.1947

McCracken, J. T., McGough, J., Shah, B., Cronin, P., Hong, D., Aman, M. G., . . . McMahon, D. (2002). Risperidone in children with autism and serious be-havioral problems. *New England Journal of Medicine, 347*(5), 314–321. https://doi. org/10.1056/NEJMoa013171

McGuire, K., Fung, L. K., Hagopian, L., Vasa, R. A., Mahajan, R., Bernal, P., . . . Whitaker, A. H. (2016). Irritability and problem behavior in autism spectrum disorder: A practice pathway for pediatric primary care. *Pediatrics, 137*(Supplement), S136–S148. https://doi. org/10.1542/peds.2015-2851L

Mezzacappa, A., Lasica, P. A., Gianfagna, F., Cazas, O., Hardy, P., Falissard, B., . . . Gressier, F. (2017). Risk for autism spectrum disorders according to period of prenatal antidepres-sant exposure: A systematic review and meta-analysis. *JAMA Pediatrics, 171*(6), 555–563. https://doi.org/10.1001/jamapediatrics.2017.0124

Mikita, N., Hollocks, M. J., Papadopoulos, A. S., Aslani, A., Harrison, S., Leibenluft, E., . . . Stringaris, A. (2015). Irritability in boys with autism spectrum disorders: An in-vestigation of physiological reactivity. *Journal of Child Psychology and Psychiatry and Allied Disciplines, 56*(10), 1118–1126. https://doi.org/10.1111/jcpp.12382

Minshew, N. J., & Williams, D. L. (2007). The new neurobiology of autism. *Archives of Neurology, 64*(7), 945. https://doi.org/10.1001/archneur.64.7.945

Nader-Grosbois, N., & Mazzone, S. (2014). Emotion regulation, personality and social adjustment in children with autism spectrum disorders. *Psychology, 5*(15), 1750–1767. https://doi.org/10.4236/psych.2014.515182

Owen, R., Sikich, L., Marcus, R. N., Corey-Lisle, P., Manos, G., McQuade, R. D., . . . Findling, R. L. (2009). Aripiprazole in the treatment of irritability in children and adolescents with autistic disorder. *Pediatrics, 124*(6), 1533–1540. https://doi.org/10.1542/peds.2008-3782

Pine, D. S., Guyer, A. E., Goldwin, M., Towbin, K. A., & Leibenluft, E. (2008). Autism spectrum disorder scale scores in pediatric mood and anxiety disorders. *Journal of the American Academy of Child and Adolescent Psychiatry, 47*(6), 652–661.

Pan, P. Y., & Yeh, C. Bin. (2016). The comorbidity of disruptive mood dysregulation disorder in autism spectrum disorder. *Psychiatry Research, 241*(2016), 108–109. https://doi.org/ 10.1016/j.psychres.2016.05.001

Piven, J., Gayle, J., Chase, G. A., Fink, B., Landa, R., Wzorek, M. M., & Folstein, S. E. (1990). A family history study of neuropsychiatric disorders in the adult siblings of autistic individuals. *Journal of the American Academy of Child & Adolescent Psychiatry, 29*(2), 177–183. https://doi.org/10.1097/00004583-199003000-00004

Rieffe, C., Oosterveld, P., Terwogt, M. M., Mootz, S., van Leeuwen, E., & Stockmann, L. (2011). Emotion regulation and internalizing symptoms in children with autism spectrum disorders. *Autism, 15*(6), 655–670. https://doi.org/10.1177/1362361310366571

Rothbart, M. K., & Bates, J. E. (1998). Temperament. In W. Damon & N. Eisenberg (Eds.), *Handbook of child psychology* (5th ed.; vol. 3). New York: Wiley.

Samson, A. C., Hardan, A. Y., Lee, I. A., Phillips, J. M., & Gross, J. J. (2015). Maladaptive behavior in autism spectrum disorder: The role of emotion experience and emotion regulation. *Journal of Autism and Developmental Disorders, 45*(11), 3424–3432. https://doi.org/10.1007/s10803-015-2388-7

Samson, A. C., Hardan, A. Y., Podell, R. W., Phillips, J. M., & Gross, J. J. (2015). Emotion regulation in children and adolescents with autism spectrum disorder. *Autism Research, 8*(1), 9–18. https://doi.org/10.1002/aur.1387

Samson, A. C., Phillips, J. M., Parker, K. J., Shah, S., Gross, J. J., & Hardan, A. Y. (2014). Emotion dysregulation and the core features of autism spectrum disorder. *Journal of Autism and Developmental Disorders, 44*(7), 1766–1772. https://doi.org/10.1007/s10803-013-2022-5

Scarpa, A., & Reyes, N. M. (2011). Improving emotion regulation with CBT in young children with high functioning autism spectrum disorders: A pilot study. *Behavioural and Cognitive Psychotherapy, 39*(4), 495–500. https://doi.org/10.1017/S1352465811000063

Siegel, M. (2012). Psychopharmacology of autism spectrum disorder: Evidence and practice. *Child and Adolescent Psychiatric Clinics of North America, 21*(4), 957–973. https://doi.org/10.1016/j.chc.2012.07.006

Siegel, M., & Beaulieu, A. A. (2012). Psychotropic medications in children with autism spectrum disorders: A systematic review and synthesis for evidence-based practice. *Journal of Autism and Developmental Disorders, 42*(8), 1592–1605. https://doi.org/10.1007/s10803-011-1399-2

Smalley, S. L., McCracken, J., & Tanguay, P. (1995). Autism, affective disorders, and social phobia. *American Journal of Medical Genetics, 60*(1), 19–26. https://doi.org/10.1002/ajmg.1320600105

Sofronoff, K., Attwood, T., Hinton, S., & Levin, I. (2007). A randomized controlled trial of a cognitive behavioural intervention for anger management in children diagnosed with Asperger Syndrome. *Journal of Autism and Developmental Disorders, 37*(7), 1203–1214. https://doi.org/10.1007/s10803-006-0262-3

Stringaris, A., Goodman, R., Ferdinando, S., Razdan, V., Muhrer, E., Leibenluft, E., & Brotman, M. A. (2012). The Affective Reactivity Index: A concise irritability scale for clinical and research settings. *Journal of Child Psychology and Psychiatry and Allied Disciplines, 53*(11), 1109–1117. https://doi.org/10.1111/j.1469-7610.2012.02561.x

Towbin, K. E., Pradella, A., Gorrindo, T., Pine, D. S., & Leibenluft, E. (2005). Autism spectrum traits in children with mood and anxiety disorders. *Journal of Child and Adolescent Psychopharmacology, 15*(3), 452–464. https://doi.org/10.1089/cap.2005.15.452

Vasa, R. A., Carroll, L. M., Nozzolillo, A. A., Mahajan, R., Mazurek, M. O., Bennett, A. E., . . . Bernal, M. P. (2014). A systematic review of treatments for anxiety in youth with autism spectrum disorders. *Journal of Autism and Developmental Disorders, 44*(12), 3215–3229. https://doi.org/10.1007/s10803-014-2184-9

Vidal-Ribas, P., Brotman, M. A., Valdivieso, I., Leibenluft, E., & Stringaris, A. (2016). The status of irritability in psychiatry: A conceptual and quantitative review. *Journal of the American Academy of Child and Adolescent Psychiatry.* https://doi.org/10.1016/j.jaac.2016.04.014

Weiss, J. A., Riosa, P. B., Mazefsky, C. A., & Beaumont, R. (2017). Emotion regulation in autism spectrum disorder. In C. A. Essau, S. S. LeBlanc, & T. H. Ollendick (Eds.), *Emotion regulation and psychopathology in children and adolescents* (pp. 235–258). New York: Oxford University Press.

White, S. W., Mazefsky, C. A., Dichter, G. S., Chiu, P. H., Richey, J. A., & Ollendick, T. H. (2014). Social-cognitive, physiological, and neural mechanisms underlying emotion regulation impairments: Understanding anxiety in autism spectrum disorder. *International Journal of Developmental Neuroscience, 39*(C), 22–36. https://doi.org/10.1016/j.ijdevneu.2014.05.012

Zelkowitz, R. L., & Cole, D. A. (2016). Measures of emotion reactivity and emotion regulation: Convergent and discriminant validity. *Personality and Individual Differences, 102,* 123–132. https://doi.org/10.1016/j.paid.2016.06.045

Zwaigenbaum, L., Bauman, M. L., Stone, W. L., Yirmiya, N., Estes, A., Hansen, R., . . . Wetherby, A. M. (2015). Early identification of autism spectrum disorder: Recommendations for practice and research. *Pediatrics, 136,* S10–S40. https://doi.org/10.1542/peds.2014-3667C

12

Irritability in Mood and Anxiety Disorders
Pablo Vidal-Ribas Belil and Argyris Stringaris

Introduction

Irritability is part of the diagnostic criteria of every pediatric mood disorder described in the fifth edition of the *Diagnostic and Statistical Manual of Mental Disorders* (DSM-5), including all types of bipolar disorder (BD), major depressive disorder (MDD), and, most recently, disruptive mood dysregulation disorder (DMDD), which is the new clinical category for severe chronic irritability (American Psychiatric Association [APA], 2013). In addition, anxiety disorders are also associated with irritable mood, with some of them, such as generalized anxiety disorder (GAD) and posttraumatic stress disorder (PTSD), also including it in their diagnostic criteria. This close relationship between irritability and mood and anxiety disorders is reflected in the psychological literature under the term "negative affectivity," a broad spectrum of negative emotions that include anger, sadness, and fear, the hallmarks of these disorders. Since irritability cuts across most emotional disorders, it is important to discuss what makes it distinctive in each of these clinical categories.

Probably the greatest effort in distinguishing irritability types across emotional disorders has come from the controversy surrounding the diagnosis of BD in children and adolescents (Leibenluft, 2011). In recent past decades in the United States, the rates of BD diagnoses in youth have increased dramatically; more than 400% in inpatient units (Blader & Carlson, 2007) between 1996 and 2004 (Figure 12.1) and a 40-fold increase in outpatient services (Moreno et al., 2007) between 1994 and 2003 (Figure 12.2). The most plausible explanation for this increase seems to be changes in how BD was diagnosed in children (Leibenluft, 2011; Mikita & Stringaris, 2013), and irritability, along with hyperarousal symptoms, played a central role in this. The idea that mania may present differently in children prompted some researchers to suggest that pediatric BD was characterized by chronic, nonepisodic irritability, as opposed to the classical episodic form of mania in

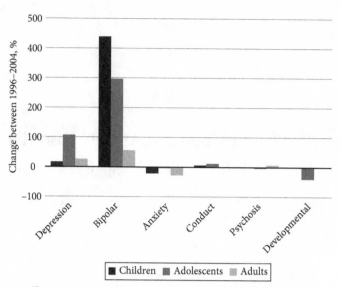

FIGURE 12.1 *Changes in US rates for groups of psychiatric disorders coded as primary diagnoses in acute US inpatient units from 1996 to 2004.*

Data from Blader & Carlson (2007).

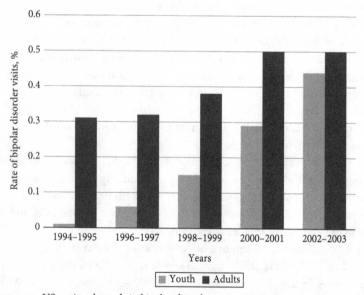

FIGURE 12.2 *US national trends in bipolar disorder visit rates in outpatient services from 1994 to 2003.*

Data from Moreno et al. (2007).

adults (Wozniak et al., 1995). Of note, the DSM criteria for mania require a "distinct period of abnormally and persistently elevated, expansive or irritable mood," which we discuss later. It seems likely that ignoring the requirement of "distinct period" led to many children with chronic irritability being misdiagnosed with BD. The increase in rates of BD diagnoses also coincided with a rise in prescription rates of antipsychotic drugs (Olfson, Blanco, Liu, Moreno, & Laje, 2006)—a recent survey from prescriptions in a US state showed that more than 10,000 children of 6 years of age or less (more than 4% of all children of that age enrolled in Medicaid) received a prescription for antipsychotic medication and that 75% of those prescriptions were for a diagnosis of BD (Lohr, Chowning, Stevenson, & Williams, 2015). The controversy about whether chronic irritability was a hallmark of pediatric BD or not motivated the definition of the severe mood dysregulation (SMD) criteria by Leibenluft et al. (Leibenluft, Charney, Towbin, Bhangoo, & Pine, 2003), which is defined by persistent negative mood and hyperarousal symptoms. The purpose of defining SMD was to facilitate the empirical comparison of youths with chronic irritability and those with classic episodic BD by using longitudinal designs, looking at family aggregation, and examining pathophysiological mechanisms. The studies that followed provided evidence against the notion that severe chronic irritability is an early-life form of BD (Leibenluft, 2011); for example, these studies showed that chronic irritability is longitudinally associated with depression and anxiety but not BD. In 2013, the American Psychiatric Association (APA)—also supported by this evidence—attempted to tackle the dramatic increase of bipolar diagnoses and consequent rise in antipsychotic prescriptions in youth by introducing DMDD in the DSM-5 (APA, 2013), which is characterized by chronic, severe, persistent irritability and frequent, severe temper outbursts.

The aim of this chapter is to describe the distinct phenomenology, epidemiology, and correlates of irritability in BD, DMDD, MDD, and anxiety disorders. Under the section of DMDD, we summarize the results of studies aimed at differentiating chronic irritability from pediatric BD, and, since DMDD is the clinical category for irritability itself, we also provide information on differential diagnosis.

Irritability in Bipolar Disorders

PHENOTYPIC PRESENTATION

BD is defined by the presence of at least one manic (BD-I)/hypomanic (BD-II) episode that may be preceded (*must be* in the case of hypomanic episodes) or followed by major depressive episodes. The DSM-5 Criterion A for manic/hypomanic episodes requires a "distinct period of abnormally and persistently elevated, expansive or irritable mood." This period of abnormal mood—either elated, irritable, or both—is associated with the onset or worsening of other symptoms (Criterion B), including inflated self-esteem or grandiosity, decreased need for sleep, more talkative than usual, pressured speech, flight of ideas, racing thoughts, distractibility, increased goal-directed activity, psychomotor agitation, and/or excessive involvement in activities that might have undesirable consequences (APA, 2013).

Two things should be noted from the definition set in Criterion A. First, the type of irritability seen in BD is *episodic*—that is, it comes as a change from the child's baseline mood, and parents describe it as something that is out of character. Therefore, in children and adolescents showing severe irritability, a diagnosis of BD should only be applied to those who have shown a "distinct period" during which the irritability clearly differed from the child's usual mood state *and* was accompanied by the onset of other manic symptoms listed in Criterion B.

Second, irritability in BD is considered a cardinal symptom alongside elated mood in both adults and children. As we will see later in this chapter, this is in contrast to the criteria for major depressive episodes, in which irritability is only considered a cardinal symptom in children and adolescents. To note, DSM guidelines differ from those in other countries, such as the United Kingdom, where the National Institute for Health and Care Excellence advises that irritability without elation or grandiosity should not allow a diagnosis of mania in children (NICE, 2014). This might partly explain the 72-fold difference in discharge rates for pediatric BD between the United States and United Kingdom in the period 2000–2010 (James et al., 2014). Nevertheless, the importance of elation over irritability in BD seems to be implicitly recognized by the DSM-5 through the requirement of four additional manic symptoms from Criterion B if the dominant mood is irritable, but *only* three symptoms if the dominant mood is elated or expansive.

Episodic irritability in BD is strongly influenced by the patient's interactions with the environment. As symptoms of disinhibition become more severe and the patient faces increasing restrictions by his or her family or mental health professionals, more and more behavioral goals are blocked, leading to frustration. Indeed, it is characteristic in such instances to observe extreme euphoria turn into very severe irritability, thus increasing the risk for aggression.

EPIDEMIOLOGY

The prevalence of pediatric BD is estimated to be 1.8% (Van Meter, Moreira, & Youngstrom, 2011). Yet this rate might be inflated by the inclusion of broad definitions of BP in some studies; studies employing narrow definitions have found rates as low as 0.1% (Costello et al., 1996; Stringaris, Santosh, Leibenluft, & Goodman, 2010). Epidemiologic studies that include BD-not otherwise specified (BD-NOS) report higher rates of BD (range 2.4–6.7%) (Van Meter et al., 2011). BD-NOS is a heterogeneous and broadly defined phenotype characterized by episodic bipolar symptoms that are too short to meet the DSM-5 duration criteria. Many children with severe chronic irritability and short temper tantrums are erroneously diagnosed with BD-NOS even though evidence shows differences with SMD in clinical presentation and longitudinal course (Towbin, Axelson, Leibenluft, & Birmaher, 2013). Moreover, recent data show that irritability as a symptom in BD-NOS is less common (46%) than in BD-I or BD-II (Van Meter, Burke, Kowatch, Findling, & Youngstrom, 2016), which further emphasizes the distinction from SMD or DMDD.

Episodic irritability is one of the most common symptoms among youth with BD, with a prevalence of 77%, along with increased energy (79%) and mood liability (76%) (Van Meter et al., 2016). However, irritability in the absence of elation is very rare; one study found that about 10% of youths with BD had *only* irritability as a cardinal symptom (Hunt et al., 2009), and most of them eventually also experienced elation in the course of 4 years (Hunt et al., 2013).

PSYCHOPATHOLOGICAL CORRELATES

Few studies have examined the correlates of episodic irritability within the context of BD. Reports from the Course and Outcome of Bipolar Illness in Youth (COBY) study, a large prospective study examining youth with BD, showed that those BD youth who only displayed irritable mood as a cardinal symptom (10%) were younger than those with elation or those with both elation and irritability (Hunt et al., 2009). In addition, they had more second-degree relatives with depressive disorders and higher risk for depressive episodes (Hunt et al., 2013). However, they did not differ from elated BD youth in BD subtype, rate of psychiatric comorbidities, severity of illness, duration of illness, family history of mania, duration of mood episodes, risk for suicidal attempts, or functional impairment. Data from the adult literature show that irritability in BD is associated with lifetime anxiety disorders as well as higher recurrence of and slower recovery from depressive episodes (Yuen, Miller et al., 2016; Yuen, Shah et al., 2016).

Irritability in Disruptive Mood Dysregulation Disorder

PHENOTYPIC PRESENTATION

DMDD is a new category in the DSM-5 classified under the section of Depressive Disorders. DMDD is characterized by persistent irritable mood and severe (i.e. out of proportion in intensity or duration) and frequent (i.e., three or more times per week) temper outbursts. These features should have been present for at least 1 year and begun before age 10, although the diagnosis should not be made before age 6 or after age 18. The irritability must be severely impairing in at least one setting (home, school, peers) and be present in a second setting. Most of our knowledge about severe chronic irritability as a category comes from research on the precursor to DMDD (i.e., SMD) (Leibenluft, 2011; Leibenluft et al., 2003). SMD and DMDD overlap substantially with two main differences. First, SMD criteria require persistent negative mood, which may be either irritability or

TABLE 12.1 Comparison of diagnostic criteria between disruptive mood dysregulation disorder (DMDD) and severe mood dysregulation (SMD)

Criteria	DMDD	SMD
Age at diagnosis[a]	6–17 years	7–17 years
Age of onset[a]	Before **10 years**	Before **12 years**
Temper outbursts	Severe and recurrent temper outbursts, inappropriate for age and/or precipitating event, manifested verbally and/or behaviorally (e.g., verbal rages, and/or aggression toward people or property.	Severe and recurrent temper outbursts, inappropriate for age and/or precipitating event, manifested verbally and/or behaviorally (e.g., verbal rages, and/or aggression toward people or property.
Frequency of temper outbursts	On average, at least three times a week	On average, at least three times a week
Mood between outburst[a]	**Irritable or angry mood** present at least half of the day most days, and is noticeable by others (e.g., parents, teachers, peers).	**Abnormal mood (specifically anger or sadness)**, present at least half of the day most days, and is noticeable by others (e.g., parents, teachers, peers).
Hyperarousal symptoms[a]	**None**	Presence of **at least three** of the following symptoms: insomnia, agitation, distractibility, racing thoughts or flight of ideas, pressured speech, intrusiveness
Duration[a]	Symptoms should have been present for at least 12 months without any symptom-free periods exceeding **3 months**.	Symptoms should have been present for at least 12 months without any symptom-free periods exceeding **2 months**.
Impact	The symptoms are present in at least two setting (i.e., at home, school, or with peers) and are severe in at least one of these.	The symptoms are present in at least two setting (i.e., at home, school, or with peers) and are severe in at least one of these.

[a] Criterion differs between DMDD and SMD; differences are highlighted **in bold**.

sadness, whereas DMDD criteria only requires irritability. Second, the definition of SMD includes a hyperarousal criterion which is omitted in the DMDD criteria. Table 12.1 highlights differences between DMDD and SMD criteria (Leibenluft et al., 2003).

DISTINGUISHING CHRONIC VERSUS EPISODIC IRRITABILITY

Although there are some studies on DMDD, most of the research aimed at differentiating chronic irritability from pediatric BD have been done using SMD criteria. The outcomes of such research provide compelling evidence against the notion that severe, chronic irritability is an early-life form of BD. We summarize some of these findings here.

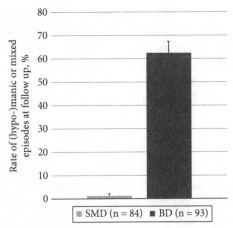

FIGURE 12.3 *Bars with standard errors show the percentage of patients with either severe mood dysregulation (SMD) or bipolar disorder (BD) who developed a (hypo-)manic or mixed episode during the follow-up period.*

Adapted from Stringaris et al. (2010).

First, follow-up studies in community samples show no associations between dimensional measures of irritability and later BD (Brotman et al., 2006; Leibenluft, Cohen, Gorrindo, Brook, & Pine, 2006; Stringaris, Cohen, Pine, & Leibenluft, 2009). The results are similar in referred samples. A clinical follow-up study (median time 28.7 months) demonstrated a clear difference in the rate of manic symptoms between youth with SMD and those with classic, episodic BD. As shown in Figure 12.3, only 1 of 84 SMD subjects (1.2%) experienced a (hypo-) manic episode during the study, whereas the frequency of such episodes was more than 50 times higher in those with narrowly defined BD (58/93, 62.4%) (Stringaris, Baroni et al., 2010). Findings were similar in other studies (Axelson et al., 2012; Deveney et al., 2015).

Second, SMD and BD also differ in family history of psychiatric disorders (Axelson et al., 2012; Brotman et al., 2007). Parents of youth with narrowly defined BD were significantly more likely to have BD (14/42, 33.3%) than parents of youth with SMD (1/37, 2.7%) (Brotman et al., 2006). Indeed, a recent study found higher rates of DMDD symptoms in offspring of parents with depression than offspring of parents with BD, and DMDD diagnoses were only present in the former (Propper et al., 2017).

Third, behavioral and functional magnetic resonance imaging (MRI) studies have found that while both youths with BD and those with SMD have impairments in labeling facial emotions (Guyer et al., 2007; Rich et al., 2008), the neural correlates of this deficit differ between the two groups (Brotman et al., 2010; Thomas et al., 2012; Wiggins et al., 2016). A similar pattern was found in their response to frustration; that is, although both SMD and BD youth displayed significantly more negative affect than healthy controls in response to negative feedback, patients with SMD differed from those with BD in their event-related potentials (Rich et al., 2007) and brain activation patterns (Rich et al., 2011). In addition, recent evidence suggests that the pathophysiological correlates of trait irritability itself differs between BD and DMDD (Wiggins et al., 2016). Chapters 3 and 8 provide more details on brain imaging and physiological studies.

EPIDEMIOLOGY

One of the main concerns about the introduction of DMDD has been pathologizing normal childhood behaviors, such as temper outbursts (Althoff et al., 2016; Axelson et al., 2012; Freeman, Youngstrom, Youngstrom, & Findling, 2016; Mayes, Waxmonsky, Calhoun, & Bixler, 2016). However, the low prevalence of DMDD in epidemiological studies suggests this was an exaggerated concern. The category of SMD, closely related to DMDD, has been estimated to occur in about 3% of the population of 9- to 16-year-olds (Brotman et al., 2006). More recently, a study by Copeland, Angold, Costello, and Egger (2013) using data from two different datasets showed that prevalence estimates of DMDD varied between 0.8% and 1.1% for children between 9 and 17 years of age. Moreover, studies using the most stringent criteria in adolescents have found rates as low as 0.12% (Althoff et al., 2016). This is relatively low compared to prevalence estimates for other conditions such as attention deficit/hyperactivity disorder (ADHD) or oppositional defiant disorder (ODD). Actually, DMDD prevalence is low (3.3%) even in youth at risk for mood disorders (Propper et al., 2017).

The temporal stability of the diagnosis and main symptoms of DMDD is low (Mayes et al., 2015), at least in community samples. For example, only 19% of children initially diagnosed with DMDD in the Longitudinal Assessment of Manic Symptoms study maintained the disorder across 12- and 24-month follow-ups (Axelson et al., 2012). This is in contrast to the moderate stability of the dimensional measure of irritability, with correlations ranging between 0.29 and 0.88 (Leadbeater & Homel, 2015; Roberson-Nay et al., 2015; Stringaris, Goodman et al., 2012; Whelan, Stringaris, Maughan, & Barker, 2013). The reasons for the low continuity are unclear but likely to be related to the arbitrarily chosen thresholds for duration of symptoms and maximum period allowed without symptoms. Indeed, most of the cases with DMDD who do not meet criteria at follow-up have significant ongoing subthreshold irritability and severe impairment (Deveney et al., 2015).

PSYCHOPATHOLOGICAL CORRELATES

DMDD co-occurs with other emotional or behavioral disorders in 65–90% of cases; these are mainly depression (~27%), anxiety (~26%), ADHD (~28%), conduct disorder (CD) (~26%), and ODD (~60%) (Althoff et al., 2016; Axelson et al., 2012;

Brotman et al., 2006; Copeland et al., 2013; Dougherty et al., 2014). However, rates of comorbidity differ across studies, probably due to the type of sample examined and age of participants. For example, rates of comorbidity are higher in referred samples and older participants, in which mood and behavioral disorders might co-occur in ~40% and ~70% of cases, respectively (Althoff et al., 2016; Axelson et al., 2012). Yet these numbers decrease to less than ~20% and ~50%, respectively, in community or younger samples (Copeland et al., 2013; Dougherty et al., 2014). In addition, some of the overlap with behavioral disorders is artificial due to item overlap (e.g., ODD) in post-hoc analyses. This is why the DSM-5 states that ODD should not be coded if DMDD criteria are met. In any case, it will be important to establish whether, after excluding such artificial overlap, DMDD shows more comorbidity than is characteristic of other established psychiatric disorders (e.g., ADHD). In addition to higher rates of comorbidities, DMDD is associated with high levels of social impairment, service use, school suspensions, and family poverty (Axelson et al., 2012; Copeland et al., 2013).

Regardless of the several associations between irritability and other disorders in cross-sectional analyses, longitudinal studies have demonstrated that irritability is a specific predictor of future depression and anxiety (Brotman et al., 2006; Leibenluft et al., 2006; Stringaris et al., 2009; Stringaris & Goodman, 2009). The results of these studies are summarized in a recent meta-analysis that included articles in which dimensional or categorical (i.e., DMDD or SMD) irritability was a predictor of any future psychiatric outcome. The analysis revealed that irritability was a significant predictor of depression and anxiety but not of BD, CD, ADHD, or substance abuse (Vidal-Ribas, Brotman, Valdivieso, Leibenluft, & Stringaris, 2016). Evidence suggests that this longitudinal association between irritability and depression/anxiety is explained by shared genetic variance rather than shared environmental risks (Savage et al., 2015; Stringaris, Zavos et al., 2012). The relation between irritability and depression is also evidenced in family studies; a family history of depression has been associated with the ODD irritability dimension (Krieger et al., 2013), and maternal depression predicts irritability in young children (Wiggins, Mitchell, Stringaris, & Leibenluft, 2014). In addition, irritability, alongside anxiety, is a major pathway to depression for children and adolescents at high risk (Rice et al., 2017; Whelan, Leibenluft, Stringaris, & Barker, 2015). Finally, DMDD and severe chronic irritability have also been associated with future functional impairment in longitudinal studies (Copeland, Shanahan, Egger, Angold, & Costello, 2014; Dougherty et al., 2016), including suicidality, independently of other psychopathology (Pickles et al., 2010).

DIFFERENTIAL DIAGNOSIS

Before diagnosing DMDD, one must exclude other conditions that may lead to tantrums and grumpiness, including medical conditions (particularly in hospital or other medical settings), drug-induced conditions, and other psychiatric problems that may be treatable in their own right.

Bipolar Disorders

Episodes are the single most reliable way to differentiate DMDD and BD-I or BD-II. Patients with DMDD do not have a course of illness with episodes that last for several days or weeks; instead, their symptoms are chronic, lasting at least a year. By contrast, patients with BD and their parents report more-or-less clearly defined periods of either mania or depression. As discussed earlier, mania is commonly characterized by elation, although irritability alone can be the predominant mood in a few cases. Such irritability should be a noticeable change from the patient's baseline mood and should be accompanied by the onset of other manic symptoms. The diagnosis of DMDD should not be assigned if the patient has ever had a manic or hypomanic episode or if elevated or expansive mood is present.

Oppositional Defiant Disorder

DSM-5 criteria for DMDD specify that ODD may not be diagnosed when both criteria are met. The intensity and frequency of temper outbursts, and the chronicity of disrupted mood between outbursts, is more severe in DMDD than in youth with ODD. For that reason, whereas most youth with DMDD will meet criteria for ODD (65–70%) the opposite is not the case; for example, rates of DMDD in youth with ODD were close to 30% in a large epidemiological study (Copeland et al., 2013). Moreover, given the significant mood component of DMDD and the specific associations among irritability, anxiety, and depression (Vidal-Ribas et al., 2016), DMDD is appropriately placed in the mood disorders section, whereas ODD is in the Disruptive Behavior Disorders section of DSM-5 (APA, 2013).

Attention Deficit/Hyperactivity Disorder

A child meeting criteria for DMDD can also be assigned a diagnosis of ADHD if the criteria are met. Rates of comorbidity of ADHD in children with DMDD are not different from those of DMDD in children with ADHD, with both close to 20% or lower (Copeland et al., 2013; Mulraney et al., 2016). One study in children with ADHD found that those who also met criteria for DMDD had higher rates of comorbidity, especially ODD and anxiety disorders, and poorer self-control and social functioning compared to those without DMDD (Mulraney et al., 2016). For the differential diagnosis, a careful history of the timing of irritability is important. In youth with ADHD, the severity of irritability commonly fluctuates as a consequence of external stimuli. Environmental events, such as the beginning of a new school year or those that place greater demands on concentration and the need to sit still, often coincide with worsening of irritability in those with ADHD.

Autism Spectrum Disorders

As further discussed in Chapter 11, the DSM-5 criteria for DMDD stipulate that if the patient's presentation is better explained by autism spectrum disorders (ASD), the diagnosis of DMDD should not be assigned. Temper outbursts in children with ASD are common and might occur as a response of change in routines or due to sensory sensitivity.

Depressive and Anxiety Disorders

Youth with depression or anxiety can be diagnosed with DMDD if the criteria for both disorders are met. However, children whose irritability is only present in the context of a depressive episode or an anxiety disorder, as discussed in detail in the next section, should not receive an additional diagnosis of DMDD. Of note, depression and anxiety in youth with DMDD is usually undiagnosed because disruptive symptoms overshadow those of low mood or anxiety. Given the evidence presented earlier about the high likelihood for irritable youth to develop these disorders as they mature, it is therefore important to assess depressive and anxiety symptoms in children with DMDD.

Irritability in Depressive Disorders

PHENOTYPIC PRESENTATION

A "major depressive episode" is defined in the DSM-5 by a period of at least 2 weeks during which there is either depressed mood or loss of interest or pleasure in most activities (Criterion A). In addition, for children and adolescents, it further notes that the mood may be irritable rather than sad.

In contrast to the criteria for BD, irritability as a cardinal symptom in depression is only allowed in young people, not in adults. This is the only difference between the diagnosis of depression in children and adults. However, similar to the irritability seen in pediatric mania, irritability in children with depression is also *episodic*; that is, it should be a change from the patient's baseline mood noticeable by parents, teachers, or friends.

EPIDEMIOLOGY

The lifetime prevalence estimate for depression in children and adolescents in the United States is 10–15% (Avenevoli, Swendsen, He, Burstein, & Merikangas, 2015; Merikangas et al., 2010). Reports from the adult literature in large community-based samples suggest that episodic irritability is a common symptom in depression, with a prevalence of around 30–55% (Fava et al., 2010; Judd, Schettler, Coryell, Akiskal, & Fiedorowicz, 2013). However, episodic irritability in the absence of depressed mood or anhedonia is extremely rare.

Evidence for irritability as a major criterion of depression in young people suggests the same profile. Using data from the Great Smoky Mountains Study, Stringaris et al. (2013) divided 9- to 16-year-old participants ($n = 1,420$) who met criteria for depression into three groups: those with depressed mood and no irritability, those with irritability and no depressed mood, and those with both depressed and irritable mood. In this study, the most common cardinal symptom in young people with depression was depressed mood (58.7%), followed by the co-occurrence of depressed and irritable mood (35.6%), while irritable mood alone was rare (5.7%). This suggests that specifying irritability as a cardinal symptom in its own right in pediatric depression does not have a significant impact in terms of identifying new cases. In this same investigation, Stringaris et al. (2013) found that boys were more likely to have depressed mood with irritability than were girls, who presented more often depressed mood only. Interestingly, there were no differences in age and pubertal stage between those with depressed and irritable mood and those with only depressed mood, suggesting that early-onset depression is not associated with higher likelihood of presenting with irritability.

PSYCHOPATHOLOGICAL CORRELATES

In terms of psychiatric correlates, Stringaris et al. (2013) found that nearly 50% of youth with depression and irritability had a comorbid ODD or CD diagnosis, more than double the rate of these comorbidities in the depressed-only group. In adults, depression with irritability is also associated with higher comorbidity rates, as well as with more severe and longer course of illness and functional impairment (Judd et al., 2013). Since most cases of adult depression have onset in adolescence (Kessler et al., 2005), it is essential to assess irritability symptoms in young people with depression, regardless of the predominant mood.

Irritability in Anxiety Disorders

PHENOTYPIC PRESENTATION

Irritable mood and temper outbursts appear in a host of anxiety disorders in children (Stoddard et al., 2014). For instance, irritability is included in the DSM-5 as an associated symptom of generalized anxiety disorder (GAD) for both adults and children. Yet, for children, it might be the only symptom needed along with excessive worry to meet criteria, whereas three additional symptoms are needed for adults. Temper outbursts are also listed in DSM-5 as associated features for selective mutism and separation anxiety. And for children, the criteria for specific and social phobia emphasize that the excessive fear and anxiety might be expressed by tantrums (APA, 2013).

Irritability is also an associated symptom of PTSD and acute stress disorder. Notably, this type of irritability that occurs after trauma is one of the most impairing symptoms of so-called *complex trauma*, a condition characterized by mood dysregulation resulting from prolonged exposure to severe stressors in developmentally vulnerable times such as early childhood or adolescence. A recent systematic review and meta-analysis found a pooled effect size of 0.37 for the association between mood dysregulation and PTSD (Villalta, Smith, Hickin, & Stringaris, 2018), suggesting that they are robustly related.

Although not listed in the DSM-5 as an associated feature, it is also common in children with obsessive compulsive disorder (OCD) to experience severe tantrums when their rituals are blocked, especially in those who also suffer from depression (Krebs et al., 2013).

In anxiety disorders, the expression of irritability is associated with the stimuli or situation that causes distress and fear, usually as a way to avoid exposure to such stimuli. For example, a child with separation anxiety might show anger toward the person who forces the separation. And an adolescent with severe social anxiety might have a tantrum in order to not attend school. When the stimulus or situation that causes distress disappears or is avoided, irritability also tends to wane. In GAD, irritability is associated with excessive worry about daily life issues. This context-dependent pattern is what differentiates the irritability seen in anxiety disorders from the more severe chronic irritable mood characteristic of DMDD.

EPIDEMIOLOGY

Anxiety disorders are the most common type of disorder in children and adolescents, with an estimated prevalence of 30%, with rates for individual disorders ranging from 2% for GAD to 19% for specific phobia (Merikangas et al., 2010). Irritability as a symptom is also very common. A study of 239 treatment-seeking youth with GAD showed that impairing irritability was present in more than 90% of cases (Comer, Pincus, & Hofmann, 2012). Moreover, the authors found that irritability was the stronger predictor of GAD even after controlling for the presence of depression, increasing the odds of having GAD in children by 12. However, irritability is also significant in other anxiety disorders. In a more recent study, Stoddard et al. (2014) found that irritability as a symptom was a problem for 50% of youth with anxiety disorders. When comparing parent- and self-reported levels of irritability across four groups—youth with anxiety disorders (including GAD, separation anxiety and social phobia), youth with SMD, youth with BD, and a healthy comparison group—the authors found that irritability was higher in those with anxiety than in the healthy group regardless of informant. Furthermore, parent-reported irritability uniquely predicted social phobia and separation anxiety disorder. In contrast, child-reported irritability was predictive of GAD.

PSYCHOPATHOLOGICAL CORRELATES

A recent study using a latent construct approach showed that the association between anxiety and irritability remained largely independent of other comorbid disorders, such as depression and ODD. Moreover, the magnitude of that association was not moderated by sex, age, or the presence of an anxiety disorder (Cornacchio, Crum, Coxe, Pincus, & Comer, 2016). In the earlier described study by Stoddard et al. (2014), parent-reported irritability was higher in children with anxiety and comorbid SMD or BD than those in the anxious-only group. Self-reported irritability was not different among the three patient groups.

Child anxiety disorders are not only associated with irritability, but also have high comorbidity rates with disorders in which irritability is a cardinal component, such as depression (Cummings, Caporino, & Kendall, 2014), ODD (Fraire & Ollendick, 2013), and DMDD (Copeland et al., 2013). In community samples, irritability is prospectively associated with GAD and specific phobias (Leibenluft et al., 2006; Stringaris et al., 2009). Similarly, as discussed earlier, DMDD has also been associated with future anxiety disorders (Copeland et al., 2014).

Conclusion

Irritability is omnipresent across mood and anxiety disorders in children and adolescents. Moreover, irritability as a disorder in its own right was recently introduced by the APA in the DSM-5 under the name of DMDD (APA, 2013). The introduction of DMDD was an attempt to hamper the dramatic rise of BD diagnoses in children presenting with severe chronic irritability. There is now compelling evidence from longitudinal, family, and pathophysiological studies showing that youth with chronic irritability differ from those with classic BD. For example, prospective epidemiological studies show that chronic irritability is specifically and robustly related to future depression and anxiety.

In this chapter, we described how irritability differs in phenomenology and course in mood and anxiety disorders. For instance, in children with depression or BD, irritability takes an episodic form and is commonly accompanied by depressed and elated mood, respectively, with very few cases presenting only irritable mood. Furthermore, in these disorders, the onset of episodic irritability should co-occur with the onset or worsening of other associated symptoms, such as grandiosity or pressured speech in the case of mania, or fatigue and excessive guilt in the case of depression, among others. In anxiety disorders, irritability is closely related to the presence or anticipation of feared situations and stimuli. In contrast, the irritability seen in DMDD is chronic and recurrent and much less influenced by changes in the environment.

Regardless of these differences, irritability seems to be associated with higher rates of comorbidity, increased risk for other mood disorders, and greater functional impairment. Therefore, clinicians should always consider assessing and, if required, treating irritability in children presenting with any mood or anxiety disorder.

References

Althoff, R. R., Crehan, E. T., He, J. P., Burstein, M., Hudziak, J. J., & Merikangas, K. R. (2016). Disruptive mood dysregulation disorder at ages 13-18: Results from the national comorbidity survey-adolescent supplement. *Journal of Child and Adolescent Psychopharmacology, 26*(2), 107–113. doi:10.1089/cap.2015.0038

American Psychiatric Association (APA). (2013). *Diagnostic and Statistical Manual of Mental Disorders* (5th ed.). Washington, DC: American Psychiatric Association.

Avenevoli, S., Swendsen, J., He, J. P., Burstein, M., & Merikangas, K. R. (2015). Major depression in the national comorbidity survey-adolescent supplement: Prevalence, correlates, and treatment. *Journal of American Academy of Child and Adolescent Psychiatry, 54*(1), 37–44.e32. doi:10.1016/j.jaac.2014.10.010

Axelson, D., Findling, R. L., Fristad, M. A., Kowatch, R. A., Youngstrom, E. A., Horwitz, S. M., . . . Birmaher, B. (2012). Examining the proposed disruptive mood dysregulation disorder diagnosis in children in the Longitudinal Assessment of Manic Symptoms study. *Journal of Clinical Psychiatry, 73*(10), 1342–1350. doi:10.4088/JCP.12m07674

Blader, J. C., & Carlson, G. A. (2007). Increased rates of bipolar disorder diagnoses among US child, adolescent, and adult inpatients, 1996–2004. *Biological Psychiatry, 62*(2), 107–114. doi:10.1016/j.biopsych.2006.11.006

Brotman, M. A., Kassem, L., Reising, M. M., Guyer, A. E., Dickstein, D. P., Rich, B. A., . . . Leibenluft, E. (2007). Parental diagnoses in youth with narrow phenotype bipolar disorder or severe mood dysregulation. *American Journal of Psychiatry, 164*(8), 1238–1241.

Brotman, M. A., Rich, B. A., Guyer, A. E., Lunsford, J. R., Horsey, S. E., Reising, M. M., . . . Leibenluft, E. (2010). Amygdala activation during emotion processing of neutral faces in children with severe mood dysregulation versus ADHD or bipolar disorder. *American Journal of Psychiatry, 167*(1), 61–69. doi:10.1176/appi.ajp.2009.09010043

Brotman, M. A., Schmajuk, M., Rich, B. A., Dickstein, D. P., Guyer, A. E., Costello, E. J., . . . Leibenluft, E. (2006). Prevalence, clinical correlates, and longitudinal course of severe mood dysregulation in children. *Biological Psychiatry, 60*(9), 991–997. doi:10.1016/j.biopsych.2006.08.042

Comer, J. S., Pincus, D. B., & Hofmann, S. G. (2012). Generalized anxiety disorder and the proposed associated symptoms criterion change for DSM-5 in a treatment-seeking sample of anxious youth. *Depression and Anxiety, 29*(12), 994–1003. doi:10.1002/da.21999

Copeland, W. E., Angold, A., Costello, E. J., & Egger, H. (2013). Prevalence, comorbidity, and correlates of DSM-5 proposed disruptive mood dysregulation disorder. *American Journal of Psychiatry, 170*(2), 173–179. doi:10.1176/appi.ajp.2012.12010132

Copeland, W. E., Shanahan, L., Egger, H., Angold, A., & Costello, E. J. (2014). Adult diagnostic and functional outcomes of DSM-5 disruptive mood dysregulation disorder. *American Journal of Psychiatry, 171*(6), 668–674. doi:10.1176/appi.ajp.2014.13091213

Cornacchio, D., Crum, K. I., Coxe, S., Pincus, D. B., & Comer, J. S. (2016). Irritability and severity of anxious symptomatology among youth with anxiety disorders. *Journal of American Academy of Child and Adolescent Psychiatry,* 55(1), 54–61. doi:10.1016/j.jaac.2015.10.007

Costello, E. J., Angold, A., Burns, B. J., Stangl, D. K., Tweed, D. L., Erkanli, A., & Worthman, C. M. (1996). The Great Smoky Mountains Study of Youth. Goals, design, methods, and the prevalence of DSM-III-R disorders. *Archives of General Psychiatry,* 53(12), 1129–1136.

Cummings, C. M., Caporino, N. E., & Kendall, P. C. (2014). Comorbidity of anxiety and depression in children and adolescents: 20 years after. *Psychology Bulletin,* 140(3), 816–845. doi:10.1037/a0034733

Deveney, C. M., Hommer, R. E., Reeves, E., Stringaris, A., Hinton, K. E., Haring, C. T., . . . Leibenluft, E. (2015). A prospective study of severe irritability in youths: 2- and 4-year follow-up. *Depression and Anxiety,* 32(5), 364–372. doi:10.1002/da.22336

Dougherty, L. R., Smith, V. C., Bufferd, S. J., Carlson, G. A., Stringaris, A., Leibenluft, E., & Klein, D. N. (2014). DSM-5 disruptive mood dysregulation disorder: Correlates and predictors in young children. *Psychological Medicine,* 1–12. doi:10.1017/s0033291713003115

Dougherty, L. R., Smith, V. C., Bufferd, S. J., Kessel, E. M., Carlson, G. A., & Klein, D. N. (2016). Disruptive mood dysregulation disorder at the age of 6 years and clinical and functional outcomes 3 years later. *Psychological Medicine,* 46(5), 1103–1114. doi:10.1017/S0033291715002809

Fava, M., Hwang, I., Rush, A. J., Sampson, N., Walters, E. E., & Kessler, R. C. (2010). The importance of irritability as a symptom of major depressive disorder: Results from the National Comorbidity Survey Replication. *Molecular Psychiatry,* 15(8), 856–867. doi:10.1038/mp.2009.20

Fraire, M. G., & Ollendick, T. H. (2013). Anxiety and oppositional defiant disorder: A transdiagnostic conceptualization. *Clinical Psychology Review,* 33(2), 229–240. doi:10.1016/j.cpr.2012.11.004

Freeman, A. J., Youngstrom, E. A., Youngstrom, J. K., & Findling, R. L. (2016). Disruptive mood dysregulation disorder in a community mental health clinic: Prevalence, comorbidity and correlates. *Journal of Child and Adolescent Psychopharmacology,* 26(2), 123–130. doi:10.1089/cap.2015.0061

Guyer, A. E., McClure, E. B., Adler, A. D., Brotman, M. A., Rich, B. A., Kimes, A. S., . . . Leibenluft, E. (2007). Specificity of facial expression labeling deficits in childhood psychopathology. *Journal of Child Psychology Psychiatry,* 48(9), 863–871.

Hunt, J., Birmaher, B., Leonard, H., Strober, M., Axelson, D., Ryan, N., . . . Keller, M. (2009). Irritability without elation in a large bipolar youth sample: Frequency and clinical description. *Journal of American Academy of Child and Adolescent Psychiatry,* 48(7), 730–739.

Hunt, J. I., Case, B. G., Birmaher, B., Stout, R. L., Dickstein, D. P., Yen, S., . . . Keller, M. B. (2013). Irritability and elation in a large bipolar youth sample: Relative symptom severity and clinical outcomes over 4 years. *Journal of Clinical Psychiatry,* 74(1), e110–e117. doi:10.4088/JCP.12m07874

James, A., Hoang, U., Seagroatt, V., Clacey, J., Goldacre, M., & Leibenluft, E. (2014). A comparison of American and English hospital discharge rates for pediatric bipolar disorder, 2000 to 2010. *Journal of American Academy of Child and Adolescent Psychiatry,* 53(6), 614–624. doi:10.1016/j.jaac.2014.02.008

Judd, L. L., Schettler, P. J., Coryell, W., Akiskal, H. S., & Fiedorowicz, J. G. (2013). Overt irritability/anger in unipolar major depressive episodes: Past and current characteristics and implications for long-term course. *JAMA Psychiatry, 70*(11), 1171–1180. doi:10.1001/jamapsychiatry.2013.1957

Kessler, R. C., Berglund, P., Demler, O., Jin, R., Merikangas, K. R., & Walters, E. E. (2005). Lifetime prevalence and age-of-onset distributions of DSM-IV disorders in the National Comorbidity Survey Replication. *Archives of General Psychiatry, 62*(6), 593–602. doi:10.1001/archpsyc.62.6.593

Krebs, G., Bolhuis, K., Heyman, I., Mataix-Cols, D., Turner, C., & Stringaris, A. (2013). Temper outbursts in paediatric obsessive-compulsive disorder and their association with depressed mood and treatment outcome. *Journal of Child Psychology Psychiatry, 54*(3), 313–322. doi:10.1111/j.1469-7610.2012.02605.x

Krieger, F. V., Polanczyk, V. G., Goodman, R., Rohde, L. A., Graeff-Martins, A. S., Salum, G., . . . Stringaris, A. (2013). Dimensions of oppositionality in a Brazilian community sample: Testing the DSM-5 proposal and etiological links. *Journal of American Academy of Child and Adolescent Psychiatry, 52*(4), 389–400 e381. doi:10.1016/j.jaac.2013.01.004

Leadbeater, B. J., & Homel, J. (2015). Irritable and defiant sub-dimensions of ODD: Their stability and prediction of internalizing symptoms and conduct problems from adolescence to young adulthood. *Journal of Abnormal Child Psychology, 43*(3), 407–421. doi:10.1007/s10802-014-9908-3

Leibenluft, E. (2011). Severe mood dysregulation, irritability, and the diagnostic boundaries of bipolar disorder in youths. *American Journal of Psychiatry, 168*(2), 129–142. doi:10.1176/appi.ajp.2010.10050766

Leibenluft, E., Charney, D. S., Towbin, K. E., Bhangoo, R. K., & Pine, D. S. (2003). Defining clinical phenotypes of juvenile mania. *American Journal of Psychiatry, 160*(3), 430–437.

Leibenluft, E., Cohen, P., Gorrindo, T., Brook, J. S., & Pine, D. S. (2006). Chronic versus episodic irritability in youth: A community-based, longitudinal study of clinical and diagnostic associations. *Journal of Child and Adolescent Psychopharmacology, 16*(4), 456–466. doi:10.1089/cap.2006.16.456

Lohr, W. D., Chowning, R. T., Stevenson, M. D., & Williams, P. G. (2015). Trends in atypical antipsychotics prescribed to children six years of age or less on Medicaid in Kentucky. *Journal of Child and Adolescent Psychopharmacology, 25*(5), 440–443. doi:10.1089/cap.2014.0057

Mayes, S. D., Mathiowetz, C., Kokotovich, C., Waxmonsky, J., Baweja, R., Calhoun, S. L., & Bixler, E. O. (2015). Stability of disruptive mood dysregulation disorder symptoms (irritable-angry mood and temper outbursts) throughout childhood and adolescence in a general population sample. *Journal of Abnormal Child Psychology, 43*(8), 1543–1549. doi:10.1007/s10802-015-0033-8

Mayes, S. D., Waxmonsky, J. D., Calhoun, S. L., & Bixler, E. O. (2016). Disruptive mood dysregulation disorder symptoms and association with oppositional defiant and other disorders in a general population child sample. *Journal of Child and Adolescent Psychopharmacology, 26*(2), 101–106. doi:10.1089/cap.2015.0074

Merikangas, K. R., He, J. P., Burstein, M., Swanson, S. A., Avenevoli, S., Cui, L., . . . Swendsen, J. (2010). Lifetime prevalence of mental disorders in US adolescents: Results from the National Comorbidity Survey Replication: Adolescent Supplement (NCS-A). *Journal of American Academy of Child and Adolescent Psychiatry, 49*(10), 980–989. doi:10.1016/j.jaac.2010.05.017

Mikita, N., & Stringaris, A. (2013). Mood dysregulation. *European Child and Adolescent Psychiatry*, 22(Suppl 1), S11–S16. doi:10.1007/s00787-012-0355-9

Moreno, C., Laje, G., Blanco, C., Jiang, H., Schmidt, A. B., & Olfson, M. (2007). National trends in the outpatient diagnosis and treatment of bipolar disorder in youth. *Archives of General Psychiatry*, 64(9), 1032–1039. doi:10.1001/archpsyc.64.9.1032

Mulraney, M., Schilpzand, E. J., Hazell, P., Nicholson, J. M., Anderson, V., Efron, D., . . . Sciberras, E. (2016). Comorbidity and correlates of disruptive mood dysregulation disorder in 6-8-year-old children with ADHD. *European Child and Adolescent Psychiatry*, 25(3), 321–330. doi:10.1007/s00787-015-0738-9

NICE. (2014). *Bipolar disorder: The assessment and management of bipolar disorder in adults, children and young people in primary and secondary care. NICE guideline (CG185).* London: National Institute for Health and Care Excellence.

Olfson, M., Blanco, C., Liu, L., Moreno, C., & Laje, G. (2006). National trends in the outpatient treatment of children and adolescents with antipsychotic drugs. *Archives of General Psychiatry*, 63(6), 679–685. doi:10.1001/archpsyc.63.6.679

Pickles, A., Aglan, A., Collishaw, S., Messer, J., Rutter, M., & Maughan, B. (2010). Predictors of suicidality across the life span: The Isle of Wight study. *Psychology Medicine*, 40(9), 1453–1466. doi:10.1017/s0033291709991905

Propper, L., Cumby, J., Patterson, V. C., Drobinin, V., Glover, J. M., MacKenzie, L. E., . . . Uher, R. (2017). Disruptive mood dysregulation disorder in offspring of parents with depression and bipolar disorder. *British Journal of Psychiatry*. doi:10.1192/bjp.bp.117.198754

Rice, F., Sellers, R., Hammerton, G., Eyre, O., Bevan-Jones, R., Thapar, A. K., . . . Thapar, A. (2017). Antecedents of new-onset major depressive disorder in children and adolescents at high familial risk. *JAMA Psychiatry*, 74(2), 153–160. doi:10.1001/jamapsychiatry.2016.3140

Rich, B. A., Carver, F. W., Holroyd, T., Rosen, H. R., Mendoza, J. K., Cornwell, B. R., . . . Leibenluft, E. (2011). Different neural pathways to negative affect in youth with pediatric bipolar disorder and severe mood dysregulation. *Journal of Psychiatric Research*, 45(10), 1283–1294. doi:10.1016/j.jpsychires.2011.04.006

Rich, B. A., Grimley, M. E., Schmajuk, M., Blair, K. S., Blair, R. J., & Leibenluft, E. (2008). Face emotion labeling deficits in children with bipolar disorder and severe mood dysregulation. *Developmental Psychopathology*, 20(2), 529–546. doi:10.1017/s0954579408000266

Rich, B. A., Schmajuk, M., Perez-Edgar, K. E., Fox, N. A., Pine, D. S., & Leibenluft, E. (2007). Different psychophysiological and behavioral responses elicited by frustration in pediatric bipolar disorder and severe mood dysregulation. *American Journal of Psychiatry*, 164(2), 309–317. doi:10.1176/ajp.2007.164.2.309

Roberson-Nay, R., Leibenluft, E., Brotman, M. A., Myers, J., Larsson, H., Lichtenstein, P., & Kendler, K. S. (2015). Longitudinal stability of genetic and environmental influences on irritability: From childhood to young adulthood. *American Journal of Psychiatry*, 172(7), 657–664. doi:10.1176/appi.ajp.2015.14040509

Savage, J., Verhulst, B., Copeland, W., Althoff, R. R., Lichtenstein, P., & Roberson-Nay, R. (2015). A genetically informed study of the longitudinal relation between irritability and anxious/depressed symptoms. *Journal of American Academy of Child and Adolescent Psychiatry*, 54(5), 377–384. doi:10.1016/j.jaac.2015.02.010

Stoddard, J., Stringaris, A., Brotman, M. A., Montville, D., Pine, D. S., & Leibenluft, E. (2014). Irritability in child and adolescent anxiety disorders. *Depression and Anxiety,* 31(7), 566–573.

Stringaris, A., Baroni, A., Haimm, C., Brotman, M., Lowe, C. H., Myers, F., . . . Leibenluft, E. (2010). Pediatric bipolar disorder versus severe mood dysregulation: Risk for manic episodes on follow-up. *Journal of American Academy of Child and Adolescent Psychiatry,* 49(4), 397–405. doi:10.1016/j.jaac.2010.01.013

Stringaris, A., Cohen, P., Pine, D. S., & Leibenluft, E. (2009). Adult outcomes of youth irritability: A 20-year prospective community-based study. *American Journal of Psychiatry,* 166(9), 1048–1054. doi:10.1176/appi.ajp.2009.08121849

Stringaris, A., & Goodman, R. (2009). Longitudinal outcome of youth oppositionality: Irritable, headstrong, and hurtful behaviors have distinctive predictions. *Journal of American Academy of Child and Adolescent Psychiatry,* 48(4), 404–412. doi:10.1097/CHI.0b013e3181984f30

Stringaris, A., Goodman, R., Ferdinando, S., Razdan, V., Muhrer, E., Leibenluft, E., & Brotman, M. A. (2012). The Affective Reactivity Index: A concise irritability scale for clinical and research settings. *Journal of Child Psychology Psychiatry,* 53(11), 1109–1117. doi:10.1111/j.1469-7610.2012.02561.x

Stringaris, A., Maughan, B., Copeland, W. S., Costello, E. J., & Angold, A. (2013). Irritable mood as a symptom of depression in youth: prevalence, developmental, and clinical correlates in the Great Smoky Mountains Study. *Journal of American Academy of Child and Adolescent Psychiatry,* 52(8), 831–840. doi:10.1016/j.jaac.2013.05.017

Stringaris, A., Santosh, P., Leibenluft, E., & Goodman, R. (2010). Youth meeting symptom and impairment criteria for mania-like episodes lasting less than four days: An epidemiological enquiry. *Journal of Child Psychology Psychiatry,* 51(1), 31–38. doi:10.1111/j.1469-7610.2009.02129.x

Stringaris, A., Zavos, H., Leibenluft, E., Maughan, B., & Eley, T. C. (2012). Adolescent irritability: Phenotypic associations and genetic links with depressed mood. *American Journal of Psychiatry,* 169(1), 47–54. doi:10.1176/appi.ajp.2011.10101549

Thomas, L. A., Brotman, M. A., Muhrer, E. J., Rosen, B. H., Bones, B. L., Reynolds, R. C., . . . Leibenluft, E. (2012). Parametric modulation of neural activity by emotion in youth with bipolar disorder, youth with severe mood dysregulation, and healthy volunteers. *Archives of General Psychiatry,* 69(12), 1257–1266. doi:10.1001/archgenpsychiatry.2012.913

Towbin, K., Axelson, D., Leibenluft, E., & Birmaher, B. (2013). Differentiating bipolar disorder-not otherwise specified and severe mood dysregulation. *Journal of American Academy of Child and Adolescent Psychiatry,* 52(5), 466–481. doi:10.1016/j.jaac.2013.02.006

Van Meter, A. R., Burke, C., Kowatch, R. A., Findling, R. L., & Youngstrom, E. A. (2016). Ten-year updated meta-analysis of the clinical characteristics of pediatric mania and hypomania. *Bipolar Disorder,* 18(1), 19–32. doi:10.1111/bdi.12358

Van Meter, A. R., Moreira, A. L., & Youngstrom, E. A. (2011). Meta-analysis of epidemiologic studies of pediatric bipolar disorder. *Journal of Clinical Psychiatry,* 72(9), 1250–1256. doi:10.4088/JCP.10m06290

Vidal-Ribas, P., Brotman, M. A., Valdivieso, I., Leibenluft, E., & Stringaris, A. (2016). The status of irritability in psychiatry: A conceptual and quantitative review. *Journal of American Academy of Child and Adolescent Psychiatry,* 55(7), 556–570. doi:http://dx.doi.org/10.1016/j.jaac.2016.04.014

Villalta, L., Smith, P., Hickin, N., & Stringaris, A. (2018). Emotion regulation difficulties in traumatized youth: A meta-analysis and conceptual review. *European Child and Adolescent Psychiatry*. doi:10.1007/s00787-018-1105-4

Whelan, Y. M., Leibenluft, E., Stringaris, A., & Barker, E. D. (2015). Pathways from maternal depressive symptoms to adolescent depressive symptoms: The unique contribution of irritability symptoms. *Journal of Child Psychology Psychiatry, 56*(10), 1092–1100. doi:10.1111/jcpp.12395

Whelan, Y. M., Stringaris, A., Maughan, B., & Barker, E. D. (2013). Developmental continuity of oppositional defiant disorder subdimensions at ages 8, 10, and 13 years and their distinct psychiatric outcomes at age 16 years. *Journal of American Academy of Child and Adolescent Psychiatry, 52*(9), 961–969. doi:10.1016/j.jaac.2013.06.013

Wiggins, J. L., Brotman, M. A., Adleman, N. E., Kim, P., Oakes, A. H., Reynolds, R. C., . . . Leibenluft, E. (2016). Neural correlates of irritability in disruptive mood dysregulation and bipolar disorders. *American Journal of Psychiatry*, appiajp201515060833. doi:10.1176/appi.ajp.2015.15060833

Wiggins, J. L., Mitchell, C., Stringaris, A., & Leibenluft, E. (2014). Developmental trajectories of irritability and bidirectional associations with maternal depression. *Journal of American Academy of Child and Adolescent Psychiatry, 53*(11), 1191–1205, 1205 e1191–1194. doi:10.1016/j.jaac.2014.08.005

Wozniak, J., Biederman, J., Kiely, K., Ablon, J. S., Faraone, S. V., Mundy, E., & Mennin, D. (1995). Mania-like symptoms suggestive of childhood-onset bipolar disorder in clinically referred children. *Journal of American Academy of Child and Adolescent Psychiatry, 34*(7), 867–876. doi:10.1097/00004583-199507000-00010

Yuen, L. D., Miller, S., Wang, P. W., Hooshmand, F., Holtzman, J. N., Goffin, K. C., . . . Ketter, T. A. (2016). Current irritability robustly related to current and prior anxiety in bipolar disorder. *Journal of Psychiatric Research, 79*, 101–107. doi:10.1016/j.jpsychires.2016.05.006

Yuen, L. D., Shah, S., Do, D., Miller, S., Wang, P. W., Hooshmand, F., & Ketter, T. A. (2016). Current irritability associated with hastened depressive recurrence and delayed depressive recovery in bipolar disorder. *International Journal of Bipolar Disorder, 4*. doi:10.1186/s40345-016-0056-2

{ SECTION V }

Treatment

13

Behavioral Interventions for Irritability in Children and Adolescents

Denis G. Sukhodolsky, Theresa R. Gladstone, Carolyn L. Marsh, and Kimberly R. Cimino

Childhood irritability, characterized by frequent and developmentally inappropriate anger outbursts, is among the most frequent reasons for outpatient mental health referrals (Costello, He, Sampson, Kessler, & Merikangas, 2014). Behavioral manifestations of irritability can range from temper tantrums and screaming matches to physical aggression that may result in harm to self or others. The mood component of irritability has been framed as enduring and intense anger. Within the current approaches to irritability, the term has been used to denote a dimension of psychopathology, as well as categorically defined symptoms (Brotman, Kircanski, & Leibenluft, 2017; Vidal-Ribas, Brotman, Valdivieso, Leibenluft, & Stringaris, 2016). In the *Diagnostic and Statistical Manual of Mental Disorders*, Fifth Edition (DSM-5), anger/irritability is an essential feature of disruptive mood dysregulation disorder (DMDD) and oppositional defiant disorder (ODD), and aggressive behavior is most commonly associated with conduct disorder (CD) (American Psychiatric Association [APA], 2013). Irritability is also a common symptom in childhood anxiety, a core symptom of depressive disorder, and an associated feature in children with attention deficit/hyperactivity disorder (ADHD). For example, in population-based studies, the prevalence rate of disruptive behavior disorders ranges from 14% to 35% in children with ADHD, from 14% to 62% in anxiety disorders, and from 9% to 45% in mood disorders (Nock, Kazdin, Hiripi, & Kessler, 2007). Children with neurodevelopmental disorders such as autism spectrum disorder (ASD) and Tourette disorder also present with high rates of co-occurring irritability, which often confers greater functional impairment than the core symptoms of the primary disorder (Sukhodolsky, Gladstone, & Marsh, 2018; Sukhodolsky et al., 2003).

This review is focused on psychosocial interventions for anger/irritability and aggression as dimensions of child psychopathology. The primary focus is on parent management training (PMT) and cognitive-behavioral therapy (CBT) because these modalities have received extensive empirical support as stand-alone interventions (Dretzke et al., 2009; Sukhodolsky, Kassinove, & Gorman, 2004). There is also evidence that these behavioral treatments can be helpful in conjunction with medication management for severe aggression (Aman et al., 2014). Then, we discuss current work on the transdiagnostic approach to CBT for irritability and aggression and recent studies of behavioral interventions for children with severe irritability or DMDD. Last, we discuss the adaptation of dialectical behavior therapy (DBT) for children with severe mood dysregulation (Perepletchikova et al., 2017).

Principles and Efficacy of Parent Management Training

PMT is one of the most studied behavioral interventions for childhood behavioral and emotional disorders (McCart & Sheidow, 2016). PMT aims to ameliorate patterns of family interactions that produce antecedents and consequences of maintaining tantrums, aggression, and noncompliance (Patterson, DeBaryshe, & Ramsey, 1989). PMT techniques stem from the fundamental principle of operant conditioning, which states that the likelihood of behavior to recur is increased or weakened based on the events that follow the behavior (Skinner, 1938). For example, a child is more likely to have another tantrum if previous anger outbursts have resulted in an escape from parental demands or the continuation of a preferred activity. Behaviors such as noncompliance, whining, or bickering may also be reinforced if the same benefits are afforded to the child.

Harsh and inconsistent discipline, such as excessive scolding and corporal punishment, has also been shown to increase aggressive behaviors (Gershoff, 2002). The broad goals of PMT are to reduce the child's aggression and noncompliance by improving parental competence in managing these maladaptive behaviors. During PMT, parents are taught to identify the function of maladaptive behavior, to give praise for appropriate behavior, to communicate directions effectively, to ignore maladaptive attention-seeking behavior, and to use consistent consequences for disruptive behaviors. The key feature of PMT is that new parenting skills are taught in a systematic and structured way via modeling, practice, role play, and feedback from the therapists. Learning new skills requires practice and repetition, and merely telling parents what to do cannot develop these skills. PMT is conducted with parents, although, for some approaches, children are invited to facilitate the practice of these new skills (Eyberg, Nelson, & Boggs, 2008). The efficacy and effectiveness of PMT have been evaluated in more than a hundred randomized controlled studies (Dretzke et al., 2009; Michelson, Davenport, Dretzke, Barlow, & Day, 2013), and excellent treatment manuals are available for clinicians (Barkley, 2013; Kazdin, 2005). There is evidence that the improvements in child behavior are stable over time and can prevent antisocial behavior in adulthood (Scott, Briskman, & O'Connor, 2014), although no studies to our knowledge have reported long-term follow-up data specifically regarding irritability after PMT. Of note, most PMT studies were conducted in children referred for disruptive behavior, and work is needed to demonstrate effectiveness of PMT in children with DMDD (Stringaris, Vidal-Ribas, Brotman, & Leibenluft, 2017).

Positive reinforcement of desirable behavior, such as getting through a frustrating situation (e.g., turning off the video game and starting homework) without whining or having an outburst, is at the core of PMT. Although intuitively appealing, reinforcement principles and techniques may be misinterpreted. For example, when social reinforcement such as attention and praise is discussed with parents, a common reaction is "we do it all the time." However, further discussions often reveal that attention may be given to disruptive behavior, and appropriate behavior may go unrecognized by praise. Attention, praise, privileges, and various tokens become positive reinforcers only when they are delivered contingently (after the behavior) and consistently (every time behavior occurs). Helping parents to focus on positive behaviors and reinforce these behaviors with social rewards (such as attention and praise, as well as tangible rewards, such as points or screen time) is the main theme of most PMT approaches. For example, Russell Barkley includes a session dedicated to helping parents schedule periods of time during the day when they can "catch their child being good" and provide frequent and developmentally appropriate prizes to their children (Barkley, 2013).

Techniques that include punishment, such as reprimands, taking away privileges, or assigning undesired chores, are also discussed during PMT. A critical point to be conveyed to the parents is that punishment alone is unlikely to change behavior. Sometimes parents who bring their children to treatment for aggression and noncompliance find themselves in what has been referred to as "punishment traps," where punishment is used excessively and thus inadvertently perpetuates a child's behavioral problems (Kazdin, 2005). A large body of research has demonstrated that harsh and inconsistent discipline, such as excessive verbal scolding and corporal punishment, increases aggression in the long term. However, because punishment may lead to immediate compliance and halt the child's aggression in the moment, this parenting practice is reinforced by the momentary cessation of misbehavior. This cycle of child tantrums and punitive parenting practices can be mutually reinforcing via the mechanisms of escape–avoidance conditioning, leading to aversive parent–child relationships (Patterson, 1982). Excessive punishment erodes family relationships and limits opportunities for fostering positive parent–child interactions. Reinforcement of "positive opposites" is an alternative to punishment that can be used for reducing inappropriate behavior. For example, a child may earn points for not swearing when frustrated. This shift from punishment to positive consequences for expected behavior is at the heart of PMT programs (NICE, 2013; Webster-Stratton & Reid, 2003).

New Directions in PMT Research

In addition to parenting interventions based on social learning and coercive family processing models, there has been increasing recognition of the roles that parental socialization of emotions can play in the development, prevention, and treatment of disruptive behavior and irritability (Dunsmore, Booker, Ollendick, & Greene, 2016; Johnson, Hawes, Eisenberg, Kohlhoff, & Dudeney, 2017). Several studies have addressed the effects of a group-based parenting program called "Tuning in to Kids," which consists of teaching parents emotional coaching skills (Havighurst, Wilson, Harley, & Prior, 2009). Emotion coaching skills were based on Gottman et al. (1997) and involve (1) awareness of the child's emotion at varying intensities, (2) considering the child's emotion as an opportunity for affection and teaching, (3) empathetic acceptance of emotions, (4) teaching the child to use words to describe how they feel, and (5) helping the child with problem-solving in the context of negative emotions. The program was first tested with groups of parents of preschool-age children in six 2-hour long weekly sessions and showed increased skills of emotional coaching in the parents and improved emotional awareness and decreased behavioral problems in the children (Havighurst, Wilson, Harley, Prior, & Kehoe, 2010). Later studies demonstrated that the emotional coaching program was also helpful for young children with emerging conduct problems (Havighurst et al., 2015) and adolescents with depression and anxiety (Duncombe et al., 2016; Kehoe, Havighurst, & Harley, 2014). When compared in a randomized trial, behavior-focused parent training (Triple P) and emotion-focused parenting training (Tuning in to Kids) were equally effective for reducing conduct problems in 4- to 9-year-old children (Salmon, Dittman, Sanders, Burson, & Hammington, 2014).

One meta-analytic review suggested that program components associated with larger effects include increased positive parent–child interactions and emotional communication skills, parental consistency with consequences, and in vivo practice of new skills with parents (Wyatt Kaminski, Valle, Filene, & Boyle, 2008). Large-sample studies are required to provide sufficient power to detect differences between active treatments and to examine moderators of differential treatment response. Of relevance to the mood/emotional aspect of irritability, one study of PMT in young children with ODD reported that children with a greater level of irritable ODD symptoms showed better response to PMT than children with a greater level of headstrong ODD symptoms (Scott & O'Connor, 2012), suggesting that PMT can be useful for children with irritability in the context of oppositional behavior.

Other developments in parent-directed interventions have included adaptations of PMT for children with specific neurodevelopmental disorders. Our work has shown that PMT can be helpful for irritability in children with Tourette syndrome (TS; Scahill et al., 2006) and in children with obsessive compulsive disorder (OCD) (Sukhodolsky, Gorman, Scahill, Findley, & McGuire, 2013). Modifications of PMT for these clinical populations required careful consideration of anger outbursts in the context of symptoms manifesting from the primary disorder. For example, irritability and noncompliance could be associated with OCD-related fears or failure of parents to provide accommodations for compulsive behaviors (Storch et al., 2012). In children with tics, disruptive behaviors have to be disentangled from complex tics that might resemble purposeful behavior (Sukhodolsky & Scahill, 2007).

Irritability in children with ASD has been a long-standing target of clinical research, including pharmacological and behavioral interventions (Fung et al., 2016; Vismara & Rogers, 2010). A recent meta-analysis reported eight randomized studies of PMT for children with autism with an average effect size of 0.59 (Postorino et al., 2017). One approach to PMT was developed to address common and unique manifestations of irritability in ASD by enhancing standard PMT techniques with functional analysis, visual schedules for routine events, and teaching communication and daily living skills (Johnson et al., 2007). A randomized trial of 124 children with ASD aged 4–13 tested this program in a comparison of risperidone alone to risperidone plus PMT and revealed greater reduction of disruptive behavior and lower drug dose in the combined condition (Aman et al., 2009). More recently, the Research Units on Behavioral Intervention (RUBI) Autism Network tested a preschool version of this program in 180 children with autism aged 3–7 relative to a parent education control condition and demonstrated significant reductions in parent-rated irritability and noncompliance in the active treatment condition (Bearss et al., 2015).

Child-Directed Cognitive-Behavioral Therapy Approaches

Child-focused CBT targets deficits in emotion regulation and social problem-solving skills that are associated with aggressive behavior (Dodge, 2003). By convention, the term "cognitive-behavioral" is used to refer to interventions that are conducted with the child and use structured strategies to produce changes in thinking, feeling, and behavior (Kendall, 2006). Common techniques of CBT for irritability and aggression include identifying the antecedents and consequences of aggressive behavior, learning strategies for recognizing and regulating anger experiences, and practicing cognitive problem-solving skills and socially appropriate behaviors that can replace angry and aggressive reactions. Although CBT is conducted with the child, parents have multiple roles in treatment, including providing information about their behavioral problems and creating a home environment where children can practice skills acquired during CBT sessions. Importantly, parents are asked to recognize their child's effort when applying frustration tolerance and emotion regulation skills learned in CBT to anger-provoking situations and to provide praise and rewards for behavioral improvements.

Various cognitive behavioral approaches place differing degrees of emphasis on each of three content areas: regulation of excessive anger, learning social problem-solving strategies, and/or developing social skills alternative to aggressive behaviors. Anger control training (ACT) was first developed for adults (Novaco, 1975) based on Meichenbaum's stress inoculation model (Meichenbaum & Cameron, 1973) and aims to improve emotion regulation and social-cognitive deficits in aggressive children (Sukhodolsky, Smith, McCauley, Ibrahim, & Piasecka, 2016). Children are taught to monitor their emotional arousal and use techniques such as cognitive reappraisal and relaxation to modulate elevated levels of anger. As part of the training, children learn to tolerate frustration associated with common anger-provoking situations, such as being teased by peers or reprimanded by adults, as well as to use other coping strategies for excessive anger. Several research programs have evaluated versions of ACT with children (Lochman, Barry, & Pardini, 2003), adolescents (Deffenbacher, Lynch, Oetting, & Kemper, 1996; Feindler & Ecton, 1986), and young adults (Kassinove & Tafrate, 2002). Compared to other CBT approaches for youth with aggressive behavior, ACT places a relatively greater emphasis on the emotional experience of anger. Several studies that included narrowly defined measures of anger as an emotional experience, such as the State Trait Anger Expression Inventory (STAXI) (Spielberger, 1999) and the Children's Inventory of Anger (Nelson & Finch, 2000), reported reduction of anger after ACT (Deffenbacher et al., 1996; Sukhodolsky et al., 2009).

Originating from research on social information processing (Dodge, Bates, & Pettit, 1990) and problem-solving in children (Shure & Spivack, 1972), hundreds of studies have examined the association between cognitions in social situations and aggressive behavior (Dodge, 2003). This model suggests that there are five steps in cognitive processing of social information: detection of cues, interpretation of cues, solution generation, analysis of consequences, and response enactment. At all steps, there could be two types of problems, cognitive deficits (not engaging a particular process) and cognitive deficiencies (making an error in processing), that are related to anger and aggressive behavior. Problem-solving skills training (PSST) addresses cognitive processes, such as faulty perceptions and decision-making, that can lead to excessive anger experience and aggressive behavior. For example, hostile attribution bias may lead to attribution of accidental events (such as tripping over a friend's foot by accident) to hostile intent of another person ("he tripped me on purpose to make fun of me in front of other kids"). In turn, unfortunate outcomes that are attributed to purposeful and hostile actions of another are more likely to lead to retaliation. Also, inability to recognize negative consequences of aggressive behavior or generate alternative solutions to interpersonal confrontations may contribute to aggressive behavior. To address these social-cognitive processes, participants of PSST are taught to analyze interpersonal conflicts, develop nonaggressive solutions, and think about the consequences of their actions in problematic situations. The efficacy of PSST has been demonstrated in several controlled studies (Guerra & Slaby, 1990; Hudley & Graham, 1993; Kazdin, Siegel, & Bass, 1992). There is also evidence that the effects of PSST on conduct problems may be mediated by a change in the targeted deficits in social information processing (Sukhodolsky, Golub, Stone, & Orban, 2005; Van Manen, Prins, & Emmelkamp, 2004).

This focus on anger and its regulation in many of the CBT approaches that have been tested in children with disruptive behavior disorders may be relevant to the treatment of chronic irritability. A recent study tested an integrative group therapy for severe mood dysregulation that consisted of 11 child group sessions of CBT for aggression and mood disorders and 11 parenting group sessions (Waxmonsky et al., 2016). This treatment was compared to community care in a randomized trial with a sample of 56 children aged 7–12 with ADHD who were stabilized on ADHD medication, but who continued to experience impairing symptoms of severe mood dysregulation. The primary outcome measure was a mood severity index (Fristad, Verducci, Walters, & Young, 2009) that combined scores from the Children's Depression Rating Scale-Revised (CDRS-R) (Poznanski & Mokros, 1996) and Young Mania Rating Scale (YMRS) (Fristad, Weller, & Weller, 1992). The outcome measure of irritability was a sum score of the three irritability items of the ODD subscale on the parent-rated Disruptive Behavior Disorders Rating Scale (DBD-RS) (Pelham, Gnagy, Greenslade, & Milich, 1992). Integrative group therapy was superior to community care for reduction of parent-rated irritability, but not for other measures of mood symptoms. Taken together, this study shows promise for combined child- and parent-focused treatments derived from those developed for children with disruptive behavior disorders for treating children with primary symptoms of irritability.

Transdiagnostic CBT Approach to Irritability

Our own approach to behavioral treatment of childhood anger and aggression has emerged over the course of three randomized controlled trials of child-focused cognitive-behavioral interventions (Sukhodolsky & Scahill, 2012) for children with disruptive behavior disorders as a primary diagnosis and several studies of parent-training for children with neurodevelopmental disorders complicated by disruptive behavior and irritability (Bearss et al., 2015; Johnson et al., 2007; Scahill et al., 2006; Sukhodolsky et al., 2013). The first study of CBT was conducted in a sample of 33 elementary school children referred by teachers for aggressive behavior (Sukhodolsky, Solomon, & Perine, 2000). Compared to the no-treatment control condition, children who received CBT displayed a reduction on teacher reports of aggression and improvement in self-reported anger control. The second study utilized a dismantling design to investigate the relative effectiveness of the social skills training and problem-solving training components of CBT in 26 children referred by their parents for high levels of aggressive behavior (Sukhodolsky et al., 2005). Children in both conditions showed a reduction in aggression, whereas the problem-solving condition resulted in a greater reduction in hostile attribution bias, and the skills-training condition resulted in a greater improvement in anger-control skills.

In the third study, we evaluated CBT for explosive anger outbursts and aggression in adolescents with TS (Sukhodolsky et al., 2009). TS is characterized by chronic motor and phonic tics which co-occur with disruptive behavior in up to 80% of referred cases (Sukhodolsky et al., 2003). We conducted the first randomized study of CBT for anger control versus treatment as usual (TAU) in 26 adolescents with TS and disruptive behavior. Assessments, which included evaluations by a blinded rater, parent reports, and child self-reports, were conducted before and after treatment as well as at 3 months post-treatment. All randomized subjects completed the endpoint evaluation. Parent ratings of disruptive behavior decreased by 52% in the CBT condition, as compared to a decrease of 11% in the control condition. The independent evaluator who was unaware of treatment assignment rated 9 of 13 subjects (69%) in the CBT condition as "much improved" or "very much improved," as compared to 2 of 13 (15%) subjects "improved" in the control condition. We have also recently illustrated application of this CBT approach to DMDD in a case report of treating a 9-year-old child with this disorder (Tudor, Ibrahim, Bertschinger, Piasecka, & Sukhodolsky, 2016). A large randomized trial of CBT for aggression versus a supportive psychotherapy control condition in children across diagnostic categories is currently under way (Sukhodolsky et al., 2016).

Here, we briefly summarize the CBT treatment that has been developed from these clinical studies and been published by the Guilford Press (Sukhodolsky & Scahill 2012). Although excellent treatment manuals are available in the area of child and adolescent anger control (Feindler & Ecton, 1986; Lochman, Wells, & Lenhart, 2008), most are written in a group therapy format for use in school or inpatient settings. Our manual has been structured for providing CBT during individual outpatient psychotherapy. The manual provides guidelines for flexible delivery by allowing therapists to select from several numbered activities that correspond to each session's treatment goals, which can be matched to targeted behavioral problems and to the child's motivation and developmental level. Last, the manual contains treatment fidelity checklists to aid in evaluating treatment adherence, an important part of implementing treatment in a reliable fashion (Perepletchikova & Kazdin, 2005).

The treatment starts with a detailed assessment of the frequency (i.e., number of episodes per week), duration (i.e., time), and intensity (i.e., risk of injury, property damage, and impact on family) of anger outbursts and aggressive behaviors. Aggression is operationalized as instances of verbal threats, physical aggression, property damage, and self-injury (Silver & Yudofsky, 1991). Based on a structured clinical interview with parent(s) and the child, two to three of the most pressing behavioral problems are identified as target symptoms and used to tailor therapeutic techniques as outlined in the treatment manual (Sukhodolsky & Scahill,

2012). The treatment manual is organized into three modules: emotion regulation, social problem-solving, and the development of social skills for preventing and resolving conflict situations. The first module starts with identifying anger triggers, developing prevention strategies, and learning emotion regulation skills, such as cognitive reappraisal, distraction, and relaxation. The emotion regulation component teaches children and their parents about the sequence of anger triggers, emotional experiences, cognitive appraisals, and behavioral expressions that can be recognized and regulated to minimize conflict and maximize positive outcomes for all involved parties. The issues of intensity and duration of emotional experiences of anger are addressed in each session via eliciting children's report of frustrating events using activities that are operationalized in the treatment manual and session handouts. Coping skills for dealing with subjective feelings of anger are built from the menu of techniques, such as distress tolerance, desensitization, and engaging in enjoyable activities. The problem-solving module covers skills, such as the generation of multiple solutions and the consideration of consequences for different courses of action in conflicts. The third treatment module is focused on practicing skills for preventing or resolving potentially anger-provoking situations with friends, siblings, parents, and teachers. For example, participants are asked to recall a situation in which they acted aggressively and to role-play behaviors that would have prevented the enactment of aggressive behaviors. Each session consists of a menu of therapeutic techniques and activities that can be used in a flexible yet reliable manner in order to achieve session goals.

Each child session also includes a parent component where parents are taught about the skills that their child has learned in the session and a plan is devised that enables the practicing of these skills before the next session. Parents are asked to serve as coaches to facilitate the acquisition of new skills by rewarding nonaggressive behaviors with praise, attention, and privileges. Three separate parent sessions are provided to identify patterns of aversive family interactions that might initiate or maintain a child's aggressive behavior. Parents are then given instruction on how to pay attention to their child's positive behavior and to provide consistent reinforcement for their child's efforts in tolerating frustration and using cognitive problem-solving strategies. Additional parenting strategies discussed in treatment include giving effective commands, ignoring minor misbehaviors, and setting up behavioral contracts.

Dialectical Behavior Therapy

DBT was first developed to treat adults at high risk for suicidal behavior (Linehan, 1987, 1993) and has been increasingly used in other disorders characterized by emotion dysregulation. DBT is a skills-training approach that includes a wide range of cognitive-behavioral strategies but also makes use of mindfulness and acceptance-based techniques to address emotion dysregulation. The dialectical framework of DBT refers to balancing therapeutic goals aimed at change with goals that are aimed at acceptance of circumstances that cannot be changed at the moment. In addition to the skill building modules that are provided in the format of individual therapy, DBT also includes extensive options for phone coaching and consultation with patients and their families. There are also clearly defined guidelines and treatment arrangements for managing crisis situations and high-risk behaviors (Linehan & Wilks, 2015). Best research support exists for DBT in adults with borderline personality disorder and/or adults with suicidal behavior and self-injury (Bohus et al., 2004; Linehan et al., 2006). Adaptations of DBT have been tested for transdiagnostic emotional dysregulation (Neacsiu, Eberle, Kramer, Wiesmann, & Linehan, 2014), as well as for children with disruptive behavior (Nelson-Gray et al., 2006), bipolar disorder (Goldstein et al., 2015; Mehlum et al., 2014) and, most recently, DMDD (Perepletchikova et al., 2017). These studies suggest that DBT may be a promising intervention for pediatric irritability.

One approach to adapt DBT from adult to child patient populations involves simplifying and condensing didactic materials to a second-grade reading level, printed in large font and including child-friendly cartoons (Perepletchikova et al., 2011). Treatment delivery of mindfulness practice was modified to support children's engagement. Use of therapeutic metaphors, one of the distinctive features of DBT, was also modified and simplified. For example, "Wise Mind ACCEPTS" and "IMPROVE the moment" DBT skills, were combined into one "DISTRACT" skill in the child modification. The resulting child-focused DBT skills are grouped into four modules: mindfulness, distress tolerance, emotion regulation, and interpersonal effectiveness. For example, the first emotion regulation skill, called "the wave," compares emotions to waves that go through six stages—event, thought, feeling, action urge, action, and after-effect. The second skill in the emotion regulation module is named "surfing your emotion" and instructs the patient to regulate emotional arousal by just attending to an emotion without trying to change its intensity. Parent training components of DBT are focused on creating a validating and change-ready environment at home, as well as helping parents learn how to give effective prompts and reinforcements for adaptive behaviors. These and other DBT skills adapted for children with emotion dysregulation are detailed in a recent review (Perepletchikova, 2017).

A recent randomized controlled trial compared DBT to TAU in a sample of 43 preadolescent children diagnosed with DMDD (Perepletchikova et al., 2017). The subjects (56% boys) aged 7–12 years were randomized to either the DBT ($n = 21$, $M = 9.19$ years, $SD = 1.86$) or the TAU cohort ($n = 22$, $M = 9.27$ years, $SD = 1.64$). The DBT condition involved 32 weekly 90-minute sessions comprised of individual counseling for children, parent training, and joint skills training with parents and children. The children randomized to the TAU condition received 32 weekly sessions that were conducted at the discretion of community clinicians. Diagnoses of DMDD and other psychiatric disorders were assigned based on the Schedule for Affective Disorders and Schizophrenia for School Aged

Children: Present and Lifetime Version (K-SADS) (Kaufman et al., 2016), and the Clinical Global Impression-Severity scales (CGI-S) (Guy, 1976) was used as a primary outcome measure. One important finding of the study was that DBT was superior to TAU in subject retention because eight subjects dropped out from the TAU condition (36.4%) compared with no drop-out in DBT. Parents and children in DBT expressed significantly higher treatment satisfaction than those in TAU. The rate of positive response on the CGI-I scale was 90.4% in DBT compared with 45.5% in TAU, and the improvements were maintained at 3-month follow-up. Of note is the relatively high rate of suicidal thoughts and behavior and relatively low rate of ADHD in this sample compared to other DMDD samples, suggesting that DBT may be particularly relevant to this patient subgroup.

Another randomized controlled study examined DBT in adolescents with suicidal and self-harming behavior (Mehlum et al., 2014). Their sample consisted of 77 adolescents, 88% girls, with a mean age of 15.6 years ($SD = 1.5$) who met criteria of borderline personality disorder and had a history of recent self-harm experiences. Participants were randomized to 19 weeks of DBT for adolescents or an enhanced usual care control condition that included weekly psychotherapy that followed psychodynamic and cognitive behavioral orientations plus medication management when needed. Co-occurring diagnoses were assigned using the Structured Clinical Interview for DSM-IV disorders (SCID) (First, Spitzer, Gibbon, & Williams, 1996), and the majority of subjects met criteria for depression or anxiety disorder. DBT was found superior to community care in reducing self-harm, suicidal ideation, and depression. Although this study did not characterize irritability symptoms such as anger and aggression in their sample, the results are relevant for consideration of DBT as a treatment for DMDD, as children with DMDD may present with co-occurring depression and/or depressed mood between anger outbursts that DBT could potentially target. Also, high-risk behaviors such as self-injury may co-occur with dimensionally defined severe irritability or the diagnosis of DMDD. A structured approach to crisis management and an excellent record of subject retention in studies of DBT can provide the safety net for preventing high-risk behaviors in children and adolescents seeking treatment for severe irritability.

Technology and Web-Based Applications

In recent years, web-based training has become an increasingly feasible approach for parents of children with disruptive behavior and irritability. As discussed earlier, during PMT, parents are taught to identify and appropriately handle maladaptive behaviors and improve communication with the child. The structured format of PMT provides a clear blueprint for developing online PMT applications, and recent research is starting to demonstrate the clinical utility of these apps (Baumel, Pawar, Mathur, Kane, & Correll, 2017). Well-designed randomized studies of web-based PMT demonstrate significant reductions in early childhood aggression and conduct problems (Baker, Sanders, Turner, & Morawska, 2017; Enebrink, Högström, Forster, & Ghaderi, 2012; Rabbitt et al., 2016; Sourander et al., 2016). However, the magnitude of treatment effects of web-based PMT range from small to medium, and the optimum number of sessions and mechanisms to assure parents' fidelity with the online treatments has not been well studied (Dittman, Farruggia, Palmer, Sanders, & Keown, 2014). Despite these limitations in currently available research support, availability of low-cost, web-based interventions offers new opportunities for stepped care treatments for children with irritability.

Interpretation bias training (IBT) is a cognitive training intervention that targets hostile interpretation bias, a tendency to interpret ambiguous social cues as hostile (Stoddard et al., 2016). Participants are presented with a stream of faces depicting emotional expressions morphed on a continuum from clearly happy to clearly angry and are asked to rate the facial expressions as happy or angry. Each training session consists of 180 trials where participants receive feedback aimed at moving the rating of ambiguous faces toward happy rather than angry interpretations. One study reported a reduction in aggressive behavior after four sessions of IBT in 46 adolescents at risk for criminal behavior (Penton-Voak et al., 2013). Stoddard and colleagues conducted an open study of four daily sessions of IBT in a sample of 14 children with DMDD (mean age [SD] = 14.1 [2.4]; 8 girls, 6 boys) and demonstrated a significant reduction of parent-rated irritability. In addition to changing behavioral ratings of irritability, there was also increased activation in the bilateral orbitofrontal cortex and left amygdala after IBT, suggesting that the treatment might engage the neural circuitry mediating responses to ambiguous social cues (Brotman et al., 2010). However, this was a small open pilot study, and replication is needed. This study and other translational research are aimed at developing more neuroscience-based psychosocial interventions for pediatric irritability (Brotman, Kircanski, Stringaris, Pine, & Leibenluft, 2017).

Conclusion

Anger/irritability and aggression are among the most frequent reasons for mental health referrals in children and adolescents. PMT is a form of behavioral therapy that aims to ameliorate patterns of family interactions that produce antecedents and consequences that maintain child anger and aggression. CBT is another well-studied psychosocial treatment for anger and aggression in children and adolescents. During CBT, children learn how to regulate their frustration, improve their social problem-solving skills, and role-play assertive behaviors that can be used during conflicts instead of aggression. Both PMT and CBT can be offered in the format of time-limited psychotherapy in outpatient mental health centers. There is also emerging support for child and adolescent adaptations of DBT for severe mood dysregulation and irritability in pediatric populations. More work is needed to understand which behavioral approaches might work best for children with particular forms of irritability symptoms and/or profiles of co-occurring psychiatric and neurodevelopmental disorders.

References

Aman, M. G., Bukstein, O. G., Gadow, K. D., Arnold, L. E., Molina, B. S. G., McNamara, N. K., . . . Findling, R. L. (2014). What does risperidone add to parent training and stimulant for severe aggression in child attention-deficit/hyperactivity disorder? *Journal of the American Academy of Child and Adolescent Psychiatry, 53*(1), 47–60.e41.

Aman, M. G., McDougle, C. J., Scahill, L., Handen, B., Arnold, L. E., Johnson, C., . . . Wagner, A. (2009). Medication and parent training in children with pervasive developmental disorders and serious behavior problems: Results from a randomized clinical trial. *Journal of the American Academy of Child and Adolescent Psychiatry, 48*(12), 1143–1154.

American Psychiatric Association (APA). (2013). *Diagnostic and Statistical Manual of Mental Disorders* (5th edition). Washington, DC: American Psychiatric Publishing.

Baker, S., Sanders, M. R., Turner, K. M. T., & Morawska, A. (2017). A randomized controlled trial evaluating a low-intensity interactive online parenting intervention, Triple P Online Brief, with parents of children with early onset conduct problems. *Behaviour Research and Therapy, 91*, 78–90. doi:10.1016/j.brat.2017.01.016

Barkley, R. A. (2013). *Defiant children: A clinician's manual for assessment and parent training* (3 ed.). New York: Guilford.

Baumel, A., Pawar, A., Mathur, N., Kane, J. M., & Correll, C. U. (2017). Technology-assisted parent training programs for children and adolescents with disruptive behaviors: A systematic review. *Journal of Clinical Psychiatry, 78*(8), e957–e969. doi:10.4088/JCP.16r11063

Bearss, K., Johnson, C., Smith, T., Lecavalier, L., Swiezy, N., Aman, M., . . . Scahill, L. (2015). Effect of parent training vs parent education on behavioral problems in children with autism spectrum disorder: A randomized clinical trial. *JAMA, 313*(15), 1524–1533. doi:10.1001/jama.2015.3150

Bohus, M., Haaf, B., Simms, T., Limberger, M. F., Schmahl, C., Unckel, C., . . . Linehan, M. M. (2004). Effectiveness of inpatient dialectical behavioral therapy for borderline personality disorder: A controlled trial. *Behaviour Research and Therapy, 42*(5), 487–499. doi:10.1016/s0005-7967(03)00174-8

Brotman, M. A., Kircanski, K., & Leibenluft, E. (2017). Irritability in children and adolescents. *Annual Review of Clinical Psychology, 13*, 317–341.

Brotman, M. A., Kircanski, K., Stringaris, A., Pine, D. S., & Leibenluft, E. (2017). Irritability in youths: A translational model. *American Journal of Psychiatry, 174*(6), 520–532. doi:10.1176/appi.ajp.2016.16070839

Brotman, M. A., Rich, B. A., Guyer, A. E., Lunsford, J. R., Horsey, S. E., Reising, M. M., . . . Leibenluft, E. (2010). Amygdala activation during emotion processing of neutral faces in children with severe mood dysregulation versus ADHD or bipolar disorder. *American Journal of Psychiatry, 167*(1), 61–69.

Costello, E. J., He, J. P., Sampson, N. A., Kessler, R. C., & Merikangas, K. R. (2014). Services for adolescents with psychiatric disorders: 12-Month data from the National Comorbidity Survey-Adolescent. *Psychiatric Services, 65*(3), 359–366. doi:0.1176/appi.ps.201100518

Deffenbacher, J. L., Lynch, R. S., Oetting, E. R., & Kemper, C. C. (1996). Anger reduction in early adolescents. *Journal of Counseling Psychology, 43*(2), 149–157.

Dittman, C. K., Farruggia, S. P., Palmer, M. L., Sanders, M. R., & Keown, L. J. (2014). Predicting success in an online parenting intervention: The role of child, parent, and family factors. *Journal of Family Psychology, 28*(2), 236–243. doi:10.1037/a0035991

Dodge, K. A. (2003). Do social information-processing patterns mediate aggressive behavior? In B. B. Lahey, T. E. Moffitt & A. Caspi (Eds.), *Causes of conduct disorder and juvenile delinquency.* (pp. 254–274). New York: Guilford.

Dodge, K. A., Bates, J. E., & Pettit, G. S. (1990). Mechanisms in the cycle of violence. *Science, 250*(4988), 1678–1683.

Dretzke, J., Davenport, C., Frew, E., Barlow, J., Stewart-Brown, S., Bayliss, S., . . . Hyde, C. (2009). The clinical effectiveness of different parenting programmes for children with conduct problems: A systematic review of randomised controlled trials. *Child and Adolescent Psychiatry and Mental Health, 3*(1), 7.

Duncombe, M. E., Havighurst, S. S., Kehoe, C. E., Holland, K. A., Frankling, E. J., & Stargatt, R. (2016). Comparing an emotion- and a behavior-focused parenting program as part of a multisystemic intervention for child conduct problems. *Journal of Clinical Child and Adolescent Psychology, 45*(3), 320–334. doi:10.1080/15374416.2014.963855

Dunsmore, J. C., Booker, J. A., Ollendick, T. H., & Greene, R. W. (2016). Emotion socialization in the context of risk and psychopathology: Maternal emotion coaching predicts better treatment outcomes for emotionally labile children with oppositional defiant disorder. *Social Development. 25*(1), 8–26. doi:10.1111/sode.12109

Enebrink, P., Högström, J., Forster, M., & Ghaderi, A. (2012). Internet-based parent management training: A randomized controlled study. *Behaviour Research and Therapy, 50*(4), 240–249. doi:10.1016/j.brat.2012.01.006

Eyberg, S. M., Nelson, M. M., & Boggs, S. R. (2008). Evidence-based psychosocial treatments for children and adolescents with disruptive behavior. *Journal of Clinical Child and Adolescent Psychology, 37*(1), 215–237.

Feindler, E. L., & Ecton, R. B. (1986). *Adolescent anger control: Cognitive-behavioral Techniques.* New York: Pergamon Press.

First, M. B., Spitzer, R. L., Gibbon, M., & Williams, J. B. W. (1996). *Structured Clinical Interview for DSM-IV Axis I Disorders, Clinician Version (SCID-CV).* Washington, DC: American Psychiatric Press.

Fristad, M. A., Verducci, J. S., Walters, K., & Young, M. E. (2009). Impact of multifamily psychoeducational psychotherapy in treating children aged 8 to 12 years with mood disorders. *Archives of General Psychiatry, 66*(9), 1013–1021. doi:10.1001/archgenpsychiatry.2009.112

Fristad, M. A., Weller, E. B., & Weller, R. A. (1992). The Mania Rating Scale: Can it be used in children? A preliminary report. *Journal of the American Academy of Child and Adolescent Psychiatry, 31*(2), 252–257. doi:10.1097/00004583-199203000-00011

Fung, L. K., Mahajan, R., Nozzolillo, A., Bernal, P., Krasner, A., Jo, B., . . . Hardan, A. Y. (2016). Pharmacologic treatment of severe irritability and problem behaviors in Autism: A systematic review and meta-analysis. *Pediatrics, 137*, S124–S135. doi:10.1542/peds.2015-2851K

Gershoff, E. T. (2002). Corporal punishment by parents and associated child behaviors and experiences: A meta-analytic and theoretical review. *Psychological Bulletin, 128*(4), 539–579.

Goldstein, T. R., Fersch-Podrat, R. K., Rivera, M., Axelson, D. A., Merranko, J., Yu, H., . . . Birmaher, B. (2015). Dialectical behavior therapy for adolescents with bipolar disorder: Results from a pilot randomized trial. *Journal of Child and Adolescent Psychopharmacology, 25*(2), 140–149. doi:10.1089/cap.2013.0145

Gottman, J. M., & DeClaire, J. (1997). *The heart of parenting: How to raise an emotionally intelligent child.* London: Bloomsbury.

Guerra, N. G., & Slaby, R. G. (1990). Cognitive mediators of aggression in adolescent offenders: 2. Intervention. *Developmental Psychology, 26*(2), 269–277.

Guy, W. (1976). *Clinical Global Impression Scales (CGI). ECDEU Assessment Manual for Psychopharmacology (Publication 76-338).* Washington, DC: Department of Health, Education, and Welfare.

Havighurst, S. S., Duncombe, M., Frankling, E., Holland, K., Kehoe, C., & Stargatt, R. (2015). An emotion-focused early intervention for children with emerging conduct problems. *Journal of Abnormal Child Psychology, 43*(4), 749–760. doi:10.1007/s10802-014-9944-z

Havighurst, S. S., Wilson, K. R., Harley, A. E., & Prior, M. R. (2009). Tuning in to Kids: An emotion-focused parenting program-initial findings from a community trial. *Journal of Community Psychology, 37*(8), 1008–1023. doi:10.1002/jcop.20345

Havighurst, S. S., Wilson, K. R., Harley, A. E., Prior, M. R., & Kehoe, C. (2010). Tuning in to Kids: Improving emotion socialization practices in parents of preschool children-findings from a community trial. *Journal of Child Psychology and Psychiatry and Allied Disciplines, 51*(12), 1342–1350. doi:10.1111/j.1469-7610.2010.02303.x

Hudley, C., & Graham, S. (1993). An attributional intervention to reduce peer-directed aggression among African-American boys. *Child Development, 64*(1), 124–138.

Johnson, A. M., Hawes, D. J., Eisenberg, N., Kohlhoff, J., & Dudeney, J. (2017). Emotion socialization and child conduct problems: A comprehensive review and meta-analysis. *Clinical Psychology Review, 54*, 65–80. doi:10.1016/j.cpr.2017.04.001

Johnson, C. R., Handen, B. L., Butter, E., Wagner, A., Mulick, J., Sukhodolsky, D. G., . . . Vitello, B. (2007). Development of a parent management training program for children with pervasive developmental disorders. *Behavioral Interventions, 22*, 201–221.

Kassinove, H., & Tafrate, R. C. (2002). *Anger management: The complete treatment guidebook for practitioners.* Atascadero, CA: Impact Publishers.

Kaufman, J., Birmaher, B., Axelson, D., Perepletchikova, F., Brent, D., & Ryan, N. (2016). Schedule for Affective Disorders and Schizophrenia for School Aged Children (6-18 Years)—Lifetime Version for DSM-V. Retrieved from https://www.pediatricbipolar.pitt.edu/resources/instruments

Kazdin, A. E. (2005). *Parent management training: Treatment for oppositional, aggressive, and antisocial behavior in children and adolescents.* New York: Oxford University Press.

Kazdin, A. E., Siegel, T. C., & Bass, D. (1992). Cognitive problem-solving skills training and parent management training in the treatment of antisocial behavior in children. *Journal of Consulting & Clinical Psychology, 60*(5), 733–747.

Kehoe, C. E., Havighurst, S. S., & Harley, A. E. (2014). Tuning in to Teens: Improving parent emotion socialization to reduce youth internalizing difficulties. *Social Development, 23*(2), 413–431. doi:10.1111/sode.12060

Kendall, P. C. (2006). Guiding theory for therapy with children and adolescents. In P. C. Kendall (Ed.), *Child and adolescent therapy: Cognitive-behavioral procedures* (3rd ed., pp. 3–30). New York: Guilford.

Linehan, M. M. (1987). Dialectical behavioral therapy: A cognitive behavioral approach to parasuicide. *Journal of Personality Disorders, 1*(4), 328–333.

Linehan, M. M. (1993). *Cognitive-behavioral treatment of borderline personality disorder.* New York: Guilford.

Linehan, M. M., Comtois, K. A., Murray, A. M., Brown, M. Z., Gallop, R. J., Heard, H. L., . . . Lindenboim, N. (2006). Two-year randomized controlled trial and follow-up of dialectical behavior therapy vs therapy by experts for suicidal behaviors and borderline personality disorder. *Archives of General Psychiatry, 63*(7), 757–766. doi:10.1001/archpsyc.63.7.757

Linehan, M. M., & Wilks, C. R. (2015). The course and evolution of dialectical behavior therapy. *American Journal of Psychotherapy, 69*(2), 97–110.

Lochman, J. E., Barry, T. D., & Pardini, D. A. (2003). Anger control training for aggressive youth. In A. E. Kazdin & J. R. Weisz (Eds.), *Evidence-based psychotherapies for children and adolescents* (pp. 263–281). New York: Guilford.

Lochman, J. E., Wells, K. C., & Lenhart, L. A. (2008). *Coping power: Child group program.* New York: Oxford University Press.

McCart, M. R., & Sheidow, A. J. (2016). Evidence-based psychosocial treatments for adolescents with disruptive behavior. *Journal of Clinical Child and Adolescent Psychology, 45*(5), 529–563. doi:10.1080/15374416.2016.1146990

Mehlum, L., Tørmoen, A. J., Ramberg, M., Haga, E., Diep, L. M., Laberg, S., . . . Grøholt, B. (2014). Dialectical behavior therapy for adolescents with repeated suicidal and self-harming behavior: A randomized trial. *Journal of the American Academy of Child and Adolescent Psychiatry, 53*(10), 1082–1091. doi:10.1016/j.jaac.2014.07.003

Meichenbaum, D., & Cameron, R. (1973). *Stress inoculation: A skills training approach to anxiety management.* Waterloo, Ontario: University of Waterloo.

Michelson, D., Davenport, C., Dretzke, J., Barlow, J., & Day, C. (2013). Do evidence-based interventions work when tested in the "real world?" A systematic review and meta-analysis of parent management training for the treatment of child disruptive behavior. *Clinical Child and Family Psychology Review, 16*(1), 18–34.

Neacsiu, A. D., Eberle, J. W., Kramer, R., Wiesmann, T., & Linehan, M. M. (2014). Dialectical behavior therapy skills for transdiagnostic emotion dysregulation: A pilot randomized controlled trial. *Behaviour Research and Therapy, 59*, 40–51. doi:10.1016/j.brat.2014.05.005

Nelson-Gray, R. O., Keane, S. P., Hurst, R. M., Mitchell, J. T., Warburton, J. B., Chok, J. T., & Cobb, A. R. (2006). A modified DBT skills training program for oppositional defiant adolescents: Promising preliminary findings. *Behaviour Research and Therapy, 44*(12), 1811–1820. doi:10.1016/j.brat.2006.01.004

Nelson, W. M., & Finch, A. J. (2000). *Children's Inventory of Anger*. Los Angeles, CA: Western Psychological Services.

NICE. (2013). *Antisocial behaviour and conduct disorders in children and young people: Recognition and management. NICE guideline (CG158)*. London: National Institute for Health and Care Excellence.

Nock, M. K., Kazdin, A. E., Hiripi, E., & Kessler, R. C. (2007). Lifetime prevalence, correlates, and persistence of oppositional defiant disorder: Results from the National Comorbidity Survey Replication. *Journal of Child Psychology and Psychiatry, 48*(7), 703–713.

Novaco, R. W. (1975). *Anger control: The development and evaluation of experimental treatment*. Lexington, MA: D. C. Health.

Patterson, G. R. (1982). *Coercive Family Process*. Eugene, OR: Castlia Press.

Patterson, G. R., DeBaryshe, B. D., & Ramsey, E. (1989). A developmental perspective on antisocial behavior. *American Psychologist, 44*(2), 329–335.

Pelham, W. E. J., Gnagy, E. M., Greenslade, K. E., & Milich, R. (1992). Teacher ratings of DSM-III-R symptoms for the disruptive behavior disorders. *Journal of the American Academy of Child and Adolescent Psychiatry, 31*(2), 210–218. doi:10.1097/00004583-199203000-00006

Penton-Voak, I. S., Thomas, J., Gage, S. H., McMurran, M., McDonald, S., & Munafò, M. R. (2013). Increasing recognition of happiness in ambiguous facial expressions reduces anger and aggressive behavior. *Psychological Science, 24*(5), 688–697. doi:10.1177/0956797612459657

Perepletchikova, F. (2017). Dialectical behavior therapy for pre-adolescent children. In M. Swales (Ed.), *The Oxford handbook of dialectical behavior theory*. New York: Oxford University Press.

Perepletchikova, F., Axelrod, S. R., Kaufman, J., Rounsaville, B. J., Douglas-Palumberi, H., & Miller, A. L. (2011). Adapting dialectical behaviour therapy for children: Towards a new research agenda for paediatric suicidal and non-suicidal self-injurious behaviours. *Child and Adolescent Mental Health, 16*(2), 116–121. doi:10.1111/j.1475-3588.2010.00583.x

Perepletchikova, F., & Kazdin, A. E. (2005). Treatment integrity and therapeutic change: Issues and research recommendations. *Clinical Psychology: Science and Practice, 12*(4), 365–383.

Perepletchikova, F., Nathanson, D., Axelrod, S. R., Merrill, C., Walker, A., Grossman, M., . . . Walkup, J. (2017). Randomized clinical trial of dialectical behavior therapy for preadolescent children with disruptive mood dysregulation disorder: Feasibility and outcomes. *Journal of the American Academy of Child and Adolescent Psychiatry, 56*(10), 832–840. doi:S0890-8567(17)31159-0 [pii]

Postorino, V., Sharp, W. G., McCracken, C. E., Bearss, K., Burrell, T. L., Evans, A. N., & Scahill, L. (2017). A systematic review and meta-analysis of parent training for disruptive behavior in children with autism spectrum disorder. *Clinical Child and Family Psychology Review, 20*(4), 391–402. doi:10.1007/s10567-017-0237-2

Poznanski, E. O., & Mokros, H. B. (1996). *Children's Depression Rating Scale-Revised (CDRS-R)*. Los Angeles, CA: Western Psychological Services.

Rabbitt, S. M., Carrubba, E., Lecza, B., McWhinney, E., Pope, J., & Kazdin, A. E. (2016). Reducing therapist contact in parenting programs: Evaluation of internet-based treatments for child conduct problems. *Journal of Child and Family Studies, 25*(6), 2001–2020. doi:10.1007/s10826-016-0363-3

Salmon, K., Dittman, C., Sanders, M., Burson, R., & Hammington, J. (2014). Does adding an emotion component enhance the Triple P-Positive parenting program? *Journal of Family Psychology, 28*(2), 244–252. doi:10.1037/a0035997

Scahill, L., Sukhodolsky, D. G., Bearss, K., Findley, D. B., Hamrin, V., Carroll, D. H., & Rains, A. L. (2006). A randomized trial of parent management training in children with tic disorders and disruptive behavior. *Journal of Child Neurology, 21*(8), 650–656.

Scott, S., Briskman, J., & O'Connor, T. G. (2014). Early prevention of antisocial personality: Long-term follow-up of two randomized controlled trials comparing indicated and selective approaches. *American Journal of Psychiatry, 171*(6), 649–657. doi:10.1176/appi.ajp.2014.13050697

Scott, S., & O'Connor, T. G. (2012). An experimental test of differential susceptibility to parenting among emotionally-dysregulated children in a randomized controlled trial for oppositional behavior. *Journal of Child Psychology and Psychiatry and Allied Disciplines, 53*(11), 1184–1193. doi:10.1111/j.1469-7610.2012.02586.x

Shure, M. B., & Spivack, G. (1972). Means-ends thinking, adjustment, and social class among elementary-school-aged children. *Journal of Consulting and Clinical Psychology, 38*(3), 348–353.

Silver, J. M., & Yudofsky, S. C. (1991). The Overt Aggression Scale: Overview and guiding principles. *Journal of Neuropsychiatry and Clinical Neuroscience, 3*(2), S22–S29.

Skinner, B. F. (1938). *The behavior of organisms: An experimental analysis.* New York: Free Press.

Sourander, A., McGrath, P. J., Ristkari, T., Cunningham, C., Huttunen, J., Lingley-Pottie, P., . . . Unruh, A. (2016). Internet-assisted parent training intervention for disruptive behavior in 4-year-old children: A randomized clinical trial. *JAMA Psychiatry, 73*(4), 378–387. doi:10.1001/jamapsychiatry.2015.3411

Spielberger, C. D. (1999). *Manual for the State-Trait Anger Expression Inventory (STAXI)* (2 ed.). Odessa, FL: Psychological Assessment Resources.

Stoddard, J., Sharif-Askary, B., Harkins, E. A., Frank, H. R., Brotman, M. A., Penton-Voak, I. S., . . . Leibenluft, E. (2016). An open pilot study of training hostile interpretation bias to treat disruptive mood dysregulation disorder. *Journal of Child and Adolescent Psychopharmacology, 26*(1), 49–57. doi:10.1089/cap.2015.0100

Storch, E. A., Jones, A. M., Lack, C. W., Ale, C. M., Sulkowski, M. L., Lewin, A. B., . . . Murphy, T. K. (2012). Rage attacks in pediatric obsessive-compulsive disorder: Phenomenology and clinical correlates. *Journal of the American Academy of Child and Adolescent Psychiatry, 51*(6), 582–592. doi:10.1016/j.jaac.2012.02.016

Stringaris, A., Vidal-Ribas, P., Brotman, M. A., & Leibenluft, E. (2017). Practitioner Review: Definition, recognition, and treatment challenges of irritability in young people. *Journal of Child Psychology and Psychiatry and Allied Disciplines.* doi:10.1111/jcpp.12823

Sukhodolsky, D. G., Gladstone, T. R., & Marsh, C. L. (2018). Irritability in autism. In F. R. Volkmar (Ed.), *Encyclopedia of autism spectrum disorders* (5th ed.). New York: Springer.

Sukhodolsky, D. G., Golub, A., Stone, E. C., & Orban, L. (2005). Dismantling anger control training for children: A randomized pilot study of social problem-solving versus social skills training components. *Behavior Therapy, 36*(1), 15–23.

Sukhodolsky, D. G., Gorman, B. S., Scahill, L., Findley, D. B., & McGuire, J. (2013). Exposure and response prevention with or without parent management training for children with obsessive-compulsive disorder complicated by disruptive behavior: A multiple-baseline design study. *Journal of Anxiety Disorders, 27*(3), 298–305.

Sukhodolsky, D. G., Kassinove, H., & Gorman, B. S. (2004). Cognitive-behavioral therapy for anger in children and adolescents: A meta-analysis. *Aggression & Violent Behavior, 9*(3), 247–269.

Sukhodolsky, D. G., & Scahill, L. (2007). Disruptive behavior in persons with Tourette Syndrome: Phenomenology, assessment, and treatment. In D. W. Woods, J. C. Piacentini & J. T. Walkup (Eds.), *Treating Tourette syndrome and tic disorders* (pp. 199–221). New York: Guilford.

Sukhodolsky, D. G., & Scahill, L. (2012). *Cognitive-behavioral therapy for anger and aggression in children.* New York: Guilford.

Sukhodolsky, D. G., Scahill, L., Zhang, H., Peterson, B. S., King, R. A., Lombroso, P. J., . . . Leckman, J. F. (2003). Disruptive behavior in children with Tourette's syndrome: Association with ADHD comorbidity, tic severity, and functional impairment. *Journal of the American Academy of Child and Adolescent Psychiatry, 42*(1), 98–105.

Sukhodolsky, D. G., Smith, S. D., McCauley, S. A., Ibrahim, K., & Piasecka, J. B. (2016). Behavioral interventions for anger, irritability, and aggression in children and adolescents. *Journal of Child and Adolescent Psychopharmacology, 26*(1), 58–64. doi:10.1089/cap.2015.0120

Sukhodolsky, D. G., Solomon, R. M., & Perine, J. (2000). Cognitive-behavioral, anger-control intervention for elementary school children: A treatment outcome study. *Journal of Child and Adolescent Group Therapy, 10*(3), 159–170.

Sukhodolsky, D. G., Vitulano, L. A., Carroll, D. H., McGuire, J., Leckman, J. F., & Scahill, L. (2009). Randomized trial of anger control training for adolescents with Tourette's Syndrome and disruptive behavior. *Journal of the American Academy of Child and Adolescent Psychiatry, 48*(4), 413–421.

Sukhodolsky, D. G., Wyk, B. C. V., Eilbott, J. A., McCauley, S. A., Ibrahim, K., Crowley, M. J., & Pelphrey, K. A. (2016). Neural mechanisms of cognitive-behavioral therapy for aggression in children and adolescents: Design of a randomized controlled trial within the National Institute for Mental Health Research Domain Criteria construct of frustrative non-reward. *Journal of Child and Adolescent Psychopharmacology, 26*(1), 38–48. doi:10.1089/cap.2015.0164

Tudor, M. E., Ibrahim, K., Bertschinger, E., Piasecka, J., & Sukhodolsky, D. G. (2016). Cognitive-behavioral therapy for a 9-year-old girl with disruptive mood dysregulation disorder. *Clinical Case Studies, 15*(6), 459–475. doi:10.1177/1534650116669431

Van Manen, T. G., Prins, P. J. M., & Emmelkamp, P. M. G. (2004). Reducing aggressive behavior in boys with a social cognitive group treatment: Results of a randomized, controlled trial. *Journal of the American Academy of Child and Adolescent Psychiatry, 43*(12), 1478–1487.

Vidal-Ribas, P., Brotman, M. A., Valdivieso, I., Leibenluft, E., & Stringaris, A. (2016). The status of irritability in psychiatry: A conceptual and quantitative review. *Journal of the American Academy of Child and Adolescent Psychiatry, 55*(7), 556–570. doi:10.1016/j.jaac.2016.04.014

Vismara, L. A., & Rogers, S. J. (2010). Behavioral treatments in autism spectrum disorder: What do we know? *Annual Review of Clinical Psychology, 6*, 447–468.

Waxmonsky, J. G., Waschbusch, D. A., Belin, P., Li, T., Babocsai, L., Humphery, H., . . . Pelham, W. E. (2016). A randomized clinical trial of an integrative group therapy for children with severe mood dysregulation. *Journal of the American Academy of Child and Adolescent Psychiatry, 55*(3), 196–207. doi:10.1016/j.jaac.2015.12.011

Webster-Stratton, C., & Reid, M. J. (2003). Treating conduct problems and strengthening social and emotional competence in young children: The Dina Dinosaur treatment program. *Journal of Emotional and Behavioral Disorders, 11*(3), 130–143.

Wyatt Kaminski, J., Valle, L. A., Filene, J. H., & Boyle, C. L. (2008). A meta-analytic review of components associated with parent training program effectiveness. *Journal of Abnormal Child Psychology, 36*(4), 567–589.

14

Pharmacological Treatment of Pediatric Irritability

Daniel P. Dickstein and Rachel E. Christensen

Introduction

Irritability is the most common reason children are brought for psychiatric evaluation (>40% of emergency room and >20% of outpatient visits) (Collishaw, Maughan, Natarajan, & Pickles, 2010; Kelly, Molcho, Doyle, & Gabhainn, 2010; Peterson, Zhang, Santa Lucia, King, & Lewis, 1996; Stringaris, Cohen, Pine, & Leibenluft, 2009). Irritability is an explicit diagnostic criterion or associated symptom for multiple diagnoses found in the *Diagnostic and Statistical Manual of Mental Disorders* (DSM), including a manic episode in bipolar disorder (BD), major depressive episode in children, generalized anxiety disorder, attention deficit/hyperactivity disorder (ADHD), oppositional defiant disorder (ODD), and the new DSM-5 disruptive mood dysregulation disorder (DMDD) (American Psychiatric Association [APA], 2013). There is no well-validated, replicated biomarker (e.g., scan or test) with sufficient sensitivity and specificity to guide clinicians in determining what disorder(s) involving irritability a child has that may hinder treatment decisions. However, effective treatment is essential as childhood irritability is linked to significant impairment in adulthood (i.e., decreased educational attainment and income and greater risk for psychopathology and suicide) (Leibenluft, Cohen, Gorrindo, Brook, & Pine, 2006; Pickles et al., 2010; Stringaris et al., 2009).

As of the writing of this chapter, three conferences have been held to address the need for greater research on irritability in children. These include the Pediatric Irritability Workshop sponsored by the National Institute of Mental Health (NIMH) and held in Bethesda, Maryland, on February 2014, and the First and Second Congresses on Pediatric Irritability held at the University of Vermont in September 2015 and 2017, respectively. Importantly, these conferences all called for greater research on the mechanisms of pediatric irritability that could improve our ability to both diagnose and treat irritability in children. Such mechanism-oriented research holds the potential to identify novel cognitive and emotional processes that might be amenable to pharmacological treatment. Furthermore, it is possible that treatments designed to address the brain/behavior processes underlying irritability may facilitate targeted treatments that are more efficacious than those that focus on a specific disorder involving irritability, which is ultimately a collection of potentially heterogeneous symptoms. Thus, a key takeaway of these conferences is that mechanism-oriented research is important to identify potential subtypes of irritability that could provide better targets for novel treatments and better indicators of treatment effect.

In that vein, this chapter seeks to provide a concise guide to the pharmacological treatment of irritability, drawing on the latest published studies. At the outset, we note that, in completing this task, we drew primarily on studies evaluating medications typically used in child psychiatric disorders that may be accompanied by irritability and aggression; these disorders include BD and unipolar major depressive disorder (MDD), ADHD, ODD, and autism spectrum disorder (ASD). Thus, this chapter covers the following major categories of medications: (1) antimanic agents, (2) ADHD stimulants, (3) α-agonists, and (4) selective serotonin reuptake inhibitors (SSRIs). Prior to going through each medication category, we provide some general principles of the pharmacological treatment of children with irritability.

We also note that the inclusion of DMDD as a new mood disorder in DSM-5 is highly relevant to treatment in several respects. First, as noted elsewhere in this book, DMDD's creation was based on more than a decade's worth of research showing that children with chronic, nonepisodic, functionally disabling irritability, without episodes of euphoria or other cardinal symptoms of mania, are distinct from those with BD (Brotman, Kircanski, & Leibenluft, 2017; Brotman, Kircanski, Stringaris, Pine, & Leibenluft, 2017; Leibenluft, Charney, & Pine, 2003; Leibenluft, Charney, Towbin, Bhangoo, & Pine, 2003; Stringaris, Vidal-Ribas, Brotman, & Leibenluft, 2017). Second, DMDD was included in the depression section rather than in the BD section of DSM-5 because studies showed that childhood-onset chronic irritability was associated with subsequent depression and/or anxiety in adulthood, rather than mania. Third, DMDD should not be used as a replacement for the DSM-IV catch-all "mood disorder not otherwise specified." In fact, the DMDD criteria are highly specific, with rule-outs for even brief euphoria or grandiosity that might be found in BD and also for other distinct causes of irritability, such as ASD. Fourth, as of now, there is no single, replicated, effective medication treatment for DMDD. However, there is considerable hope that its inclusion in DSM-5 will lead to treatment trials for DMDD, including medication, psychotherapy, and novel brain-mechanism targeted treatments, such as cognitive remediation and brain stimulation.

In the future, fueled by these NIMH conferences and the NIMH Research Domain Criteria (RDoC) Project, we expect growth in treatment studies involving mechanism-driven, transdiagnostic samples of children exhibiting a range of irritability, rather than from a single DSM-oriented categorical disorder (Insel et al., 2010). We also hope for more studies using big data approaches to leverage information from electronic medical records and the millions of prescriptions for psychotropic medications written for children and adolescents. Such studies could address important questions about the potential benefits and side effects/risks of extant medications for pediatric irritability.

General Treatment Principles

The medication treatment of children and adolescents struggling with irritability should be guided by standard approaches to child psychiatric disorders generally. This includes the following principles.

First, proper treatment requires a good assessment. That means careful evaluation of the child for the main presenting problem, such as irritability. It also means screening for major forms of psychopathology, including ADHD, ASD, ODD, MDD, BD, anxiety disorders, learning disorders, substance use disorders, and psychosis. It also requires evaluating the family environment and history, including relatives' history of psychiatric medication treatment response and side effects. Moreover, evaluation for medical issues, including allergies, concussions, seizures, and cardiac issues, is essential. The goal is to derive a working hypothesis of treatment targets based on a biological, psychological, and social formulation.

Second, assessment should guide treatment. Practitioners should treat what they see as part of their working diagnosis, but they will have to be especially collaborative with the family to address common gray areas and use psychoeducation to ensure that families understand why they are focusing first on some problems rather than others. For example, a child with depression who has a first-degree relative with BD should be treated for the depression they have, not for the BD or mania they might have in the future due to biological risk or side effects of antidepressant medication. This will require that families understand this approach, as they may wonder why the clinician is not treating the child's risk for BD. Like all patients, that patient and their family should be informed of signs of worsening, such as symptoms of mania. However, the patient with a family history of BD should be monitored more closely for such worsening than a patient without such a history. Similarly, treating comorbid anxiety with an SSRI in a child who has a confirmed diagnosis of BD after antimanic treatment has already been started also requires careful monitoring for clinical worsening. If irritability worsens, is it due to worsening mania, or depression from BD, or worsening anxiety? All three of these can involve irritability. Additionally, assessment should continue over the course of treatment because a working diagnosis may change over time. In fact, it often changes as practitioners develop a stronger relationship with the patient and his or her family and are able to observe treatment response.

Third, medication management is only one aspect of treatment. Even in time-limited visits that include medication management and brief therapy, physicians should address other aspects of the child's life, including diet, exercise, sleep hygiene, and socialization, that may be modified to reduce irritability. Practitioners can also help families learn communication skills that promote neutral (or positive) communication and hence reduce irritability (Scott & O'Conner, 2012).

Fourth, treatment is an iterative process—working with families to identify treatment targets, monitoring progress, evaluating side effects, and then again identifying new treatment targets (Stringaris et al., 2017).

Aligning with this approach, we will now discuss what is known about the medication treatment of irritability in children. We will cover the following major categories of medications: (1) antimanic agents, (2) ADHD stimulants, (3) α-agonists, and (4) SSRIs. For each, we provide context by identifying the DSM-oriented disorders associated with irritability in which these agents have been studied, including BD, MDD, DMDD, ADHD, ODD, and ASD. We also provide information about potential mechanisms, side effects, and monitoring.

Antimanic Agents

OVERVIEW

We start this chapter about the medication treatment of irritability with a discussion of agents commonly referred to as "mood stabilizers," not because every child presenting with irritability has BD. Rather, all too often, these medications are used to treat "moody" or "irritable" children—the terms used interchangeably by clinicians and parents. Unfortunately, this approach is often not helpful because it obscures the fact that irritability is not a solitary construct. In fact, a very careful diagnostic approach is needed to ascertain if an individual child has features of specific disorders (e.g., BD, MDD, ADHD, ODD, ASD, etc.) or combinations of these disorders for which a more tailored approach would be better. Concern has been raised that this lack of precision contributed to overuse of second-generation antipsychotics (SGAs) in "moody" children and other patients who did not meet threshold for specific diagnoses (Goodwin, Gould, Blanco, & Olfson, 2001; Olfson, Blanco, Liu, Moreno, & Laje, 2006).

In fact, the term "mood stabilizer" is a marketing term used by the pharmaceutical industry to sell SGAs in the 1990s to physicians and directly to consumers as medications that could be used without the need for blood draws for serum levels or other monitoring, unlike lithium or antiepileptic drugs (AEDs). Moreover, this general term should be contrasted with that of other medication categories that are specific either to a diagnosis, or a mechanism of action, or both, such as SSRI antidepressants (Bauer & Mitchner, 2004; Keck, McElroy, Richtand, & Tohen, 2002).

Thus, we use the term "antimanic agent" rather than the term "mood stabilizer." There are three major types of antimanic agents: (1) SGAs, (2) lithium, and (3) AEDs. Importantly, it is clear that all of these agents require periodic blood draws to monitor for side effects. Moreover, as will be described later, these medications have been studied in patients with disorders besides BD. Thus, this section is not just germane to children with BD, but to those with irritable mood more broadly.

SECOND-GENERATION ANTIPSYCHOTICS

Currently, SGAs have an indication from the US Food and Drug Administration (FDA) to treat mania or mixed states associated with BD in 7- to 17-year-olds and also to treat irritability associated with ASD. It remains unknown if SGAs would be effective in treating DMDD. However, it was hoped that providing a "diagnostic home" for children with chronic, functionally impairing irritability other than BD would result in decreased numbers of prescriptions for SGAs (Frazier & Carlson, 2005). However, that outcome remains unknown. SGAs include a number of medications, many of which are currently generic, such as risperidone, aripiprazole, olanzapine, and quetiapine.

Use in Disorders Involving Irritability

SGAs have been studied in several disorders involving irritability, including ASD, BD, and ADHD (Geller et al., 2012; McCracken et al., 2002; van Schalkwyk et al., 2017). One hallmark study, which led to the FDA indication for risperidone in the treatment of irritability associated with ASD, was the Research Unit on Pediatric Psychopharmacology (RUPP) autism network 8-week randomized controlled trial (RCT) showing that children with autism treated with risperidone (mean dose 0.75 mg) had significant reductions in irritability, defined as at least a 25% reduction in the Aberrant Behavior Checklist (ABC) irritability subscale score and with the Clinical Global Impressions-Improvement (CGI-I) for irritability rated "much" or "very much" improved at 8 weeks, with two-thirds maintaining that response at 5 months (McCracken et al., 2002).

A recent random effects meta-analysis by Van Schalkwyk of 14 RCTs of SGAs in children across a range of diagnoses including ADHD, ODD, low IQ, conduct disorder (CD), ASD, and BD using multiple outcome measures including the ABC-Irritability scale, the Child Behavior Checklist (CBCL), and Overt Aggression Scale (OAS), showed that SGAs were effective in reducing irritability and aggression. While individual medications did not differ significantly from one another in either efficacy or specific diagnostic indication, both aripiprazole and risperidone demonstrated significant benefit versus placebo. They did not find a significant association between SGA dose and antiaggressive effects from rating scales and did not examine the effect of SGA dose on irritability (van Schalkwyk et al., 2017). It should also be noted that, while very helpful, this meta-analysis did not capture all SGA RCTs, potentially due to inherent limitations related to identification of appropriate published studies. For example, a negative 6-week RCT comparing 20 mg and 60 mg of lurasidone versus placebo (n = 50, 49, and 51, respectively) in ASD youth was not included (Loebel et al., 2016). Thus, future studies directly comparing multiple SGAs to one another and also to placebo may ultimately suggest a rank-order of how effective individual SGAs are in treating irritability associated with ASD and other disorders.

Several interesting RCTs of SGAs have been conducted in BD youth. While not specifically focused on irritability, they are important when thinking about how these agents are tolerated in children struggling with severe forms of psychopathology and how they may or may not work on more global constructs like mania and depression. For example, the Treatment of Early Onset Mania (TEAM) study compared risperidone, lithium, and divalproex sodium in BD youth (Geller et al., 2012). This study enrolled 279 antimanic-naïve children aged 6–15 years (mean age 10.1 + 2.8 years, 50.2% female) to receive lithium carbonate (maximum serum level 1.1–1.3 mEq/L), divalproex sodium (maximum serum level 111–125 mUg/mL), or risperidone (maximum dose 4–6 mg/day). Overall, they found a significantly higher response rate for risperidone than for either lithium or divalproex sodium. They also found a significantly higher discontinuation rate for lithium than for risperidone. From this, the authors concluded that risperidone was more efficacious than either lithium or divalproex sodium.

Mechanism of Action and Pharmacology

At present, we do not fully understand the SGAs' mechanism of action in reducing irritability. We know that their primary mechanism of action involves both dopamine and serotonin receptors, distinguishing them from "typical" antipsychotics or neuroleptics that act primarily through effects on dopamine receptors. Specifically, SGAs block type-2 dopamine receptors (D_2) in the central nervous system resulting in reduced positive symptoms of psychosis. They also block 5-HT2A serotonin receptors resulting in reduced risk for extrapyramidal symptoms (EPS) compared to "typical" antipsychotics, such as akathisia ("inner sense of restlessness") or acute dystonic reactions (sudden muscle spasms such as tongue thrusting). However, SGAs affect other receptors, including histamine and α-adrenergic, potentially accounting for variation in both symptom reduction and side effects. Better understanding of the cellular mechanism of action in reducing irritability in children is important to precision in our treatment of irritability.

Side Effects and Monitoring

Common side effects of SGAs include risk for metabolic syndrome, which includes extreme and rapid weight gain out of proportion to typical development. More precisely, metabolic syndrome is defined as body mass index (BMI, defined as weight in kilograms divided by height in meters squared) greater than 95%, fasting triglycerides greater than 110 mg/dL, HDL less than 40 mg/dL, and glucose more

TABLE 14.1 Metabolic syndrome: definition, prevention, and monitoring

Definition	Extreme and rapid weight gain out of proportion to typical development
Defining laboratory parameters	BMI greater than 95% Fasting triglycerides greater than 110 mg/dL, HDL <40 mg/dL, and glucose >110 mg/dL Blood pressure greater than 90%
Prevention	Appropriate pretreatment consent and warning about risk Pretreatment fasting laboratory screening and body measurements Encouragement of daily mild/moderate exercise and nutrition counseling
Monitoring	Measure height, weight, and abdominal circumference at every visit Fasting lipid panel and glucose, as well as liver function tests twice per year

BMI, body mass index (weight in kilograms [kg] divided by height in meters [m] squared [kg/m^2])

than 110 mg/dL, or blood pressure greater than 90%. At its most extreme, metabolic syndrome can result in type 2 diabetes (see Table 14.1). Despite pharmaceutical industry marketing claims that some SGAs have no or low risk for metabolic syndrome, studies from Correll et al. have demonstrated that all SGAs have the potential to cause metabolic syndrome, with weight gain of 5–10 kilograms over 3 months in first-time users across several examples of these agents, including aripiprazole, risperidone, quetiapine, and olanzapine. Moreover, several studies have shown that while no SGA has no risk of metabolic syndrome, olanzapine has the greatest risk (Correll et al., 2009).

Current recommendations include warning patients and parents about this risk prior to initiating treatment with an SGA and obtaining a fasting lipid profile and measurements of height, weight, and abdominal circumference. After initiating treatment, it is recommended that those measurements be repeated at each follow-up visit and that fasting laboratory measurements be repeated at least twice per year (Correll, 2007; Correll et al., 2006).

Summary of Second-Generation Antipsychotics

SGAs, in particular risperidone and aripiprazole, appear to have a role in treating irritability in children and adolescents. However, metabolic syndrome is a serious consideration, not just because it impairs the physical health of the child, but also because of its potential mental health impact, including decreased self-esteem and increased teasing or bullying due to obesity. At all visits, families should be warned of these risks and should be encouraged to monitor for them and to try prevention strategies with increased mild/moderate daily exercise and decreased calorie-dense foods. There is also some data suggesting that the addition of metformin, a medication that can reduce the liver's production of glucose and that was originally developed for type 2 non–insulin-dependent diabetes may be helpful when combined with these strategies in reducing the risk of obesity and metabolic syndrome in children treated with SGAs (Klein, Cottingham, Sorter, Barton, & Morrison, 2006; McDonagh, Selph, Ozpinar, & Foley, 2014).

LITHIUM

Lithium's role in treating irritability stems from its role as the hallmark antimanic agent used to treat BD. But it also has a role in treating unipolar MDD, as well as in treating adolescents hospitalized for aggression. Lithium has an FDA indication to treat mania in patients as young as 12 years.

Use in Disorders Involving Irritability

There are compelling data showing the efficacy of lithium in youth hospitalized for aggression, regardless of BD diagnosis. Specifically, three of four studies by Campbell et al. showed that lithium effectively reduced aggression as measured by the aggression subscale of the Children's Psychiatric Rating Scale in these youth (Campbell et al., 1984, 1995; Malone, Delaney, Luebbert, Cater, & Campbell, 2000; Rifkin et al., 1997). One study has examined the use of lithium in treating children with severe mood dysregulation—the forerunner of DMDD. While small, this double-blind placebo-controlled RCT found that 6 weeks of lithium ($n = 14$) was neither superior to placebo ($n = 11$) in clinical effect nor in affecting brain level of N-acetyl aspartate or myo-inositol (Dickstein et al., 2008, 2009).

Studies of children with BD, in which irritability is one aspect of both depression and mania, have yielded mixed results. For example, in one of the largest multiagent RCTs, the above-mentioned data from the TEAM study of 279 children aged 6–15 years with BD showed that lithium was not significantly better in treating mania than either risperidone or divalproex but did result in higher discontinuation than risperidone (Geller et al., 2012). Several other studies have compared lithium either to placebo or to divalproate, but the data are far more mixed than in adults with BD, where the data about lithium's use as an antimanic agent are more compelling. In one such study, BD type I youth who were manic or mixed, who were randomized to lithium ($n = 53$) had a greater reduction in symptoms than those randomized to placebo ($n = 28$) though this failed to meet the statistical threshold for significance (Findling et al., 2015).

Mechanism of Action and Pharmacology

Lithium's mechanism of action is thought to include increased intracellular signaling via decreases of the second-messenger myo-inositol, which may be measured via magnetic resonance spectroscopy (MRS) (Manji, Moore, & Chen, 2000; Moore et al., 2000; Zarate, Singh, & Manji, 2006).

Side Effects and Monitoring

Common side effects of lithium include increased thirst, nausea/vomiting, diarrhea, headache, acne, bedwetting, and impaired concentration or attention. Additionally, lithium use may cause renal or thyroid dysfunction, requiring regular monitoring of both. Moreover, patients should be warned that many common side effects of lithium vary with the magnitude of serum lithium level over 1 mEq/

TABLE 14.2 Relationship between lithium serum levels and side effects

Serum Level (milli-equivalents/liter [mEq/L])	Symptoms
1.5–2.0	Dry mouth Increased thirst (polydipsia) or urination (polyuria) Fine tremor Impaired concentration/memory Weakness
2.0–2.5	Above symptoms <u>PLUS</u>: Skin changes: acne, psoriasis, rash Metallic taste T-wave changes on EKG Hypothyroidism Weight gain Alopecia
>2.5	Mental status changes: confusion, impaired concentration/memory, lethargy, seizures, or coma Trouble speaking or forming words (dysarthria) Nephrotoxicity Muscle twitches or coarse tremor Hyperreflexia Nystagmus Nausea or vomiting

L (see Table 14.2). Since lithium is excreted by the kidneys, patients should be cautioned to avoid dehydration because it could result in elevated lithium levels, and thus, side effects. They should also be cautioned not to use nonsteroidal antiinflammatory drugs (NSAIDs), such as ibuprofen, that alter blood flow to the afferent renal arteriole and thus, alter lithium excretion.

Patients who might become pregnant should be cautioned that lithium use in the first trimester of pregnancy is associated with a 1/1,000 risk of Ebstein's anomaly. This results in the posterior displacement of the septal and posterior leaflets of the tricuspid valve between the right atrium and ventricle, causing cyanosis and arrhythmias in newborns.

Summary of Lithium

Taken as a whole, the data are not compelling with regard to using lithium to treat irritability in children, including those with DMDD. However, we do not know enough about potential subtypes of irritability that might benefit from lithium, including irritability in children with ASD or potential age or gender windows when lithium might be of benefit.

ANTIEPILEPTIC DRUGS

AEDs are medications originally used to manage seizures or epilepsy. This was then extended to BD by virtue of what has been called the "kindling hypothesis of mania," which essentially held that mania was like a "seizure of emotions" largely based on a widely circulated case series of fewer than a dozen adult patients (Post, Uhde, Putnam, Ballenger, & Berrettini, 1982). However, research has not demonstrated substantial seizure disorders or specific electroencephalogram (EEG) seizure alterations in children or adults with BD. Nevertheless, AEDs continue to be used for and studied in the treatment of BD, anger, aggression, and irritability via their effect on increasing GABA-ergic inhibitory neurotransmission.

Of all AEDs, only valproate has an FDA indication for the treatment of acute BD manic episodes, with text providing cautions about hepatotoxicity in children, especially those under 2 years old, without clear age cutoffs for this indication. None has an indication for irritability.

Use in Disorders Involving Irritability

Several large studies have examined AEDs in treating children with BD, with most focusing on potential benefit in mania, though irritability is a component of both mania and depression in children, with the gestalt view suggesting that these agents are less effective in treating mania than are SGAs. These data include several large RCTs, such as a study by Wagner et al. showing that oxcarbazepine was not superior to placebo in 300 BD youth (Wagner et al., 2006) and also that valproate was not superior to placebo in 150 BD youth (Wagner et al., 2009).

Valproate has been shown in an RCT ($n = 20$) to reduce anger in children with either ODD or CD (Donovan et al., 2000). Divalproex augmentation of ADHD stimulants has also been shown to reduce aggression in children with ADHD and chronic aggression unremitting to psychostimulant treatment alone, with 8/14 (57%) meeting remission criteria versus 2/13 (15%) randomized to placebo for 8 weeks (Blader, Schooler, Jensen, Pliszka, & Kafantaris, 2009). Similarly, in a 12-week RCT, ASD youth randomized to valproate showed significant reductions on the ABC-Irritability subscale and CGI-I for irritability compared to those treated with placebo ($N = 27$) (Hollander et al., 2010). Coccaro et al. conducted a 12-week RCT with adults with intermittent explosive disorder (IED) (mean age 34 years) randomized to placebo, fluoxetine, or divalproex ($n = 9$, 10, and 11, respectively), but failed to find significant between-group differences in reduction of irritability or aggression (Coccaro, Lee, Breen, & Irwin, 2015).

Mechanism of Action and Pharmacology

Overall, AEDs work to boost inhibitory mechanisms affecting cell signaling so as to reduce risk of seizures. This may include combinations of increasing GABA-ergic inhibition (valproate, gabapentin) or decreasing glutamate excitation (topiramate). It may also include inhibition of sodium channels, resulting in decreased action potential firing (carbamazepine, oxcarbazepine, lamotrigine).

Side Effects and Monitoring

Side effects common to AEDs include sedation and weight gain. Importantly, all AEDs result in hepatic autoinduction, meaning that concomitant use of

AEDs with other medications that are also metabolized by the liver results in increased breakdown and decreased efficacy of those other medications. In addition, there are several side effects that are specific to particular AEDs. For example, valproate may result in polycystic ovary syndrome (PCOS) resulting in irregular menses and increased levels of androgens and neural tube defects in babies born to mothers on valproate. Valproate has an FDA black box warning for potential hepatotoxicity that is especially more common in children under 2 years old.

Lamotrigine, particularly rapid dose changes, is associated with increased risk of rash, ranging from benign to Stevens-Johnson syndrome, the latter of which is associated with nonpruritic (not itchy) erythematous (red) target-shaped maculopapular lesions, fever, blood pressure instability, altered level of consciousness, and, at its extreme, death. Increased risk for lamotrigine-induced Stephens-Johnson syndrome is associated with patient age less than 12 years or coadministration with hepatically metabolized medications. Prevention, via slow titrations by 25 mg every 3–4 weeks, is the best strategy to manage this risk.

Summary of Antiepileptic Drugs

While there is some limited data supporting the use of valproate and divalproex to reduce irritability, the field is ripe for studies that can better understand mechanisms underlying subtypes of irritability that could be amenable to specific types of AEDs. For example, irritability in children with ADHD or in primary DMDD who may respond to the combination of an ADHD stimulant and AED—although, again, this needs to be tested before it is used clinically.

ADHD STIMULANTS

While irritability is not an explicit diagnostic criterion for ADHD in DSM-IV or in DSM-5, it is a common associated feature—thus, a discussion about ADHD treatments is included in this chapter on the pharmacological treatment of irritability. Stimulants are the primary type of medication used to treat children with ADHD since the pioneering studies of Charles Bradley who, in 1937, used D,L-amphetamine to decrease motor hyperactivity, increase compliance, and improve academic performance in children (Strohl, 2011). They are among the most studied of all medication treatments for child psychiatric disorders. Among the most notable studies is the Multimodal Treatment of ADHD (MTA) study, which showed that stimulants by themselves or combined with behavioral treatment led to stable long-term improvements in ADHD symptoms (MTA Cooperative Group, 1999).

FDA indications for the use of stimulants include (1) methylphenidate for treating patients with ADHD 6–65 years of age and (2) dextroamphetamine for treating ADHD for patients as young as 3 years of age.

Use in Disorders Involving Irritability

The effect of stimulants on irritability in patients with ADHD remains unclear. On the one hand, many individual double-blind RCTs of stimulant medication for ADHD report that irritability may be a common side effect occurring in 5–10% of children with ADHD (Childress, Kollins, Cutler, Marraffino, & Sikes, 2017; Newcorn et al., 2017; Robb et al., 2017). On the other hand, other RCTs show improvements in irritability following stimulant medication treatment (Childress, Sallee, & Berry, 2011). Stuckelman et al. conducted a meta-analysis of 32 double-blind RCTs involving 3,664 children with ADHD that reported data on irritability as a side effect of stimulant medication. They found that methylphenidate-based ADHD stimulants had a significantly decreased risk of irritability versus placebo (relative risk [RR] = 0.89), whereas amphetamine-based ADHD stimulants had a significantly increased risk of causing irritability (RR = 2.90). From this, the authors concluded that the potential increased risk for irritability due to stimulants may be confined to amphetamine-based ADHD stimulants, though large head-to-head trials are necessary to fully flesh this out (Stuckelman et al., 2017).

We need far more research on the mechanisms and treatment of irritability in children with ADHD. As one example of an important study, Fernandez de la Cruz et al. conducted a secondary data analysis from the MTA that specifically evaluated irritability among 144 ADHD participants treated with stimulant medication versus 144 receiving only behavioral treatment. In treating irritability, they found that the combination of stimulant medication and behavioral treatment was superior to community care and to behavioral treatment alone, but not to medication management alone. They concluded that targeting ADHD symptoms with stimulant medication can reduce irritability in children with ADHD, although irritability did not itself moderate parent or teacher ratings of ADHD symptom response, and the effect size for the response of irritability symptoms was less than that of ADHD symptoms (Fernandez et al., 2015). Related smaller studies show that dose optimization may be the key to reducing irritability in those whose irritability appears initially to not respond to stimulants (Blader, Pliszka, Jensen, Schooler, & Kafantaris, 2010).

Several other examples show the potential benefit of stimulants in treating irritability in youth with ADHD. For example, Connor et al. conducted a meta-analysis testing the effect of stimulants on overt and covert aggression in children with ADHD beyond effects on ADHD core features of hyperactivity, impulsivity, and inattention. Using published studies from 1970 to 2001, they found 28 studies of overt and 7 studies of covert aggression. They found that the effect size for the decrease in aggression was 0.84 for overt and 0.69 for covert aggression—similar benefit to the effect sizes reported for stimulants' effect on core ADHD symptoms (Connor, Glatt, Lopez, Jackson, & Melloni, 2002).

Waxmonsky et al. studied the effects of methylphenidate (0.15 mg/kg three times per day, 0.3 mg/kg, and 0.6 mg/kg each three times per day) or placebo combined with behavior modification therapy (none, low-, and high-intensity) among 33 children aged 5–15 with severe mood dysregulation (SMD) and ADHD compared to children with ADHD alone (*n* = 68). They found that both groups had substantial improvement in externalizing behaviors on the Disruptive Behavior Scale and behavioral observations from a therapeutic treatment program, with no difference in side effects. SMD youth were more likely to remain impaired at home and to have elevated ODD/CD symptoms than were non-SMD youth (Waxmonsky et al., 2008). This suggests that ADHD stimulants have a role in reducing externalizing behavior, including aggression and irritability, in youth with SMD plus ADHD, and also in those with ADHD alone.

Comparisons to nonstimulant ADHD treatments, including the norepinephrine reuptake inhibitor atomoxetine, are also worth noting. In one of the largest such studies, Cortese et al. used data from the Italian ADHD Registry and found that 753 children with ADHD treated with atomoxetine had a significantly higher incidence rate ratio (IRR) of irritability compared to the 1,350 children with ADHD receiving only methylphenidate (Cortese et al., 2015). Thus, the authors suggest that the nonstimulant atomoxetine increased irritability, rather than decreasing it.

Mechanism of Action and Pharmacology

ADHD stimulants are thought to work by causing the release of dopamine and norepinephrine catecholamines from dopamine axons, as well as blocking their reuptake. Methylphenidate releases catecholamines from long-term stores, whereas amphetamines release them from newly formed storage granules on the presynaptic neuron. Stimulants also bind to dopamine transporters in the striatum, blocking reuptake of dopamine and norepinephrine and leading to an increase in dopamine within the synapse. This, in turn, enhances prefrontal cortex (PFC) function, which is thought to improve executive control over thought, behavior, and emotions (Posner et al., 2011; Schweren, de Zeeuw, & Durston, 2013).

Side Effects and Monitoring

Common side effects include decreased appetite, delayed sleep onset, headache, and jitteriness. Stimulants also potentially bring out a child's vulnerability to motor or vocal tics. However, as studies have shown that ADHD, tics, and anxiety disorders all involve alterations in fronto-striato-thalamic circuits, physicians often have to balance out treatment of ADHD with treatment of tics. Concern has been raised that stimulants could potentially increase either mania or irritability. Carlson et al. showed in a 20-year follow-up study that ADHD stimulant treatment did not increase risk for mania (Carlson, Loney, Salisbury, Kramer, & Arthur, 2000), although, as indicated earlier, it can lead to increased irritability, particularly amphetamine-based medications (Stuckelman et al., 2017).

Concern has also been raised for potential cardiac effects of stimulant medication, specifically increased risk for arrhythmia and sudden cardiac death. However, guidelines from the American Academy of Pediatrics state that while all patients should be screened for personal and familial history of cardiac illness, including arrhythmia, prior to initiation of ADHD stimulants, evaluations including electrocardiograms (EKGs) are only required for children with elevated risk (Denchev, Kaltman, Schoenbaum, & Vitiello, 2010; Perrin et al., 2008).

Summary of ADHD Stimulants

Overall, methylphenidate-based ADHD stimulants in children with ADHD combined with behavioral treatments may be helpful for improving function and reducing irritability. However, as always, the more complex the child, the more complex the treatment. When treating children who have ADHD plus other psychiatric disorders, like mood or anxiety problems, physicians need to set clear treatment targets and monitor for side effects, and they may need to use more than just ADHD stimulants to achieve the right balance.

α_2 AGONISTS

α_2 Adrenergic agonists, including clonidine and guanfacine, have FDA indications for the treatment of ADHD as both a monotherapy and in combination with stimulant medication in patients as young as 6 years of age. Their use in treating ADHD stems from their mechanism in norepinephrine neurotransmission, as they were originally developed to treat abnormally elevated blood pressure. Clinically, they are often used to treat many other conditions for which they do not have an official FDA indication, including irritability and aggression.

Use in Disorders Involving Irritability

Despite myriad review articles listing α-agonists as potential treatments for children or adolescents with disorders involving irritability, aggression, or disruptive behavior, including ADHD, ASD, IED, and ODD, there are surprisingly few RCTs that have explicitly tested their use for those behavioral/emotional outcomes.

An 8-week RCT conducted by the Research Units on Pediatric Psychopharmacology Autism Network (RUPP-Autism) in 62 children with ASD showed that extended-release guanfacine (modal dose at week 8 was 3 mg/day) resulted in a significant reduction in hyperactivity. However, irritability was reported as a side effect more frequently in children in the guanfacine condition than in those randomized to placebo (Scahill et al., 2015). Similarly, a 9-week RCT pharmaceutical study showed that, compared to placebo, extended-release guanfacine reduced ADHD symptoms in 324 children with ADHD (five groups: placebo, 1-, 2-, 3-, and 4-mg extended-release guanfacine, with about $n = 65$ randomly assigned to each arm and about $n = 40$ completers in each). Again, more children given guanfacine reported irritability as a side effect (5%) than did those on placebo (Sallee et al., 2009).

Mechanism of Action and Pharmacology

α₂ agonists' mechanism of action involves G-protein coupled second-messenger signaling, which reduces adenylate cyclase and simultaneously inhibits calcium channels while activating potassium channels, ultimately, reducing overall sympathetic nervous system activity (reducing fight-or-flight behaviors). The main site of α₂ receptors is in the locus ceruleus, which is the center of noradrenergic neurotransmission. However, α₂ receptors are located throughout the brain, including in the striatum, amygdala, hippocampus, cerebral cortex, and cerebellum.

Studies suggest that cognitive benefits of α₂ agonists may be due to stimulation of postsynaptic α₂ₐ-andrenoreceptors in cortex (Arnsten & Goldman-Rakic, 1985; Robbins & Arnsten, 2009). Calming effects may be due to inhibition of norepinephrine release in the locus ceruleus by presynaptic α receptors.

Side Effects and Monitoring

Common side effects of α₂ agonists include sedation, dizziness, weakness, and dry mouth. Because they are blood pressure lowering medications, it is important to monitor blood pressure and heart rate before initiating treatment, with dose increases, and with any complaint that might indicate blood pressure or heart rate changes, such as dizziness or weakness.

As with ADHD stimulants, practitioners should carefully review individual cardiac risk factors prior to initiating treatment, including history of arrhythmia and bradycardia (slow heart rate) in particular. This should include asking about symptoms that might be classified as neurological that could have a cardiac cause, such as syncope or fainting. Recommendations for pretreatment EKGs for α agonists either alone or in combination with ADHD stimulants are mixed. This is clearly an important research topic ripe for the use of electronic medical records and a big data approach. To avoid cardiovascular effects, these medications should be tapered slowly during dose increases and decreases (i.e., by 0.05 mg clonidine or 0.5 mg guanfacine every 4–5 days). Because these medications undergo both renal and hepatic metabolism, baseline screening to ensure normal kidney and liver function is recommended.

Summary of Alpha Agonists

On the one hand, well-conducted, reasonably large studies suggest that α₂ agonists may not be helpful in the treatment of irritability. On the other hand, it is possible that future work may identify particular children who might benefit from α₂ agonists, such as those with a particular subtype of irritability (possibly episodic, such as seen with BD or MDD; or chronic, as in association with DMDD) or type of child (younger vs. older; male vs. female). Until this is sorted out via more research, α agonists should not be used as the first agent when trying to reduce irritability and aggression.

SELECTIVE SEROTONIN REUPTAKE INHIBITOR ANTIDEPRESSANT/ ANTIANXIETY AGENTS

SSRIs, including fluoxetine, citalopram, and sertraline, are commonly used to treat depression and anxiety disorders in children and adolescents, both of which involve irritability. FDA indications for the use of SSRIs in children include (1) fluoxetine for the treatment of children aged 8–18 with MDD and 7–17 with obsessive compulsive disorder (OCD) and (2) sertraline for the treatment of OCD. Despite these official FDA indications, first-line SSRIs in children also include citalopram, fluoxetine, and sertraline, with first-degree relatives' history of response being the most useful guide in selecting a particular medication for an individual patient (Bertilsson, Dahl, Dalen, & Al-Shurbaji, 2002).

However, these same medications may also increase irritability, agitation, and aggression in children, and they also have the potential to cause mania or suicidality. Thus, treating an individual child with an SSRI agent requires a careful assessment to ensure that current symptoms and possible risk for depression, anxiety, and mania are evaluated and discussed with the child and his or her parents. It is also important to monitor for those treatment-emergent symptoms, especially in the first 3 months of treatment, following the FDA's black box warning on SSRI medications issued in 2004 and applicable to all patients under age 25 (Hammad, Laughren, & Racoosin, 2006).

There are other forms of antidepressant or antianxiety medication, including combined serotonergic/noradrenergic agents. However, these medications are not considered first-line treatment, and a full discussion is beyond the scope of this chapter.

Use in Disorders Involving Irritability

While there are multiple studies that have focused on the use of SSRIs in the treatment of irritability, they have all focused on adult samples. For example, Coccaro et al. conducted a double-blind placebo-controlled trial with fluoxetine in 100 adults with IED and found a significant and sustained reduction in the Overt Aggression Scale-Modified (OAS-M) for outpatient use, including the irritability subscale of the OAS-M, as well as the CGI-I, versus placebo (Coccaro, Lee, & Kavoussi, 2009). Full or partial remission of impulsive-aggressive behaviors occurred in 46 of those treated with fluoxetine, an effect independent of changes in anxiety or depressive symptoms. In another, smaller 12-week RCT among adults with IED, Coccaro et al. reported negligible changes in levels of aggression and irritability scores in response to fluoxetine ($n = 10$), divalproex ($n = 11$), or placebo ($n = 9$) (Coccaro et al., 2015).

Other studies have shown SSRIs' efficacy in reducing irritability and aggression in adults with other conditions, perhaps more distal to typical child/adolescent psychiatric issues. For example, several studies have shown that SSRIs can reduce irritability and anger associated with premenstrual syndrome (PMS) and premenstrual dysphoric disorder (PMDD). Marjoribanks et al. conducted a Cochrane database meta-analysis harnessing data from 31 placebo-controlled RCTs of women with PMS, and found that the SSRIs, including fluoxetine, paroxetine, sertraline, escitalopram, and citalopram, effectively reduced reported levels of psychological symptoms and irritability. In a placebo-controlled RCT of sertraline by Yonkers et al., 125 women with PMDD showed greater improvements in ratings of anger and irritability after treatment (Marjoribanks, Brown, O'Brien, & Wyatt, 2013; Yonkers et al., 2015). In another example, George et al.'s 12-week, double-blind, placebo-controlled study showed that fluoxetine significantly lowered irritability among alcoholic perpetrators of domestic violence (George et al., 2011). Similarly, several large, double-blind, placebo-controlled studies have shown that citalopram may reduce irritability among adults with Alzheimer's dementia (Leonpacher et al., 2016; Porsteinsson et al., 2014).

Mechanism of Action and Pharmacology

In general, SSRI medications' mechanism of action involves blocking the presynaptic reuptake and recycling of serotonin, resulting in increased levels of serotonin in the synaptic cleft and increased postsynaptic serotonin-mediated neurotransmission.

SSRIs differ in the presence or absence of active metabolites that may prolong the overall elimination half-life. Fluoxetine, sertraline, and citalopram all have active metabolites (norfluoxetine, des-methyl-sertraline, and des-methyl-citalopram, respectively). Fluoxetine has the longest half-life of any SSRI at approximately 7 days, with sertraline and citalopram having half-lives of approximately 1 day, and fluvoxamine at 18 hours. This results in fluvoxamine often being dosed twice daily, while the others are typically dosed once daily.

Side Effects and Monitoring

Like many medications, SSRIs are metabolized by cytochrome p450 enzymes in the liver. The emerging field of pharmacogenomics seeks to identify how genetic alterations in these hepatic enzymes, which may be inherited, affect the metabolism of specific medications. Moreover, specific ethnoracial groups may characteristically share patterns of cytochrome p450 enzyme activity (see Moore, Hill, & Panguluri, 2014, for a review). While tests to evaluate an individual patient's pharmacogenetic profiles are commercially available, at present, data do not support these tests as part of the standard evaluation for the majority of psychiatric patients across ages and diagnoses (see the Evaluation of Genomic Applications in Practice and Prevention [EGAPP] Working Group Statement, 2007). However, clinicians should inquire about first-degree relatives' history of either response to or intolerance/side effects of specific SSRIs and use that information in selecting a specific SSRI for an individual patient.

Common side effects from SSRIs include gastrointestinal (e.g., nausea, vomiting, diarrhea, or constipation) mediated via serotonin receptors throughout the gastrointestinal tract, drowsiness or fatigue, or exacerbation of depression or anxiety. Importantly, since 2004, all antidepressant and antianxiety medications have had an FDA black box warning related to their use. In brief, pooled data from 4,400 child/adolescent patients in 24 short-term trials of nine antidepressant medications and more than 77,000 adults in 295 trials of 11 antidepressant medications showed an increased risk of thoughts of suicide in those on one of these antidepressants versus placebo (overall 4% vs. 2% risk, respectively). In addition to the black box warning placed on product labeling, guidelines have supported the role for better informed consent from parents about this risk and more regular monitoring for suicidality and other side effects, especially in the first 3 months.

Summary of SSRIs

Studies of SSRIs for the treatment of MDD, OCD, or other anxiety disorders have reported on irritability as an adverse event rather than as a potential beneficial outcome or treatment target. These studies have yielded mixed results, showing that irritability may occur among children treated with SSRIs for depression or anxiety, and, if it does occur, it may result in patients' discontinuing their medications (Hughes et al., 2007; Reid et al., 2015).

However, these data clearly show the need for greater reporting about irritability in SSRI treatment trials in children and adolescents. They also show the need for more such trials, including among youth with DMDD, given that DMDD is incorporated in the mood disorders section of DSM-5. There is also a great need to evaluate the safe and effective treatment of depression and anxiety among youth with BD. Specifically, each of these disorders (depression, anxiety, mania) alone, as well as in combination, can involve irritability as a symptom. Studies that are adequately powered and designed to sort this out are very important to our most common and impairing disorders, as well as to the field of irritability more broadly.

Conclusion

In conclusion, irritability is a common and disabling symptom associated with numerous child psychiatric disorders. Current studies support the role of medications in treating irritability, starting with using specific medications to address common disorders involving irritability, including SGAs for BD and ASD, ADHD stimulants for ADHD, and SSRIs for anxiety and depression. There is a great need to identify optimal medication treatment for other conditions, including for DMDD and for children who present with more than one disorder. Improved ways to monitor for irritability in children are crucial when paired with these medication trials so that we can sort out which particular medications improve irritability and which may worsen it in particular children. Future mechanism-oriented research needs to address cost-effective ways to identify which medication (or medications) will work for an individual child's needs, how to prevent or to treat any related side effects, and how these mechanisms affect brain development.

References

A 14-month randomized clinical trial of treatment strategies for attention-deficit/hyperactivity disorder. The MTA Cooperative Group. Multimodal Treatment Study of Children with ADHD. (1999). *Archives of General Psychiatry, 56*(12), 1073–1086.

American Psychiatric Association (APA). (2013). *Diagnostic and Statistical Manual of Mental Disorders* (5th edition). Arlington, VA: American Psychiatric Association.

Arnsten, A. F., & Goldman-Rakic, P. S. (1985). Alpha 2-adrenergic mechanisms in prefrontal cortex associated with cognitive decline in aged nonhuman primates. *Science, 230*(4731), 1273–1276.

Bauer, M. S., & Mitchner, L. (2004). What is a "mood stabilizer"? An evidence-based response. *American Journal of Psychiatry, 161*(1), 3–18.

Bertilsson, L., Dahl, M. L., Dalen, P., & Al-Shurbaji, A. (2002). Molecular genetics of CYP2D6: Clinical relevance with focus on psychotropic drugs. *British Journal of Clinical Pharmacology, 53*(2), 111–122.

Blader, J. C., Pliszka, S. R., Jensen, P. S., Schooler, N. R., & Kafantaris, V. (2010). Stimulant-responsive and stimulant-refractory aggressive behavior among children with ADHD. *Pediatrics, 126*(4), e796–e806. doi:10.1542/peds.2010-0086

Blader, J. C., Schooler, N. R., Jensen, P. S., Pliszka, S. R., & Kafantaris, V. (2009). Adjunctive divalproex versus placebo for children with ADHD and aggression refractory to stimulant monotherapy. *American Journal of Psychiatry, 166*(12), 1392–1401. doi:10.1176/appi. ajp.2009.09020233

Brotman, M. A., Kircanski, K., & Leibenluft, E. (2017). Irritability in children and adolescents. *Annual Review of Clinical Psychology, 13*, 317–341. doi:10.1146/ annurev-clinpsy-032816-044941

Brotman, M. A., Kircanski, K., Stringaris, A., Pine, D. S., & Leibenluft, E. (2017). Irritability in youths: A translational model. *American Journal of Psychiatry, 174*(6), 520–532. doi:10.1176/appi.ajp.2016.16070839

Campbell, M., Adams, P. B., Small, A. M., Kafantaris, V., Silva, R. R., Shell, J., . . . Overall, J. E. (1995). Lithium in hospitalized aggressive children with conduct disorder: A double-blind and placebo-controlled study. *Journal of the American Academy of Child and Adolescent Psychiatry, 34*(4), 445–453.

Campbell, M., Small, A. M., Green, W. H., Jennings, S. J., Perry, R., Bennett, W. G., & Anderson, L. (1984). Behavioral efficacy of haloperidol and lithium carbonate. A comparison in hospitalized aggressive children with conduct disorder. *Archives of General Psychiatry, 41*(7), 650–656.

Carlson, G. A., Loney, J., Salisbury, H., Kramer, J. R., & Arthur, C. (2000). Stimulant treatment in young boys with symptoms suggesting childhood mania: A report from a longitudinal study. *Journal of Child and Adolescent Psychopharmacology, 10*(3), 175–184. doi:10.1089/10445460050167287

Childress, A. C., Kollins, S. H., Cutler, A. J., Marraffino, A., & Sikes, C. R. (2017). Efficacy, safety, and tolerability of an extended-release orally disintegrating methylphenidate tablet in children 6-12 years of age with attention-deficit/hyperactivity disorder in the laboratory classroom setting. *Journal of Child and Adolescent Psychopharmacology, 27*(1), 66–74. doi:10.1089/cap.2016.0002

Childress, A. C., Sallee, F. R., & Berry, S. A. (2011). Single-dose pharmacokinetics of NWP06, an extended-release methylphenidate suspension, in children and adolescents with ADHD. *Postgraduate Medicine, 123*(5), 80–88. doi:10.3810/pgm.2011.09.2462

Coccaro, E. F., Lee, R., Breen, E. C., & Irwin, M. R. (2015). Inflammatory markers and chronic exposure to fluoxetine, divalproex, and placebo in intermittent explosive disorder. *Psychiatry Research, 229*(3), 844–849. doi:10.1016/j.psychres.2015.07.078

Coccaro, E. F., Lee, R. J., & Kavoussi, R. J. (2009). A double-blind, randomized, placebo-controlled trial of fluoxetine in patients with intermittent explosive disorder. *Journal of Clinical Psychiatry, 70*(5), 653–662. doi:10.4088/JCP.08m04150

Collishaw, S., Maughan, B., Natarajan, L., & Pickles, A. (2010). Trends in adolescent emotional problems in England: A comparison of two national cohorts twenty years apart. *Journal of Child Psychology and Psychiatry, 51*(8), 885–894. doi:10.1111/j.1469-7610.2010.02252.x

Connor, D. F., Glatt, S. J., Lopez, I. D., Jackson, D., & Melloni, R. H., Jr. (2002). Psychopharmacology and aggression. I: A meta-analysis of stimulant effects on overt/covert aggression-related behaviors in ADHD. *Journal of the American Academy of Child and Adolescent Psychiatry, 41*(3), 253–261. doi:10.1097/00004583-200203000-00004

Correll, C. U. (2007). Weight gain and metabolic effects of mood stabilizers and antipsychotics in pediatric bipolar disorder: A systematic review and pooled analysis of short-term trials. *Journal of the American Academy of Child and Adolescent Psychiatry, 46*(6), 687–700. doi:10.1097/chi.0b013e318040b25f

Correll, C. U., Manu, P., Olshanskiy, V., Napolitano, B., Kane, J. M., & Malhotra, A. K. (2009). Cardiometabolic risk of second-generation antipsychotic medications during first-time use in children and adolescents. *JAMA, 302*(16), 1765–1773.

Correll, C. U., Penzner, J. B., Parikh, U. H., Mughal, T., Javed, T., Carbon, M., & Malhotra, A. K. (2006). Recognizing and monitoring adverse events of second-generation antipsychotics in children and adolescents. *Child and Adolescent Psychiatric Clinics of North America, 15*(1), 177–206. doi:10.1016/j.chc.2005.08.007

Cortese, S., Panei, P., Arcieri, R., Germinario, E. A., Capuano, A., Margari, L., . . . Curatolo, P. (2015). Safety of methylphenidate and atomoxetine in children with attention-deficit/hyperactivity disorder (ADHD): Data from the Italian National ADHD Registry. *CNS Drugs, 29*(10), 865–877. doi:10.1007/s40263-015-0266-7

Denchev, P., Kaltman, J. R., Schoenbaum, M., & Vitiello, B. (2010). Modeled economic evaluation of alternative strategies to reduce sudden cardiac death among children treated for attention deficit/hyperactivity disorder. *Circulation, 121*(11), 1329–1337. doi:10.1161/CIRCULATIONAHA.109.901256

Dickstein, D. P., Towbin, K. E., Van Der Veen, J. W., Rich, B. A., Brotman, M. A., Knopf, L., . . . Leibenluft, E. (2009). Randomized double-blind placebo-controlled trial of lithium in youths with severe mood dysregulation. *Journal of Child and Adolescent Psychopharmacology, 19*(1), 61–73. doi:10.1089/cap.2008.044

Dickstein, D. P., van der Veen, J. W., Knopf, L., Towbin, K. E., Pine, D. S., & Leibenluft, E. (2008). Proton magnetic resonance spectroscopy in youth with severe mood dysregulation. *Psychiatry Research, 163*(1), 30–39. doi:10.1016/j.pscychresns.2007.11.006

Donovan, S. J., Stewart, J. W., Nunes, E. V., Quitkin, F. M., Parides, M., Daniel, W., . . . Klein, D. F. (2000). Divalproex treatment for youth with explosive temper and mood lability: A double-blind, placebo-controlled crossover design. *American Journal of Psychiatry, 157*(5), 818–820. doi:10.1176/appi.ajp.157.5.818

Evaluation of Genomic Applications in Practice and Prevention Working Group. (2007). Recommendations from the EGAPP Working Group: Testing for cytochrome P450 polymorphisms in adults with nonpsychotic depression treated with selective serotonin reuptake inhibitors. *Genetic Medicine, 9*(12), 819–825. doi:10.1097GIM.0b013e31815bf9a3

Fernandez, d. l. C., Simonoff, E., McGough, J. J., Halperin, J. M., Arnold, L. E., & Stringaris, A. (2015). Treatment of children with attention-deficit/hyperactivity disorder (ADHD) and irritability: Results from the Multimodal Treatment Study of Children with ADHD (MTA). *Journal of the American Academy of Child and Adolescent Psychiatry, 54*(1), 62–70.

Findling, R. L., Robb, A., McNamara, N. K., Pavuluri, M. N., Kafantaris, V., Scheffer, R., . . . Taylor-Zapata, P. (2015). Lithium in the acute treatment of bipolar I disorder: A double-blind, placebo-controlled study. *Pediatrics, 136*(5), 885–894. doi:10.1542/peds.2015-0743

Frazier, J. A., & Carlson, G. A. (2005). Diagnostically homeless and needing appropriate placement. *Journal of Child and Adolescent Psychopharmacology, 15*(3), 337–342. doi:10.1089/cap.2005.15.337

Geller, B., Luby, J. L., Joshi, P., Wagner, K. D., Emslie, G., Walkup, J. T., . . . Lavori, P. (2012). A randomized controlled trial of risperidone, lithium, or divalproex sodium for initial treatment of bipolar I disorder, manic or mixed phase, in children and adolescents. *Archives of General Psychiatry, 69*(5), 515–528. doi:10.1001/archgenpsychiatry.2011.1508

George, D. T., Phillips, M. J., Lifshitz, M., Lionetti, T. A., Spero, D. E., Ghassemzedeh, N., . . . Rawlings, R. R. (2011). Fluoxetine treatment of alcoholic perpetrators of domestic violence: A 12-week, double-blind, randomized, placebo-controlled intervention study. *Journal of Clinical Psychiatry, 72*(1), 60–65. doi:10.4088/JCP.09m05256gry

Goodwin, R., Gould, M. S., Blanco, C., & Olfson, M. (2001). Prescription of psychotropic medications to youths in office-based practice. *Psychiatric Services, 52*(8), 1081–1087. doi:10.1176/appi.ps.52.8.1081

Hammad, T. A., Laughren, T., & Racoosin, J. (2006). Suicidality in pediatric patients treated with antidepressant drugs. *Archives of General Psychiatry, 63*(3), 332–339. doi:10.1001/archpsyc.63.3.332

Hollander, E., Chaplin, W., Soorya, L., Wasserman, S., Novotny, S., Rusoff, J., . . . Anagnostou, E. (2010). Divalproex sodium vs placebo for the treatment of irritability in children and adolescents with autism spectrum disorders. *Neuropsychopharmacology, 35*(4), 990–998. doi:10.1038/npp.2009.202

Hughes, C. W., Emslie, G. J., Crismon, M. L., Posner, K., Birmaher, B., Ryan, N., . . . Texas Consensus Conference Panel on Medication Treatment of Childhood Major Depressive, D. (2007). Texas Children's Medication Algorithm Project: Update from Texas Consensus Conference Panel on Medication Treatment of Childhood Major Depressive Disorder. *Journal of the American Academy of Child and Adolescent Psychiatry, 46*(6), 667–686. doi:10.1097/chi.0b013e31804a859b

Insel, T., Cuthbert, B., Garvey, M., Heinssen, R., Pine, D. S., Quinn, K., . . . Wang, P. (2010). Research domain criteria (RDoC): Toward a new classification framework for research

on mental disorders. *American Journal of Psychiatry, 167*(7), 748–751. doi:10.1176/appi.
ajp.2010.09091379

Keck, P. E., Jr., McElroy, S. L., Richtand, N., & Tohen, M. (2002). What makes a drug a primary mood stabilizer? *Molecular Psychiatry, 7*(Suppl 1), S8–S14.

Kelly, C., Molcho, M., Doyle, P., & Gabhainn, S. N. (2010). Psychosomatic symptoms among schoolchildren. *International Journal of Adolescent Mental Health, 22*(2), 229–235.

Klein, D. J., Cottingham, E. M., Sorter, M., Barton, B. A., & Morrison, J. A. (2006). A randomized, double-blind, placebo-controlled trial of metformin treatment of weight gain associated with initiation of atypical antipsychotic therapy in children and adolescents. *American Journal of Psychiatry, 163*(12), 2072–2079. doi:10.1176/ajp.2006.163.12.2072

Leibenluft, E., Charney, D. S., & Pine, D. S. (2003). Researching the pathophysiology of pediatric bipolar disorder. *Biological Psychiatry, 53*(11), 1009–1020.

Leibenluft, E., Charney, D. S., Towbin, K. E., Bhangoo, R. K., & Pine, D. S. (2003). Defining clinical phenotypes of juvenile mania. *American Journal of Psychiatry, 160*(3), 430–437. doi:10.1176/appi.ajp.160.3.430

Leibenluft, E., Cohen, P., Gorrindo, T., Brook, J. S., & Pine, D. S. (2006). Chronic versus episodic irritability in youth: A community-based, longitudinal study of clinical and diagnostic associations. *Journal of Child and Adolescent Psychopharmacology, 16*(4), 456–466. doi:10.1089/cap.2006.16.456

Leonpacher, A. K., Peters, M. E., Drye, L. T., Makino, K. M., Newell, J. A., Devanand, D. P., . . . Cit, A. D. R. G. (2016). Effects of citalopram on neuropsychiatric symptoms in Alzheimer's dementia: Evidence from the CitAD study. *American Journal of Psychiatry, 173*(5), 473–480. doi:10.1176/appi.ajp.2016.15020248

Loebel, A., Brams, M., Goldman, R. S., Silva, R., Hernandez, D., Deng, L., . . . Findling, R. L. (2016). Lurasidone for the treatment of irritability associated with autistic disorder. *Journal of Autism and Developmental Disorders, 46*(4), 1153–1163. doi:10.1007/s10803-015-2628-x

Malone, R. P., Delaney, M. A., Luebbert, J. F., Cater, J., & Campbell, M. (2000). A double-blind placebo-controlled study of lithium in hospitalized aggressive children and adolescents with conduct disorder. *Archives of General Psychiatry, 57*(7), 649–654.

Manji, H. K., Moore, G. J., & Chen, G. (2000). Lithium up-regulates the cytoprotective protein Bcl-2 in the CNS in vivo: A role for neurotrophic and neuroprotective effects in manic depressive illness. *Journal of Clinical Psychiatry, 61*(Suppl 9), 82–96.

Marjoribanks, J., Brown, J., O'Brien, P. M., & Wyatt, K. (2013). Selective serotonin reuptake inhibitors for premenstrual syndrome. *Cochrane Database of Systematic Reviews*(6), CD001396. doi:10.1002/14651858.CD001396.pub3

McCracken, J. T., McGough, J., Shah, B., Cronin, P., Hong, D., Aman, M. G., . . . Research Units on Pediatric Psychopharmacology Autism, N. (2002). Risperidone in children with autism and serious behavioral problems. *New England Journal of Medicine, 347*(5), 314–321. doi:10.1056/NEJMoa013171

McDonagh, M. S., Selph, S., Ozpinar, A., & Foley, C. (2014). Systematic review of the benefits and risks of metformin in treating obesity in children aged 18 years and younger. *JAMA Pediatrics, 168*(2), 178–184. doi:10.1001/jamapediatrics.2013.4200

Moore, G. J., Bebchuk, J. M., Hasanat, K., Chen, G., Seraji-Bozorgzad, N., Wilds, I. B., ... Manji, H. K. (2000). Lithium increases N-acetyl-aspartate in the human brain: In vivo evidence in support of bcl-2's neurotrophic effects? *Biological Psychiatry, 48*(1), 1–8.

Moore, T. R., Hill, A. M., & Panguluri, S. K. (2014). Pharmacogenomics in psychiatry: Implications for practice. *Recent Patents in Biotechnology, 8*(2), 152–159.

MTA Cooperative Group. (1999). A 14-month randomized clinical trial of treatment strategies for attention-deficit/hyperactivity disorder. The MTA Cooperative Group. Multimodal Treatment Study. *Archives of General Psychiatry, 56*, 1073–1086.

Newcorn, J. H., Nagy, P., Childress, A. C., Frick, G., Yan, B., & Pliszka, S. (2017). Randomized, double-blind, placebo-controlled acute comparator trials of lisdexamfetamine and extended-release methylphenidate in adolescents with attention-deficit/hyperactivity disorder. *CNS Drugs, 31*(11), 999–1014. doi:10.1007/s40263-017-0468-2

Olfson, M., Blanco, C., Liu, L., Moreno, C., & Laje, G. (2006). National trends in the outpatient treatment of children and adolescents with antipsychotic drugs. *Archives of General Psychiatry, 63*(6), 679–685. doi:10.1001/archpsyc.63.6.679

Perrin, J. M., Friedman, R. A., Knilans, T. K., Black Box Working, G., Section on, C., & Cardiac, S. (2008). Cardiovascular monitoring and stimulant drugs for attention-deficit/hyperactivity disorder. *Pediatrics, 122*(2), 451–453. doi:10.1542/peds.2008-1573

Peterson, B. S., Zhang, H., Santa Lucia, R., King, R. A., & Lewis, M. (1996). Risk factors for presenting problems in child psychiatric emergencies. *Journal of the American Academy of Child and Adolescent Psychiatry, 35*(9), 1162–1173.

Pickles, A., Aglan, A., Collishaw, S., Messer, J., Rutter, M., & Maughan, B. (2010). Predictors of suicidality across the life span: The Isle of Wight study. *Psychological Medicine, 40*(9), 1453–1466. doi:10.1017/S0033291709991905

Porsteinsson, A. P., Drye, L. T., Pollock, B. G., Devanand, D. P., Frangakis, C., Ismail, Z., ... Cit, A. D. R. G. (2014). Effect of citalopram on agitation in Alzheimer disease: The CitAD randomized clinical trial. *JAMA, 311*(7), 682–691. doi:10.1001/jama.2014.93

Posner, J., Maia, T. V., Fair, D., Peterson, B. S., Sonuga-Barke, E. J., & Nagel, B. J. (2011). The attenuation of dysfunctional emotional processing with stimulant medication: An fMRI study of adolescents with ADHD. *Psychiatry Research, 193*(3), 151–160. doi:10.1016/j.pscychresns.2011.02.005

Post, R. M., Uhde, T. W., Putnam, F. W., Ballenger, J. C., & Berrettini, W. H. (1982). Kindling and carbamazepine in affective illness. *Journal of Nervous and Mental Disorders, 170*(12), 717–731.

Reid, A. M., McNamara, J. P., Murphy, T. K., Guzick, A. G., Storch, E. A., Goodman, W. K., ... Bussing, R. (2015). Side-effects of SSRIs disrupt multimodal treatment for pediatric OCD in a randomized-controlled trial. *Journal of Psychiatr Research, 71*, 140–147. doi:10.1016/j.jpsychires.2015.10.006

Rifkin, A., Karajgi, B., Dicker, R., Perl, E., Boppana, V., Hasan, N., & Pollack, S. (1997). Lithium treatment of conduct disorders in adolescents. *American Journal of Psychiatry, 154*(4), 554–555. doi:10.1176/ajp.154.4.554

Robb, A. S., Findling, R. L., Childress, A. C., Berry, S. A., Belden, H. W., & Wigal, S. B. (2017). Efficacy, safety, and tolerability of a novel methylphenidate extended-release oral suspension (MEROS) in ADHD. *Journal of Attention Disorders, 21*(14), 1180–1191. doi:10.1177/1087054714533191

Robbins, T. W., & Arnsten, A. F. (2009). The neuropsychopharmacology of fronto-executive function: Monoaminergic modulation. *Annual Review of Neuroscience, 32,* 267–287. doi:10.1146/annurev.neuro.051508.135535

Sallee, F. R., McGough, J., Wigal, T., Donahue, J., Lyne, A., Biederman, J., & Spd503 Study, G. (2009). Guanfacine extended release in children and adolescents with attention-deficit/ hyperactivity disorder: A placebo-controlled trial. *Journal of the American Academy of Child and Adolescent Psychiatry, 48*(2), 155–165. doi:10.1097/CHI.0b013e318191769e

Scahill, L., McCracken, J. T., King, B. H., Rockhill, C., Shah, B., Politte, L., . . . Research Units on Pediatric Psychopharmacology Autism, N. (2015). Extended-release guanfacine for hyperactivity in children with autism spectrum disorder. *American Journal of Psychiatry, 172*(12), 1197–1206. doi:10.1176/appi.ajp.2015.15010055

Schweren, L. J., de Zeeuw, P., & Durston, S. (2013). MR imaging of the effects of methylpheni-date on brain structure and function in attention-deficit/hyperactivity disorder. *European Neuropsychopharmacology, 23*(10), 1151–1164. doi:10.1016/j.euroneuro.2012.10.014

Scott, S., & O'Connor, T. G. (2012). An experimental test of differential susceptibility to parenting among emotionally-dysregulated children in a randomized controlled trial for oppositional behavior. *Journal of Child Psychology and Psychiatry, 53*(11), 1184–1193. doi:10.1111/j.1469-7610.2012.02586.x. Epub 2012 Aug 6.

Stringaris, A., Cohen, P., Pine, D. S., & Leibenluft, E. (2009). Adult outcomes of youth irri-tability: A 20-year prospective community-based study. *American Journal of Psychiatry, 166*(9), 1048–1054. doi:10.1176/appi.ajp.2009.08121849

Stringaris, A., Vidal-Ribas, P., Brotman, M. A., & Leibenluft, E. (2017). Practitioner Review: Definition, recognition, and treatment challenges of irritability in young people. *Journal of Child Psychology and Psychiatry.* doi:10.1111/jcpp.12823

Strohl, M. P. (2011). Bradley's Benzedrine studies on children with behavioral disorders. *Yale Journal of Biological Medicine, 84*(1), 27–33.

Stuckelman, Z. D., Mulqueen, J. M., Ferracioli-Oda, E., Cohen, S. C., Coughlin, C. G., Leckman, J. F., & Bloch, M. H. (2017). Risk of irritability with psychostimulant treat-ment in children with ADHD: A meta-analysis. *Journal of Clinical Psychiatry, 78*(6), e648–e655. doi:10.4088/JCP.15r10601

van Schalkwyk, G. I., Lewis, A. S., Beyer, C., Johnson, J., van Rensburg, S., & Bloch, M. H. (2017). Efficacy of antipsychotics for irritability and aggression in children: A meta-analysis. *Expert Reviews in Neurotherapy, 17*(10), 1045–1053. doi:10.1080/ 14737175.2017.1371012

Wagner, K. D., Kowatch, R. A., Emslie, G. J., Findling, R. L., Wilens, T. E., McCague, K., . . . Linden, D. (2006). A double-blind, randomized, placebo-controlled trial of oxcarbazepine in the treatment of bipolar disorder in children and adolescents. *American Journal of Psychiatry, 163*(7), 1179–1186. doi:10.1176/ajp.2006.163.7.1179

Wagner, K. D., Redden, L., Kowatch, R. A., Wilens, T. E., Segal, S., Chang, K., . . . Saltarelli, M. (2009). A double-blind, randomized, placebo-controlled trial of divalproex extended-release in the treatment of bipolar disorder in children and adolescents. *Journal of the American Academy of Child and Adolescent Psychiatry, 48*(5), 519–532. doi:10.1097/ CHI.0b013e31819c55ec

Waxmonsky, J., Pelham, W. E., Gnagy, E., Cummings, M. R., O'Connor, B., Majumdar, A., . . . Robb, J. A. (2008). The efficacy and tolerability of methylphenidate and beha-vior modification in children with attention-deficit/hyperactivity disorder and severe mood dysregulation. *Journal of Child and Adolescent Psychopharmacology, 18*(6), 573–588. doi:10.1089/cap.2008.065

Yonkers, K. A., Kornstein, S. G., Gueorguieva, R., Merry, B., Van Steenburgh, K., & Altemus, M. (2015). Symptom-onset dosing of sertraline for the treatment of premenstrual dysphoric disorder: A randomized clinical trial. *JAMA Psychiatry, 72*(10), 1037–1044. doi:10.1001/jamapsychiatry.2015.1472

Zarate, C. A., Jr., Singh, J., & Manji, H. K. (2006). Cellular plasticity cascades: Targets for the development of novel therapeutics for bipolar disorder. *Biological Psychiatry, 59*(11), 1006–1020. doi:10.1016/j.biopsych.2005.10.021

{ INDEX }

Tables and figures are indicated by an italic *t* and *f*, respectively, following the page number.